THE
PATIENT

Biological, Psychological,
and Social Dimensions
of Medical Practice

THE PATIENT

Biological, Psychological, and Social Dimensions of Medical Practice

HOYLE LEIGH, M.D., F.A.P.A.

Associate Professor of Psychiatry
Yale University School of Medicine and
Director, Psychiatric Consultation-Liaison and Outpatient Services
Yale-New Haven Hospital, New Haven, Connecticut

and

MORTON F. REISER, M.D., F.A.P.A.

Charles B. G. Murphy Professor of Psychiatry and
Chairman, Department of Psychiatry
Yale University School of Medicine
New Haven, Connecticut

PLENUM MEDICAL BOOK COMPANY
NEW YORK AND LONDON

Library of Congress Cataloging in Publication Data

Leigh, Hoyle.
   The patient.

   Includes bibliographies and index.
   1. Sick — Psychology. 2. Physician and patient. I. Reiser, Morton F., joint
author. II. Title. [DNLM: 1. Psychiatry. 2. Patients. WM100.3 L528p]
R726.5.L44   610.69'6   79-9518
ISBN 0-306-40207-6

Plenum Publishing Corporation
227 West 17th Street, New York, N.Y. 10011

Plenum Medical Book Company is an imprint of Plenum Publishing Corporation

Printed in the United States of America

FOR VINNIE AND LYNN

Foreword

The old-fashioned doctor, whose departure from the modern medical scene is so greatly lamented, was amply aware of each patient's personality, family, work, and way of life. Today, we often blame a doctor's absence of that awareness on moral or ethical deficiency either in medical education or in the character of people who become physicians.

An alternative explanation, however, is that doctors are just as moral, ethical, and concerned as ever before, but that a vast amount of additional new information has won the competition for attention. The data available to the old-fashioned doctor were a patient's history, physical examination, and "personal profile," together with a limited number of generally ineffectual therapeutic agents. A doctor today deals with an enormous array of additional new information, which comes from X rays, biopsies, cytology, electrographic tracings, and the phantasmagoria of contemporary laboratory tests; and the doctor must also be aware of a list of therapeutic possibilities that are both far more effective and far more extensive than ever before.

The old-fashioned doctor could concentrate on the patient's personal profile, therefore, because it was one of the few sources of available information and because it had a major therapeutic role. Unable to rely on powerful drugs and other treatments, the old-fashioned doctor made himself into an agent of treatment, using his skillful knowledge of people, human reactions, and communication as the basis for the "iatrotherapy." What the doctor learned about a patient's personal status was a guide to the way the iatrotherapy was planned and delivered.

Today's doctor must contend not only with all the additional data and treatments of modern technology, but also with the scientific advances that provide pathophysiologic explanations for the data, pharmacologic and other bases for the treatment, and a coordinated rationale for the practice. Struggling to keep abreast of all the new data, treatments, and advances, and often having restricted a specialized focus to only some of them, the doctor may not find time or make time for the personal features that were once so preeminent and predominant in medical practice.

And yet, despite all the technologic changes, people have not changed. They still have personalities, families, work, and a way of life. Those "psychological and social dimensions" influence the course of illness and also act as important determinants of gratification, distress, hope, anxiety, and the diverse joys and sorrows of human existence. When seeking medical aid today, people want all the benefits of modern medical technology, but they still want (and still need) attention to their attributes as people.

As technology brought its powerful new revelations and interventions for ailments of the soma, the concomitant psyche of the patient became increasingly detached from concomitant medical consideration. Instead, a patient's personal problems and psychic discomforts became relegated to a separate group of specialists who had their own ideas about psychodynamic patterns in pathophysiology, about treatments that usually emphasized talking, and about scientific explanations for the observed phenomena and therapeutic tactics.

With psychiatry developing in one set of directions and "organic medicine" in another, patients become increasingly partitioned among modern specialists. This trend seems to have crested about a decade ago, however, and remedial action has already begun. For "somatic medicine," a new emphasis or renascence has occurred for the generalist, whose job is sometimes named with a bewildering array of titles (*general practitioner, family practitioner, general internist, ambulatory pediatrician, primary care physician,* etc.), but whose medical role clearly includes a return of attention to the patient as a person. For psychiatry, the new developments have been a powerful set of "psychotropic" drugs, which are often more promptly effectual than years of talking, and a more open approach to pathophysiology, which has liberalized the constraints of a dominant emphasis on older psychodynamic formulations.

As this progress was occurring in the individual domains of both soma and psyche, a reunion of the two seemed logical as well as necessary. The conjunction has now begun to happen with the development of liaison services, in which psychiatrists work directly with somaticists in the care of patients in medical, surgical, and other nonpsychiatric sections of medical institutions. This book emanates from two authors who have been both prominent and successful in developing this type of liaison.

From their professional familiarity with conventional psychiatry as well as their extensive experience in medical liaison work, Drs. Leigh and Reiser have integrated the biological aspects of the soma with the psychological and social attributes of the psyche. The authors have identified a series of important clinical features that seldom receive enough medical attention and discussion: the *iatrotropic stimulus* and other reasons why patients seek medical help; the expectations and behavior patterns of sick people; and the communication mechanisms that can help or hinder the relationship between doctors and patients. Separate chapters are provided for clinical phenomena that commonly occur in ordinary medical practice: problems in anxiety, defense mechanisms, depression, pain, and sleep.

An outstanding part of the book is a "patient evaluation grid," which demonstrates how personal-profile information can be organized chronologically in a manner analogous to the family history, past history, and present illness of the routine medical record. This new grid also coordinates the personal profile as an "environmental" concomitant of the "biological dimensions" that are usually the main constituent of medical records.

A particularly attractive feature of the book is the "vignettes" used to introduce each chapter. These brief case reports, which represent problems that are constantly encountered in medical practice, have been carefully chosen to illustrate the themes of each chapter and to provide direct clinical relevance for the discussions. In the last part of the book, the authors make use of the vignettes, previous discussions, and patient evaluation grid to demonstrate and help solve a series of professional and pharmaceutical challenges in the management of patients.

The book should be especially worthwhile for medical students and for house staff who want to transcend modern technocratic wisdom by developing their own talents as skillful iatrotherapists. The comments and suggestions will also appeal to both psychiatric and medical practitioners whose main clinical concerns are with helping patients rather than maintaining professional paradigms. The perceptions cited in the text were formerly available only to the small group of physicians and students who encountered the authors during the activities of a psychiatric department and liaison service. With this book, the authors have made their useful and important ideas accessible to everyone else.

Alvan R. Feinstein, M.D., F.A.C.P.
Professor of Medicine and Epidemiology
Yale University School of Medicine
New Haven, Connecticut

Preface

The primary subject matter of medicine is the patient. Diagnosis and treatment of disease is an integral part of the patient's care, but the latter includes, in addition, an understanding of the behavioral aspects of the patient and of the surrounding environment, including the family and the health care personnel. Until recently, behavioral aspects of patient care have been relegated by many physicians to the "art of medicine" rather than the "science of medicine," and much of the information relevant to the care of a patient as a person came from researchers in nonmedical disciplines, often through the study of normal healthy persons rather than patients. This led to conceptual and practical gaps between behavioral science and the practice of medicine.

In our work with medical students as lecturers and seminar leaders in a basic behavioral science course, as teachers and preceptors of medical student clinical clerks both in psychiatry and medicine, and as faculty members intimately involved in curriculum development at the Yale University School of Medicine, we became acutely aware that many students were bemoaning the lack of a good practical and relevant textbook that would bridge the gap between the behavioral sciences and medicine. Initially, our plan was to present information relevant to medicine gleaned primarily from behavioral sciences under the tentative title "Behavioral Foundations of Medical Practice." In the course of actual writing, however, we came to realize that straight presentations of behavioral science knowledge, however relevant, would be of limited value to the student of medicine. We have found in our liaison consultation practice and teaching that the clinician's best use of behavioral science data is achieved when it can be integrated with the biological clinical data of medicine. We also realized that integration of behavioral and biological foundations of medicine was not taught anywhere in the medical curriculum. Although many experienced physicians have, on their own, achieved such an integration, many others never even attempt it. Without basic behavioral science information, this integration is haphazard even when there is motivation for it. Thus, we decided to attempt a practical demonstration of integration between behavioral science knowledge and the biological underpinnings of medicine and to focus on patient care. The practice of medicine involves, for each physician, the challenge of achieving such integration. The care of patients provides an opportunity for linking the spheres of medical biology and the behavioral sciences.

Some basic principles concerning patient care will be the same for some time to come, even though facts and data bases may change. One of the basic principles we refer to is the principle referrable to good patient care—that comprehensiveness and thoroughness are essential. Simple as it may seem, this involves the simultaneous addressing of three dimensions of information—that of the disease, the patient as a person, and the surrounding environmental system.

This book is intended to challenge medical students in the preclinical years and those who are preparing for their first clinical clerkships. The challenge is to think about the patients as entities in their own right and to integrate the basic knowledge that they are in the process of gaining into an approach to the care of patients. This book, if successful, should also challenge serious students at all levels of experience, including house staff and attending physicians in nonpsychiatric clinical specialties as well as psychiatrists who work and teach in the field of consultation liaison psychiatry.

A few words on what this book is not:

> This book is *not* a conventional textbook of behavioral science.
> This book is *not* a conventional textbook of medicine.
> This book is *not* an introduction to clinical psychiatry.

This book *is* intended to be a practical book. Many people have expounded on the need for the biopsychosocial perspective in medicine, but few have shown how this perspective could actually be used in practice. The patient evaluation grid (PEG) (Chapter 9) is a concrete and practical method through which the reader may plan the management of his or her patient in the biological, personal,* and environmental dimensions. In integrating behavioral sciences with medical practice, we used as an organizing principle the general systems approach.†

---

*We use the term "personal" here to denote all the attributes of the whole person as a unit. This, of course, includes the psychological dimension, but also includes behavioral characteristics such as habits.

†For a comprehensive and authoritative exposition on general systems theory of living things, we recommend James G. Miller's *Living Systems* (New York, McGraw-Hill, 1978). For a concise introduction, we recommend Miller's chapter, General systems theory, in *Comprehensive Textbook of Psychiatry, II,* Vol. 1, edited by A. M. Freedman, H. I. Kaplan, and B. J. Sadock (Baltimore, Williams & Wilkins, 1975), pp. 75–78.

References are given in order that the reader may read further about the topic being discussed. Thus, our references do not necessarily refer to the original source; review papers and original papers are referred to without distinction.

Much impetus for writing this book came from our students and colleagues. In the course of our work, we learned more from our students than from anyone else. Many versions of various chapters of this book have been read by them in various contexts, and their incisive and thoughtful comments and suggestions have served as stimuli to improve the work. Student interest (and encouragement) served as powerful support when the progress of the book seemed to lag. Our first thanks, then, are due our students, past and present.

Many friends and colleagues have read portions of this book and given us valuable advice. It is impossible to name all of them, but we owe special thanks to the following: Malcolm Bowers, Jr., M.D., Robert Byck, M.D., William Collins, M.D., Marshall Edelson, M.D., Ph.D., Alvan R. Feinstein, M.D., Stephen Fleck, M.D., Earl Giller, M.D., Ph.D., Richard Goldberg, M.D., Eugene Redmond, M.D., Richard Ross, M.D., and Gary Schwartz, Ph.D.

We are also indebted to Ms. Hilary Evans of Plenum Publishing Corporation for editorial assistance and to Mss. Erica Fritz, Judy Guy, and Jacqueline Collimore for typing innumerable drafts and for other secretarial work.

Hoyle Leigh, M.D.
Morton F. Reiser, M.D.

New Haven, Connecticut

Contents

Chapter 3. Expectations in the Consulting Room   23

PART II. ON BEING A PATIENT:
PSYCHOPHYSIOLOGIC CONSIDERATIONS

Chapter 4. Anxiety   39

PART III. ON ASSESSING A PATIENT:
A CLINICAL SYSTEMS APPROACH

Chapter 9. Approach to Patients: The Systems–Contextual
Framework and the Patient Evaluation Grid

Chapter 10. The Current Context of Help-Seeking Behavior

PART IV. ON MANAGING A PATIENT

List of Figures and Tables

PART I

ON BECOMING A PATIENT
Psychosocial Considerations

CHAPTER 1

Illness and Help-Seeking Behavior

In the past, the term *patient* used to mean a person who was suffering or enduring pain, related to the word *patience* (*Webster's Third New International Dictionary*). Modern usage of the term *patient* denotes a person who is seeking or is being given medical care. Although an illness usually leads an individual to seek medical help, not all who are ill become patients nor are all patients necessarily ill.

1. A man, age 39, has been experiencing occasional sharp pain in his chest for the last two months. Being a pressured junior executive, he has put off seeing a doctor, attributing the pain to indigestion associated with pressure at work. In fact, Alka Seltzer seemed to help it somewhat. Last night, during an argument with his wife, he had another bout of chest pain which took several hours to subside despite Alka Seltzer. He called his doctor this morning for an urgent appointment.

2. Three months ago, a 30-year-old woman developed severe headaches and fainting spells following a "head cold." She told her close friends, who then arranged a prayer meeting to chase away the "evil spirits" that they felt were causing her problems. Today, after the prayer meeting, she felt much better.

3. A 45-year-old woman decided to do something about her varicose veins, which she had had for 20 years. She told her doctor today that she wanted to have the operation as soon as possible, even tomorrow.

4. A coal-mine worker came to see the company physician, complaining of chest pain and difficulty in breathing. Careful medical workup was negative for any physical disease. The physician felt that psychological factors might be involved in his coming for medical evaluation when he

3

*learned that a co-worker of the patient had recently been found to have
"black lung" disease and had been given a sizable compensation.*

All four patient vignettes presented above involve help-seeking behavior, but
how each individual perceived the symptoms and when and how each went
about getting help were quite dissimilar.

How is help-seeking behavior to be conceptualized, and how can the wide
variations in the form it may take in different persons be understood? Medical
sociologists have studied these questions and developed concepts, definitions,
and data that are useful to the physician in his efforts to understand the
circumstances that brought the patient for help and to facilitate development of
a productive relationship with his patient from the very start.

Concepts and Definitions: Help-Seeking
Behavior and Illness Behavior

Help-seeking behavior consists of an individual deciding to do something
about a symptom or distress, and this behavior may be subcategorized into
medical and nonmedical. In *medical* help-seeking behavior, a patient–doctor
contact is made, and this initiates a process whereby a small health care system
forms around the patient. Calling the doctor to make an appointment, visiting
the doctor in his office, or presenting oneself to the emergency room of a
hospital are examples (vignettes 1 and 3 above). *Nonmedical* help-seeking
behaviors include going to a clergyman or a variety of nonprofessional people
such as "root workers" and faith healers or asking a relative or friend for advice
(vignette 2). Of course, nonmedical help-seeking behaviors often lead to
medical contacts through advice and referral, and many patients engage in
medical and nonmedical help-seeking behaviors at the same time, for example, mobilizing family support and visiting a doctor. Quasimedical behaviors,
such as self-medications or discussing symptoms with a druggist, while nonmedical by definition since they do not involve the immediate formation of
doctor–patient contact, may also lead to it eventually. (In vignette 1, buying
Alka Seltzer, a quasimedical help-seeking behavior, was an intermediate step
toward medical help-seeking behavior.)

Help-seeking behavior is closely related to its antecedent, *illness behavior.*
Illness behavior, described by Mechanic (1962), consists of the ways in which
given symptoms may be perceived, evaluated, and acted (or not acted) upon
by different individuals. Illness behavior may or may not lead to help-seeking
behavior. Help-seeking behavior occurs in the presence of a symptom motivated and influenced by the severity and quality of the symptom. It is to be
expected that the more acute, severe, distressful, frightening, and persistent
the symptoms are, the more likely will medical help-seeking behavior occur.
But these common-sense expectations are overly simple. Help-seeking

Table 1. Factors Affecting
Help-Seeking Behavior

Symptoms and signs
  Commonality, familiarity, predictability, threat

Demography
  Socioeconomic class, religion, ethnicity

Stress

Previous Experience
  Personal, others

phenomena as they actually occur in practice may be far more complex and hard to understand. Even in the presence of severe persistent and frightening symptoms like fainting spells, an individual often does not engage in a medical help-seeking behavior (vignette 2). A patient's response to symptoms is modified considerably by a variety of factors which influence the individual's ultimate decisions and actions, for example, whether or not to initiate help-seeking behavior, and, if so, when and what kind (Table 1).

Factors Influencing Help-Seeking Behavior

Factors Affecting Perception of a Symptom

Four dimensions of an illness (and/or symptom) are important in influencing how symptoms are perceived. They are (1) the frequency with which it occurs in a given population *(commonality);* (2) the familiarity of the symptoms to the average member of the community *(familiarity);* (3) the predictability of the outcome of the illness; and (4) the amount of threat and loss likely to result from the illness (Mechanic, 1962). For example, with the common cold—being familiar, easily recognized, self-limited, and carrying minimal risk of major loss—help-seeking behavior is unlikely to occur. Coughing up blood, on the other hand, is uncommon, unfamiliar, unpredictable, and threatening, increasing the probability of contact with a physician.

Naturally, the patient's personality also is important in determining help-seeking behavior. These factors are taken up in Chapter 15.

Demographic Factors

Socioeconomic Class. Whether or not symptoms lead to help-seeking behavior may be influenced by the patient's socioeconomic class. For example, upper-class persons tend to report themselves ill more often than lower-class persons (Koos, 1954). This class difference has been considered to be related to realistic economic considerations—the upper classes more easily affording medical bills and losing a day's work to see a doctor—as well as to the higher educational level and greater awareness of methods of getting help. The very poor on public assistance can afford to engage in help-seeking behavior more readily than the working poor as they do not have to lose hourly pay to make use of the medical facility in the community, but there is some evidence that these social class differences in medical care utilization are diminishing (Ross, 1962).

Orientations toward illness differ according to social class (Mechanic, 1968). In general, lower-class populations are more fatalistic about contracting disease and thus less likely to be oriented toward preventive medicine (Deasy, 1956; Rosenstock, 1969) and toward consultation with medical professionals when ill (Koos, 1954; Redlich *et al.*, 1955; Brightman *et al.*, 1958).

There is some evidence to suggest that similar disease processes may present differently in patients in different socioeconomic classes. Upper-class persons with coronary disease often present themselves to the medical facility with angina pectoris, while lower-class persons are more likely to present themselves with acute myocardial infarction or sudden death (Shekelle and Ostfeld, 1969). It is not clear why this is so, although upper-class persons might be readier to come to a medical facility with a milder distress.

Diagnoses of neuroses and personality disorders have been made with higher frequency in upper-class persons, while diagnoses of psychoses, "psychosomatic" reactions, or hysterical reactions have been more commonly made in lower-class populations. (Hollingshead and Redlich, 1958). This difference may indicate actual prevalence difference, and doctors may tend to diagnose more benign conditions in the upper-class persons because of their own biases. The greater prevalence of schizophrenia (psychosis) in lower-class populations may be explained in one of two ways: Either (1) lower-class environment and genetic pool contribute to the development of the disorder ("origin hypothesis") or (2) schizophrenic individuals wind up in lower classes because of the disability caused by the illness ("drift hypothesis").

Religion and Ethnic Origin. Religion and ethnic origin are related to illness behavior probably through different cultural attitudes and expectations. Some cultural groups (e.g., the Spanish-speaking people in the Southwest) are more likely than others (English-speaking people in the same area) to seek family care and support and to rely on folk medicine when ill (Saunders, 1954). English-speaking people in the same area tend to seek modern medical treatment. In a questionnaire study in a large university, Jews and Episcopalians reported that they would have a higher inclination to use medical facilities for various hypothetical symptoms than did Christian Scientists and Catholics

(Mechanic, 1962). Religious differences appear to influence illness behavior independently of social class.

Zborowski (1952, 1969) studied attitudes and responses to pain of patients belonging to different ethnic groups. His subjects consisted of "Old American," Irish, Jewish, and Italian male patients. The Old American and Irish patients tended to minimize pain, delay seeking consultation with a physician, and respond to pain stoically, while the Jewish and Italian patients tended to exaggerate pain and react to it more emotionally. The Jewish and Old American patients were more concerned about pain as a "warning signal," that is, its implication as a symptom; the Irish were more concerned about its crippling indications; and the Italians were more concerned about the immediate consequences of the painful experience and its instant relief. Ethnic differences were also related to help-seeking behavior and attitude toward doctors. The Old Americans tended to consult druggists, osteopaths, chiropractors, etc., before finally consulting the doctor but had implicit trust in the professional competence of the doctor on the basis of his being an M.D., once he was consulted. The Jewish patients, on the other hand, tended to consult the doctor quite readily and also check into the doctor's qualifications and "doctor shop." The attitude and warmth of the doctor rather than his professional skills were seen to be of overriding importance to the Italian patients.

Although these findings represent a cross-sectional picture of illness behavior in the recent past and their validity at present is uncertain, they nevertheless demonstrate the importance of socioethnic milieu with respect to the development of pscyhological sets concerning symptoms, illness, and the medical profession.

The Role of Stress

Psychosocial stress plays a major role in transforming illness behavior into help-seeking behavior (Mechanic, 1962).

The type of stress is particularly important. By and large, *interpersonal stresses* such as difficulties with loved ones are more likely to lead illness behavior into medical help-seeking behavior than are noninterpersonal stresses such as financial hardship. This may be because communication, interaction, and nurturance usually expected from a doctor are especially (and unconsciously) sought after by persons in interpersonal difficulty. People often can initiate a personal interaction with the physician more easily than with someone with whom the contact is less structured and the role less defined. Interaction with the physician can usually be initiated with little difficulty and does not usually require complex and subtle cues and responses necessary in social relationships. In other words, social skills on the part of the patient are not as necessary in interaction with physicians as in other social situations.

Interpersonal difficulties are also frequent precipitating events of anxiety, depression, and grief, and these are probably accompanied by physiological states that may precipitate an illness or exacerbate a symptom (see Chapters 4, 6, and 9).

Finally, it should be remembered that somatic symptoms themselves are emotional stressors, and the stress they generate may finally push the illness behavior toward help-seeking behavior.

The Role of Previous Experience ("Priming Factors")

Previous personal experiences as a patient with illness and health care may strongly influence subsequent help-seeking behavior. Positive memories of a hospital experience, such as uneventful recovery from an appendectomy, make it easier to initiate contact with a doctor the next time. On the other hand, exposure to negative experiences, such as complications arising from medical treatment, prolonged recovery, and exposure to impersonal and brusque behavior on the part of health care personnel, will discourage and/or introduce delay into future medical help-seeking behavior. Even when a patient with negative past experiences does contact the physician, he is likely to do so with negative expectations, and this may result in a self-fulfilling prophecy.

Exposure to the *experiences of relatives or friends* with medical systems in the community may also have its effects, shaping the expectations that the person might bring to the system when he becomes ill. Similarly, such exposure may influence attitudes toward a particular illness or set of symptoms.

> A woman was convinced that she had cancer of the breast when she developed pains in her joints. This conviction persisted in the face of her doctor's repeated reassurances that she had arthritis. As it turns out, a friend had suffered bone pain from spread of breast cancer to the bone. The conviction was strong enough to make her delay return visits to the doctor for fear that she would have to undergo mutilating breast surgery as had her friend.

In these ways, direct and/or indirect personal exposure to illness and health care systems affects help-seeking attitudes and behavior. Additionally, it may "prime" a patient for psychological complications such as depression based on unfounded or fantasized expectations. Similarly, educational programs, reading medical books or magazine articles, watching television programs about medical matters, etc., may also set the stage for unfounded fears, although it is our impression that their impact is somewhat weaker than the personal exposures discussed above.

Community attitudes toward health care provide an explicit and implicit background against which an individual contemplates the possibility of seeking care. We have observed that when a hospital which originally had been used for chronic and terminally ill patients was converted to a modern, acute-care, general hospital, many patients admitted to that hospital as long as ten years later expressed uneasiness because of the lingering reputation of the hospital as "a place to die." Community and peer-group myths and superstitions also influence the type of help that is sought, for example, physician or hospital emergency room.

Taxonomy of Medical Help-Seeking Behavior

McWhinney (1972) proposed a taxonomy of medical help-seeking be-behavior which he calls *"patient behavior,"* using the doctor—patient contact as the reference point. This classificatory scheme is useful in assessing clinical situations. It consists of five mutually exclusive categories as immediate precipitating causes of the doctor—patient contact.

Limit of Tolerance. The patient initiates contact with the doctor because the discomfort, pain, or disability has become intolerable. A subcategory is limit of tolerance for unhappiness.

Limit of Anxiety. The patient initiates contact with the doctor because of anxiety concerning the implications of the symptom. The symptom itself may be quite tolerable, but the implications are not. An example is bloody urine.

Heterothetic, or Problems of Living Presenting as a Symptom. "Heterothetic" presentation means "putting forward other things." The patient initiates contact with a physician ostensibly because of symptoms which are minor (exceed neither the limit of tolerance nor anxiety) but in the context of disturbing emotional difficulties which are the underlying but unrecognized motive for the help-seeking action. An example is a woman who, at the time of painful interpersonal conflict with her boss, comes to the doctor complaining of back pain which she has had occasionally for many years.

Here, the underlying reason for the doctor—patient contact is an *attempt to establish a supportive interpersonal relationship* and find *relief from the emotional distress.* Many patients who present with vague and long-standing symptoms (20 years in vignette 3 above) and many patients who experience unexplained delay in recovering from illness will often on further inquiry be found to have some major emotional problems.

Conversely, some patients who present with *emotional problems* to mental health personnel or nonmedical counselors may turn out to be suffering from *serious medical disorders,* and it is important that the *medical condition* of the patient be checked before assuming that the symptoms are indeed psychological in origin.

The next two categories are doctor–patient contacts that are not help-seeking in the usual medical sense:

Administrative. These doctor–patient contacts are for administrative reasons only, whether or not the patient is ill, for example, insurance examination.

No Illness. This includes all visits for preventive purposes, as well as routine physical examinations, for example, antenatal care.

In this scheme of classification, all patients who present with symptoms should be classified as belonging in one of the first three categories. If the visit cannot be categorized as due to either limit of anxiety or to limit of tolerance, the physician should consider the possibility that he is dealing with *problems of living presenting as a symptom.* Heterothetic presentations are often motivated by an unrecognized wish to hide the true nature of suffering, and it is therefore necessary for the physician to inquire about personal problems and psychosocial aspects of the patient's life.

Patient behavior is often a result of complex interpersonal interactions between the patient and his immediate environment (Figure 1). There are instances when the patient comes to the doctor not by choice but because he is forced by others. This is especially true in the case of mental disorders. For example, a schizophrenic patient may not have been brought to a doctor had it not been for his bizarre behavior which others could not tolerate. Although McWhinney's classification system of patient behavior is primarily oriented toward the individual patient, we can use the same scheme to classify patient behavior instigated by others, for example, limit of tolerance—family; limit of anxiety—employer; problems of living—family, etc.

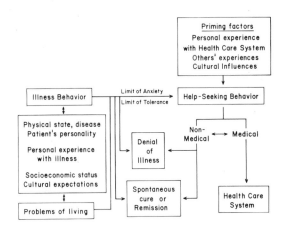

Figure 1. Help-seeking behavior.

Example 1. The patient comes to the doctor because his wife is concerned about his weight loss and change in behavior (social withdrawal), although the patient himself feels that he is just tired because of overwork. He comes only because his wife insisted. Here, the behavorial diagnosis would be limit of anxiety—wife; the patient's clinical diagnosis may be depressive syndrome (see Chapter 6).

Example 2. The patient, a seven-year-old boy, is brought in by the parents because of frequent fights at school and minor accidents. Further inquiry reveals that these problems started a year ago when the father lost his job after an industrial accident. This, in turn, had led to financial difficulties and frequent fights between the parents. Behavioral diagnosis: heterothetic problems of living on the part of parents. Clinical diagnosis (child): transient situational reaction of childhood related to problems of living.

The use of a behavioral diagnostic taxonomy in parallel with medical diagnosis will alert the physician to the fact that the help-seeking behavior which was instrumental in initiating the doctor—patient contact is linked with the patient's and the family's implicit expectations—that the physician will attempt to relieve symptoms and so render them more tolerable, and/or that he will reduce anxiety by explanation and treatment, and/or that he will provide a supportive interpersonal relationship at times of emotional stress. The supportive relationship may lead to more focused psychotherapeutic work or direct intervention in problems of living.

Summary

What one does in the presence of symptoms (illness behavior) is determined not only by the nature of the symptom(s) but also by demographic factors, presence or absence of stress, and, most importantly, previous experience with or exposure to similar symptoms and/or the health care system (priming experiences).

Help-seeking behavior occurs when a person does something to get help for his symptom or distress. This may be medical (seeing a doctor) or nonmedical (talking with a friend, attending a prayer meeting). In medical help-seeking behavior, the immediate reason for the patient—doctor contact may be the patient's (or the family's) having reached the limit of tolerance for the symptoms or for the associated anxiety. On the other hand, the patient (family) may be emotionally distressed and more in need of *interpersonal support* than elimination of a benign symptom; this would be an example of problems of living presenting as a physical symptom.

Implications

For the Patient

The presence of a symptom is not a sufficient condition for seeking medical help. The interpretation of the symptom by the patient in the light of his own unique background and personal experience, together with the prevailing community expectations, determines the action. Many patients engage in nonmedical help-seeking behavior before consulting a physician. Contact with the physician represents, for many patients, a last resort—having reached the limit of anxiety or tolerance concerning the symptom. It may also be an indication of problems of living about which the patient is unaware.

For the Physician

Patients are different. What they do in the hospital or consulting room is determined by a number of factors that are not directly involved in the disease process and its associated symptoms. *Demographic data* concerning the patient are important in enabling the physician to understand the patient's behavior in the context of the normative attitudes and expectations of his cultural and social groups. Information concerning the patient's *previous medical experiences,* exposure to similar symptoms, and to the health care system (doctors, hospitals) may also be essential for understanding the patient and for effective communication with him. It is often necessary to clarify misunderstandings and misconceptions carried over by the patient from priming experiences before the patient can attend to the words and recommendations of the doctor. Recognition of *heterothetic help-seeking behavior* will enable the physician to avoid unnecessary laboratory tests and medical procedures and to provide more effective support, such as simple listening and follow-up or referral to a psychiatrist. Remember that problems of living may not be apparent unless the patient is queried about his life situation. For example, it turned out that the woman in vignette 3 was undergoing menopause and had recently separated from her husband. It was these difficulties that had motivated her seeking help in the form of a request for surgery on her varicose veins. The operation, which was unnecessary, was postponed by her doctor, and she was referred for counseling and followed at regular intervals by the physician. In six months, she had resolved the difficulties with her husband, and her (initially urgent) request for operation was dropped.

For the Community and Health Care System

The underutilization of health care services by lower socioeconomic classes calls for community efforts to increase their accessibility and acceptability, especially the preventive and educational facilities. Since cultural and ethnic factors play a role in help-seeking behavior, hospitals should, if possible, have members of various cultural and ethnic groups available to assist in communication between the health care personnel and patients in need of their services. Nonmedical personnel (clergy, teachers, etc.) should be educated to be alert to the possible presence of medical disorders and to facilitate medical help-seeking behavior when it is indicated.

Recommended Reading

Hollingshead AP, Redlich FC: *Social Class and Mental Illness.* New York, John Wiley & Sons, 1958. A classic study on the relationship between social class and the prevalance of mental disorders in the psychiatric patient population in the New Haven area in 1950.

McWhinney IR: Beyond diagnosis. *N Engl J Med* **287**:384–387, 1972. The author proposes a taxonomy of medical help-seeking behavior which includes "heterothetic" presentation, or problems of living presenting as a symptom. In addition, he proposes a taxonomy of social factors in illness and medical help-seeking behavior, such as loss, conflict, and change.

Mechanic D: The concept of illness behavior. *J Chronic Dis* **15**:189–194, 1962. A relatively brief but succinct exposition of the concept of illness behavior. The author developed the concept on the basis of his findings concerning how students in a large university behaved differently according to demographic and psychosocial variables in the presence of a symptom.

Mechanic D: Social psychologic factors affecting the presentation of bodily complaints. *N Engl J Med* **286**:1132–1139, 1972. A brief but comprehensive review of cultural and social factors in illness behavior. There is also a brief discussion on the "medical students' disease."

Srole L, Langner T, Michael ST, *et al.: Mental Health in the Metropolis: The Midtown Manhattan Study.* New York, Harper Torch Books, 1975. Originally published in 1962, this study, somewhat similar in scope to the New Haven study, utilized home-interview techniques also. An important study showing a high prevalence of emotional distress (80%) in the general population. Demographic data are shown to be associated with prevalance and type of mental disorders. Low socioeconomic class and increasing age are related to higher prevalence of mental illness.

Zborowski M: *People in Pain.* San Francisco, Jossey-Bass, 1969. An easily readable, sometimes dramatic presentation of the ethnic differences in how people behave in the presence of pain. The author studied "Old Americans," Italian, Jewish, and Irish Americans who were being treated for pain in a Veterans Administration Hospital in New York City. Somewhat stereotyped and oversimplified.

References

Brightman I, Notkin H, Brumfield W, *et al.*: Knowledge and utilization of health resources by public assistance recipients. *Am J Public Health* **48**:188–199, 319–327, 1958.

Deasy L: Socioeconomic status and participation in the poliomyelitis vaccine trial. *Am Social Rev* **21**:185–191, 1956.

Hollingshead AP, Redlich FC: *Social Class and Mental Illness.* New York, John Wiley & Sons, 1958.

Koos E: *The Health of Regionville: What the People Thought and Did about It.* New York, Columbia University Press, 1954.

McWhinney IR: Beyond diagnosis. *N Engl J Med* **287**:384–387, 1972.

Mechanic D: The concept of illness behavior. *J Chronic Dis* **15**:189–194, 1962.

Mechanic D: *Medical Sociology: A Selective View.* New York, The Free Press, 1968.

Redlich F, Hollingshead A, Bellis E: Social class differences in attitudes toward psychiatry. *Am J Orthopsychiatry* **25**:60–70, 1955.

Rosenstock I: Prevention of illness and maintenance of health, in Kosa J, Antonovsky A, Zola IK (eds): *Poverty and Health.* Cambridge, Harvard University Press, 1969, pp. 168–190.

Ross J: Social class and medical care. *J Health Hum Behav* **2**:35–40, 1962.

Saunders L: *Cultural Differences and Medical Care.* New York, Russell Sage Foundation, 1954.

Shekelle R, Ostfeld AM: Social status and incidence of coronary heart disease. *J Chronic Dis* **22**:381–394, 1969.

Zborowski M: Cultural components in response to pain. *J Soc Issues* **8**:16–30, 1952.

Zborowski M: *People in Pain.* San Francisco, Jossey-Bass, 1969.

CHAPTER 2

The Sick Role

1. *An epidemic of Hong Kong flu swept through town. Absenteeism was highest among students, followed by white-collar workers, and lowest among the blue-collar workers at the steel mill, especially those with least seniority.*

2. *[A newspaper excerpt] Policemen in the city today called in sick in droves as negotiations broke down between the city and the police union.*

3. *A 35-year-old secretary, who had never missed a day's work, became noticeably pale and seemed to have trouble walking but would not miss work to see a doctor. Since she lived alone, there was no one to be alarmed when she started vomiting in the evening or when excruciating pains kept her awake at night. She would, however, invariably show up at work with a smile on her white parched lips. Then, one day she did not come to work. She had died of massive stomach bleeding in the early hours of the morning.*

4. *[Senator Hubert Humphrey, upon returning to the Senate after discovery of inoperable cancer] "I must believe that I am going to win this battle. . . . I have to do it, nobody else can. The doctors can't do it for me, although they can help."*

5. *A 25-year-old white man was admitted to the hospital when he came to the emergency room vomiting blood. All tests were negative, and he was discovered stealing a test tube of blood from a technician's cart. Upon discovery, he immediately walked out of the hospital. Two days later, he was admitted to another hospital in an adjacent city after coming to that hospital's emergency room vomiting blood.*

6. *[In a bedroom] "No, not tonight. I have a terrible headache."*

7. *Having been found incompetent to stand trial, the defendant was committed to the mental hospital.*

Sick Role Expectations

Society assigns specific expectations to the ill person by virtue of his being ill. These expectations comprise what is known as the "sick role."

Talcott Parsons, a sociologist, formulated the sick role as consisting of four aspects. The first is an *exemption from normal social role responsibilities* (Parsons, 1951). The degree of such exemption is, of course, dependent on the nature and severity of the illness. This exemption, according to Parsons, is a right of the sick. In order to prevent abuse of this right (malingering), society also requires that this right be legitimized by others. The physician is most often the key person in this legitimizing process, both as a direct legitimizing agent and as a "court of appeal." The sick role may be assumed by some persons without having engaged in medical help-seeking behavior or having been recognized as ill (vignettes 2 and 6). In these instances, the legitimacy of the exemption from social responsibilities may be seen as tenuous, and, further, should such persons eventually engage in medical help-seeking behavior (after having assumed the sick role for prolonged periods without medical legitimization), the physician may be reluctant to grant legitimization. Thus, patients suspected of being "crocks" or "hysterics" tend not to be taken seriously by doctors even when their complaints might otherwise stimulate further investigation.

The second aspect of the sick role is *recognition* "that the sick person cannot be expected by 'pulling himself together' to get well by an act of decision or will. In this sense also he is exempted from responsibility—he is in a condition that requires being 'taken care of.' His 'condition' must be changed, not merely his 'attitude.' Of course the process of recovery may be spontaneous, but while the illness lasts he can't 'help it.' This element in the definition of being ill is obviously crucial as a bridge to the acceptance of 'help'" (Parsons, 1951).

Parsons goes on to say that "the third element is the definition of the state of *being ill* as *itself undesirable with its obligation to want to 'get well.'*" According to Parsons, the first two elements of the sick role, the exemption from normal role responsibilities and legitimization of dependency on others, are contingent on the acceptance of the idea that the assumption of the sick role is an undesirable and unfortunate necessity which should be relinquished as soon as possible (vignette 4). Although the sick person cannot be expected to "pull himself together" to get well, he may be seen as responsible for his condition if he does not show motivation to get well, to get out of the sick role.

The fourth aspect of the sick role is the *obligation*—in proportion to the severity of the condition, of course—*to seek technically competent help,* usually from a physician, and to cooperate with him in the process of trying to get well. It is here, of course, that the role of the sick person as patient becomes articulated with that of the physician in a complementary role structure.

Parsons attached great importance to motivational factors concerning the sick role, realizing that the privileges and exemptions of the sick role would give rise to attempts by some to assume the role for "secondary gain." The balance between the pull toward the sick role and the push toward relinquishing it is of utmost importance.

The sick role, Parsons states further, is a "contingent" role which anyone may assume regardless of his status in other respects.

In essence, then, the sick role consists of two rights and two obligations: the rights of exemption from normal responsibilities and the recognition that the ill person is not to blame for his illness, and the obligations of a desire to get well and to seek competent medical help.

The sick role is seen as being "universalistic"; that is, "generalized objective criteria determine whether one is or is not sick, and with what kind of sickness" (Parsons, 1951).

When the physician recognizes a person as being ill, that person becomes a *patient,* legitimately assuming the sick role, exempted from normal responsibilities such as going to work, and expected to want to get well and to cooperate with the physician and other health care personnel.

Sick Role Performance by Patients

The sick role expectations are obviously shared by the doctors and other health care personnel. The patients who fail to conform to the sick role are considered to be "bad" patients. When a patient fails to conform, the legitimacy of the illness itself is often questioned—that is, the patient may be suspected of malingering. An uncooperative patient may be denied continuation of hospitalization by premature discharge because the physicians become angry with him for not living up to the fourth expectation. A convalescing patient who repeatedly complains of minor symptoms is seen as not fulfilling the third expectation to regard the sick role as an undesirable one that should be relinquished as soon as possible. This may even tempt the physician to withdraw legitimization of the sick role from such a patient. Some patients, on the other hand, may foster approved prolongation of the sick role by being "good" patients, that is, by extreme cooperativeness (sometimes even volunteering to participate in experimental procedures, etc.).

The way an individual actually behaves when he becomes sick may be conceptualized as *sick role performance.* Sick role performance is influenced by socioeconomic and ethnic–cultural factors (vignette 1). Persons of deprived economic status might be reluctant to assume the sick role because of loss of income and increased financial hardship. For individuals involved in industrial accidents, assumption of the sick role (for a legitimate injury) may mean prolonged exemption from work and secure income as long as the sickness continues. Students in training for careers may be reluctant to assume the sick role due to possible disruption of studies and delay in career achievement.

Personal experiences are also important in sick role performance. Exposure to persons who derived benefit from being sick may predispose one to seek out sick role exemptions and secondary gains whenever the opportunity presents itself. For example, a friend of a patient who received a large compensation after an industrial accident may come to the doctor with exaggerated lingering symptoms of a minor injury. Patients who seem to want to prolong the sick role have often been exposed to and envied the prerogatives of persons who had been seriously ill for long periods of time.

How a particular illness is *viewed in the society* also affects whether a person is more or less likely to be motivated to assume the sick role for the illness. Patients suffering from socially stigmatized illnesses such as venereal disease or mental illness may be reluctant to assume the sick role. Stigmatized illnesses are not treated with neutral attitudes (as Parsons formulated), and they often carry an assumption of responsibility for the illness on the patient's part (such as venereal disease and alcoholism). Heterothetic presentation of symptoms (McWhinney; see Chapter 1) may be seen as an attempt on the part of the patient with emotional difficulties to assume some elements of the sick role.

The concept of the sick role as formulated by Parsons does not apply to all illnesses. Specifically, it is *inadequate* to deal with (1) minor illnesses in which no exemption from normal social roles is granted and no requirement to contact the physician is made; (2) incurable illnesses which require adjustment rather than a motivation to recover; and (3) legitimate "ill" roles which do not require continuing attention by a physician or exemption from normal responsibilities or motivation toward recovery, such as in the handicapped (Freidson, 1962). More recently, physicians are becoming more and more aware of the fact that many illnesses occur due to neglect of clearly preventive measures on the part of potential patients. Such neglect may be active, such as smoking despite respiratory symptoms, or passive, such as not consulting a physician after discovering a lump in the breast. In this sense, society's sick role expectations concerning responsibility for illness may need revision.

Role conflict problems are relatively frequent. For example, an elderly person may become very sick with a viral illness that usually runs a mild course. He may find that he will feel guilty if he assumes the sick role, and yet he may be chided by others if he does not.

We often see patients with incurable illnesses such as advanced cancer attempting to recover from the illness completely through the use of irrational methods of treatment such as Laetrile—and spending enormous amounts of money and energy in the attempt. This would be an example of conflict between the third and fourth expectations.

In psychiatric illnesses, there are divergent role expectations depending upon the physician's orientation to the illness, with varying degrees of modification from Parsons' sick role. A biologically oriented psychiatrist using mainly a medical model of psychiatric illness may legitimize the full assumption of the sick role for the mentally ill patient. On the other hand, psychiatrists with a more sociopsychological orientation may be reluctant to grant their patients exemptions from social role responsibilities and to expect them to work at getting well through their own efforts assisted by the psychotherapist. Then, there are some who still believe that mental illness is a condition for which the patients are totally responsible, that they could "pull themselves together" if they really wanted to. This attitude contributes to the continuing stigmatization of mental illness and, consequently, the reluctance of the patients to seek help.

The sick role, as any other newly assumed role, requires a period of adjustment. In newly hospitalized patients, conflicts often arise between the patient and the staff because of the inability or difficulty of some patients to accept the sick role, which leads to the patient being perceived as uncooperative rather than inexperienced in the role.

The personality of the patient has a major bearing on how the sick role is perceived and accepted by the patient (see Chapter 15).

Summary

Society's expectations of a person who becomes ill constitute the "sick role." Parsons describes four components of the sick role: (1) exemption from normal role responsibilities; (2) recognition that the sick person cannot be expected to get well by an act of will or decision on his part; (3) definition of the state of being ill as an undesirable state; and thus (4) the obligation to seek technically competent help by a physician.

As generalized social expectations, they are generally shared by both physicians and patients. The "sick role performance," that is, how a patient actually behaves when he becomes sick, is determined by many factors besides the "sick role expectations." These factors include the realities of economics, personal experiences with illness, the context of being ill, and the personality of the patient, to list a few. The sick role performance of specific patients may be at variance with the sick role expectations of the society or of the physicians, resulting in misunderstandings or conflicts between patients and the health care personnel.

Implications

For the Patient

The generalized sick role expectations form the basis or "ground rules" for persons when they become ill. Thus, patients "know" that they can and should stay home from work in the presence of high fever and, if it continues, that they should go to the doctor; also, that they should take the medications prescribed by the doctor to get well. The sick role performance in individual patients, however, is influenced by a number of individualized or class-dependent factors, including unique personal experience with illness or ill persons. Thus, some patients behave in ways at variance with the way they should behave according to society's expectations. For example, some patients may not seek help in the presence of serious symptoms (as in vignette 3); and some may "assume" parts of the sick role as a means to a goal (e.g., the policemen in vignette 2), or as an excuse to be exempted from normal role expectations (e.g., that of a spouse in vignette 6), or as a legitimate reason for such an exemption (vignette 7).

For the Physician

The physician should first *understand what his expectations are of the sick persons he is treating,* as they may influence his attitudes or generate prejudices concerning a particular patient. Then, the physician should attempt to understand the determinants of the patient's sick role performance—the influence of socioeconomic class, personal experiences, contexts of the assumption of the sick role, etc. For example, did the patient delay seeking help (assumption of sick role) because of economic reasons? Is the patient seeking certain aspects of the sick role (e.g., exemption from normal responsibilities) because of psychological needs (being unable to cope with a severe emotional stress)? *Many problem patients can be understood if the problem is analyzed in terms of the sick role expectations of the physician and the sick role performance of the patient.* For example, in vignette 5, we see a patient who is "addicted" to the sick role performance, assuming it by deception. Part of the sick role expectation is that it is an "undesirable state" and should not be voluntarily assumed in the absence of illness. Physicians, in general, tend to be angry at such patients. However, once the physician recognizes that the anger is directed at the sick role performance of the patient (not playing by the rules) and also that it gives the doctor a sense of being "cheated" by the patients, the physician can then recognize that the person's need to be hospitalized is itself an illness requiring treatment in its own right. With this perspective, the physician can then endeavor to understand the personal determinants of the sick role performance of the patient, including the meaning of hospitalization.

For the Community and Health Care System

The generalized sick role expectations as described by Parsons may be modified in specific communities and health care systems. For example, in certain communities, the expectation that an ill person should seek professional help may not apply (e.g., a community of Christian Scientists). In certain hospitals for chronic or terminal diseases, the expectation of hoping to get well may not be appropriate. A community may have latent prejudice against certain minority members who do not share the sick role expectations of the larger community. It may also show prejudice against persons who cannot fulfill the community's sick role expectations when they become sick. For example, patients with chronic or terminal diseases or some geriatric patients often are not treated with the same degree of compassion and caring that more acutely ill persons receive in the community.

Generalized sick role expectations of the community change as we become more aware that certain diseases might, but for the patients' inaction— for example, failing to stop smoking—have been prevented or might have been precipitated by patients' actions—for example, becoming malnourished because of a dietary fad.

In understanding "problem" patients in a given health care system, it is important to understand what the sick role expectations of that system are and how they interact with the patient's sick role performance. Many problems may turn out to be a conflict between the expectations of the health care system as to how patients should behave and the patient's expectations (determined by his own unique experiences) as to how he should behave and be treated.

Recommended Reading

Parsons T: *The Social System*. New York, The Free Press, 1951, chap X (Social structure and dynamic process: The case of modern medical practice), pp 428–479. This chapter by Parsons is a classic which lucidly formulates the concept of the sick role and the social expectations of the doctor's role; it also contains a thoughtful functional analysis of the institution of medicine. Very highly recommended.
Twaddle AC: The concepts of sick role and illness behavior, in Lipowski ZJ (ed): *Advances in Psychosomatic Medicine*. Vol 8: *Psychosocial Aspects of Physical Illness*. Basel, Karger, 1972,

pp 162–179. This is a succinct summary of the concepts and controversies concerning the sick role and illness behavior. With extensive references.

References

Freidson E: The sociology of medicine. *Curr Sociol* **x/xi**:3, 1962.
Parsons T: *The Social System*. New York, The Free Press, 1951.

CHAPTER 3

Expectations in the Consulting Room

1. A 32-year-old woman came to her doctor for low back pain of one month's duration. Physical examination was within normal limits except for a small hard lump in her left breast. The physician suspected a malignant breast tumor and referred her to a surgeon, who admitted her to the hospital for breast biopsy. Upon admission, the patient was noted to be anxious and reticent. When the admitting intern asked why she came to the hospital, she said, "I don't know. I've had this back pain for a month or so —after straining it lifting a heavy suitcase. I guess you want to do surgery to straighten my back." When the intern asked about the lump in her breast, she said, "Yes, my doctor told me about that. It doesn't hurt or anything, and I told him not to bother. He said it should be checked just to be sure, though. But my question is what are you going to do about my back pain." The chart revealed the following note by the intern: "This 32-year-old white female was admitted to the hospital with the chief complaint of a lump in the breast."

2. A conversation at the bedside of a patient in a community hospital. Intern: "This is the 58-year-old gentleman with possible mitotic lesions of the liver." Attending: "Hello, Mr. X. How are you this morning?" Patient: "I am fine . . . er, much better, I think, Doc. I think I am getting a little less yellow now . . . maybe the X rays yesterday helped." Attending: "Fine, I think things are moving along O.K., Mr. X." Intern to the Attending: "Mr. X. had chest X rays yesterday for possible mets —negative." Attending to Intern: "Ought to repeat the LFT, lytes and bilirubin and get a GI consult."

3. A 38-year-old woman visited her family doctor complaining of severe migraine headaches. She had had migraine for more than ten years, but both the frequency and intensity had increased during the past three months. The intensity had increased to the point where she had nearly collapsed on several occasions. She made three visits to the doctor's office in three weeks, urgently asking him to "do something" about the headaches. Careful physical examination was within normal limits, and the headaches did not respond to the usual antimigraine regimen despite good results in the past. Finally, her doctor decided to ask her specific questions about any changes in her life during the past several months. Initially, she denied any major changes, but when questioned about personal habits, including sexual activity, she revealed that she had been involved in an extramarital affair for four months and that she felt intensely guilty and worried. Having shared her concerns about the affair, she was assured that the physician would help her to deal with her personal problems. The migraine headaches decreased in frequency and intensity.

A patient brings to the consultation with the physician both overt and covert expectations of the doctor. Conversely, the physician holds expectations of the patient consonant with societal expectations about the *sick role* and automatically expects the patient to behave according to them (see Chapter 2). Especially important is the expectation that the patient will *cooperate* with the doctor in order to get well. Often there is an associated implicit idea that patients should and will be *candid* with physicians and that they will *volunteer* pertinent information. Because of this implicit expectation, some *doctors may fail to inquire* into personal situations and matters that may be relevant to help-seeking behavior. In vignette 3, if the doctor had *not* specifically asked about the patient's sexual life, a successful outcome would not have been likely.

Some of the patient's expectations in the consulting room manifest themselves only when they are not met, that is, when the patient is frustrated. An important conscious attitude shared by patient and doctor alike is that of *hope:* the patient's expectant hope that the doctor can help him, and the doctor's hopeful expectation that he can do something for the patient (Freidson, 1970). *Relief from distress* usually holds top priority for the immediate help that the patient wishes and seeks to gain by consulting the physician. Implicit in this hope, of course, is the expectation that the doctor will be competent and that he will be interested.

In this chapter, we will discuss some of the expectations brought to the consulting room and examine how divergence or incongruity of such expectations between patient and doctor can interfere with optimal medical care. In the course of the discussion, expectations of the physician, that is, the "doctor role," will also be examined.

Relief from Distress

As noted above, the immediate expectation of the patient is that the doctor will relieve his distress. This may, in fact, occur to a considerable degree simply by the experience of visiting the physician, even before the symptom or underlying disease has been changed. Freidson states that, because of the mutual hope that the doctor can and will do something to help the patient, both patient and doctor are motivated to believe that something effective has occurred during the doctor–patient contact (Freidson, 1970). Consequently, according to Freidson, the patient may feel better and the physician may consider his ministrations to have been responsible (whether or not this was actually the case). But if the patient does not, in follow-up contacts, perceive that specific procedures to alleviate or remove the symptom are being instituted or planned, the distress may again increase.

The physician's expectations generally focus on a related but somewhat differently timed process, that is, to relieve the patient's distress *by treating the underlying disease.* This means that his inclination is first to identify and then to treat the underlying disease, with relief following naturally. Here then is the potential for a covert difference in priorities between the patient (relief from distress) and the doctor (treatment of underlying disease). Such a situation is particularly well illustrated when the physician diagnoses a serious medical condition unrelated to the immediate (coincidental benign) distress that brought the patient to him and then understandably subordinates the treatment of the immediately distressing, but minor, condition to the treatment of the serious one (vignette 1).

Depending on the nature of the symptom and the level of sophistication, most patients, of course, also expect treatment of the underlying cause. This may hold first priority for some patients, particularly those coming because of "limit of anxiety," but it most often takes second place to more immediate relief of discomfort. Covert differences in expectations can, of course, lead to difficulties in the doctor–patient relationship and interfere with the treatment process. Clearly, problems of this nature can be prevented and/or corrected by effective and open *communication,* and it is the doctor's responsibility to be alert to this phenomenon and to take the initiative in dealing with it.

Physicians expect their patients to cooperate with recommended diagnostic and treatment regimens, and patients do, indeed, expect to render such cooperation and compliance with the doctor's instructions. This cooperation, however, is *conditional* on their understanding that such cooperation will eventually result in relief from distress.

Physicians expect (and require) that patients will provide them with information concerning past history, history of present illness, etc., to aid in the diagnosis and assessment of the illness, but patients do not know the relevant details and kinds of information that are needed. Yet some patients carry an *implicit expectation* that the doctor will *divine* the source of their distress and do not expect to give detailed specific descriptions and history. Furthermore, body sensations are difficult to describe in words, even when the sensations are not threatening. Such communication problems can only be ameliorated by the physician's skill and patience in taking a medical history. This is an art that the good physician works an entire lifetime to perfect. Patients expect the physician to *communicate* diagnostic findings and therapeutic plans as well as to manifest an *interest* in providing relief. Communicating about diagnosis and treatment may be difficult and often requires considerable thought and planning. It can be misleading to assume that it is sufficient to convey only as much as the patient appears to be interested in and capable of understanding. Patients' interest in information, and their capacity for understanding, tend to be underestimated by physicians (Pratt *et al.*, 1957), and the amount of information received from the physician seems to influence the patient's readiness to comply with the physician's orders—the less information furnished by the doctor relative to the amount provided by the patient, the less compliance the patient is likely to show (Davis, 1968).

The physician may overestimate the strength of the patient's blind trust or the extent of his understanding. Overestimating the patient's trust leads to the unwarranted assumption that the patient will understand that every procedure and advice the doctor gives is aimed at relief from distress in the long run. The physician may then fail to make connections for the patient and express the intent to eventually relieve his distress. Overestimating the patient's level of understanding and sophistication leads to an assumption that the explanations are unnecessary, again resulting in neglect of full communication.

Many studies indicate that there is a higher level of dissatisfaction on the part of patients about the amount of information physicians provide than about any other aspect of medical care (Cartwright, 1964; Duff and Hollingshead, 1968; Waitzkin and Stoeckle, 1972). In addition to the factors discussed above, Waitzkin and Stoeckle (1972) postulate that the feeling of power arising from keeping the patient uncertain and uninformed may (unwittingly) motivate some physicians to withhold information.

The problems of frustrated expectations generally arise from problems in communication. In essence, both patient and doctor have the same and/or mutually syntonic central expectations, but the physician's intentions are often *implicit* and need to be made explicit. Treating the underlying illness first will lead to relief of symptoms; there is no inherent conflict, and, in fact, one follows the other. The patient, however, does not understand how an immediately distressful and seemingly irrelevant procedure like a breast biopsy (vignette 1) might eventually help relieve the felt distress of low back pain *unless* the physician explains *explicitly* that (1) the lump in the breast may be unrelated to the back pain but needs to be evaluated before it becomes a problem; (2) although unlikely, the back pain may be related to the lump in the breast (metastatic cancer); in which case, both need to be treated; and (3) in any case, the doctor *will treat* the *back pain* with medications. Physicians do attend exclusively to relief of symptoms when it is necessary, that is, when prompt treatment of the underlying cause is not possible.

Inaccurate estimation of patients' desire to receive information is particularly problematic in dealing with patients of *lower socioeconomic status.* Cartwright (1964) reports that professional white-collar workers obtained most of their medical information by asking their physicians and nurses direct questions, while blue-collar workers received such information through a passive process not involving active asking, and, consequently, they tended to receive less information than the upper classes. He attributes this diffidence of the lower class concerning the medical personnel to four factors: (1) their sense that the doctors do not expect them to ask questions; (2) a problem of language which results from their unfamiliarity with technical terms the doctors use; (3) the awe with which they regard physicians; and (4) their social distance from the physicians' higher social class. This reluctance to engage in active information-seeking behavior is often misinterpreted by the physician as a lack of interest. But it should be emphasized that there is *no* general class difference *in patients' desire for as much medical information as possible* presented in nontechnical language. "Good explanation" of illness is considered to be one of the most important qualities of a "good doctor" by a majority of hospitalized patients (Skipper and Leonard, 1965).

Differences in language skills and pattern of *linguistic use* may also contribute to the phenomenon of the lower-class patients receiving inadequate information from physicians. Bernstein distinguishes two basic linguistic codes differentially used by the middle and working classes (Bernstein, 1964). The *elaborated code* refers to the mode of speech in which the speaker selects from a wide range of syntactic alternatives, and it renders itself more easily to descriptions and reasoning based on the content of the speech. The *restricted code,* on the other hand, has a reduced range of alternatives and syntactic options, and the vocabulary tends to be drawn from a narrow range. The restricted code tends to discourage verbal elaboration and discussion. The elaborated code also often involves "expression of intent," while nonverbal signals are usually used for this purpose in the restricted code. The elaborated code uses higher levels of abstractions than the restricted code. The elaborated code, then, is the linguistic style used by the middle class, while the lower class tends to use the restricted code.

Physicians, using an elaborated code, are likely to expect patients to express intent verbally, while lower-class patients, using a restricted code, are not accustomed to making such verbal requests. Thus, their expectations, expressed nonverbally, are likely to be frustrated.

The physician often concludes incorrectly on the basis of the restricted-code language used by lower class patients, with its usage of a lower level of abstraction and a lack of verbal expression of intention, that the patient lacks the *competence* to understand his explanations and that the patient also lacks the desire to know about his disease processes and plans for its treatment (Waitzkin and Stoeckle, 1972).

Actually, this difference in language use between the classes is largely one of *performance* rather than of competence. Chomsky uses the term "performance" to refer to language use in concrete, specific situations, while "competence" is used to refer to the person's actual knowledge of language (Chomsky, 1965). Although a lower-class person is more accustomed to the restricted code in speaking, influenced by early experiences and current practice of his social station, he is nevertheless usually able to understand the elaborated code of the upper classes.

Communication of Information

Reference was made above to the patients' desire to know about illness in nontechnical language. Even if a patient belongs to the middle class, with its elaborated code, he still has a class difference from the physician—doctors belong to a special closed class whose members habitually speak in a language comprehended only by its own members. Technical language or jargon serves several useful *functions*. One, among others, is setting the context of meaning (in this case, medical) and being specific. For example, carcinoma of the cervix refers to a particular form of cancer arising from a specific area of the female genital organ, and it is clear that this term is used in a medical context.

When communicating with a nonmedical person (patient and/or family), however, problems may arise in attempting to translate medical jargon into nontechnical language. One problem with such translations is the loss of *specificity*. In the example given above, translation of "carcinoma of the cervix" to "cancer of the womb" clearly loses the specificity concerning the type and the exact site of the lesion. This can give rise to confusion in the mind of the lay person who might have heard of the same term being applied to such diverse conditions as endometrial carcinoma, fibroadenoma (considering that "tumor" is often used synonymously with cancer), ovarian tumor (some lay people may confuse the womb and ovaries), carcinoma of the vagina, etc. Of course, marked differences obtain in the course, treatment, and prognoses of these conditions.

Translation to nontechnical language is nonetheless desirable, as the use of jargon results in both noncommunication and misinterpretation. It is important to recognize that in translating medical jargon to lay terms, specificity is very often lost and that the person is likely to have his *own fantasies and ideas* about what the doctor is telling him. For information to be communicated accurately, therefore, it is essential that the physician attempt to be as specific as possible and that he *ask* the lay person what he *understood* from the explanation provided. This will provide an opportunity for prompt clarification of misunderstandings and misinterpretations which may have occurred.

Medical jargon is sometimes used deliberately when physicians are communicating with each other in the presence of the patient. This can be very risky. *If the patient is not provided with sufficient information, he will attempt to construct his own meaning out of whatever he heard.* Just imagine for yourself the fantastic notions the patient in vignette 2 might have developed from sounds he overheard!

Another problem with translations of medical terms into lay terms is that "affective neutrality" (see below) might be lost by the loss of medical context. This is obvious when one considers the nontechnical terms denoting body organs, such as uterus, vagina, and esophagus. With the popularization of the medical terminology in nonmedical populations, however, this particular problem has largely abated. Nonetheless, some terms may still run into difficulties in translation ("mortality rate," "prognosis," etc). Medical context should be kept in translations as much as possible.

Effect of Priming Factors on Expectations

Previous experiences with illness, physicians, and hospitals also determine the patient's expectations in the consulting room. This is especially so if the present illness to be treated is in any way related to the previous experience—for example, same symptoms, same body organ, or same physician.

The physician's expectations are also influenced by his own previous experiences with the particular type of disease, symptoms, and even with the type of personality of the patient.

The Physician's Covert Expectations

In addition to the shared expectations of the doctor and patient, some physicians have additional covert expectations of patients. For example, some expect that the patient *should be suffering* to see a doctor and that the suffering must be *physical*. In such a case, if a patient visits the physician with a minor symptom from which little suffering is evident, he may be viewed with suspicion or even derision because of this expectation. When the expectation is that the suffering must be physical, there is a tendency not to consider the possibility that the presenting symptoms might be heterothetic, that is, problems of living presenting as a symptom. Such expectations on the physician's part, then, may result in *inadequate or delayed diagnosis* through the lack of vigilance and concern.

Society's Expectations about the Physician— The "Doctor Role"

Society places certain expectations on the conduct of physicians just as it does on ill persons. These will be referred to as the "doctor role" to complement the "sick role" of the patient.

Parsons (1951) elucidated the role of the physician together with the sick role in his book *The Social System.* According to Parsons, there are five essential aspects to the role of the physician. They are as follows.

Technical Competence

The physician is expected to facilitate the patient's recovery from illness to the best of his ability. In order to meet this responsibility, he is expected to acquire and practice high technical competence in "medical science" and the techniques based upon it.

Parsons points out that this can be a cause of frustration for the physician because of the inherent uncertainties in medicine and because scientific advances do not necessarily result in an increase in the ability of the physician to facilitate recovery from illness.

In the context of "doing everything possible," the physician is *exempted from certain social prohibitions.* These include the need to invade the patient's *privacy* in handling and examining his body (physicians are allowed to look and feel and otherwise explore another person's body in ways barred even to a spouse or lover), to acquire confidential and personal information from the patient, and to subject the patient's body to discomfort and injury (such as surgical procedures).

Universalism of the Medical Role

Parsons characterized the doctor role as being "universalistic," as opposed to "particularistic," in two senses. First, this role is *open to anyone* who meets the performance criteria. This tends to reduce nepotism and to facilitate interdisciplinary communication and thus the furtherance of medical science. Second, the universalism of the role *protects the physician* from "assimilation to the nexus of personal relationships in which the patient is placed." This particular aspect also implies that the treatment the physician renders is universal; that is, he renders his professional services to *any patient*, not just to friends and relatives. This is clearly related to the functional specificity and affective neutrality described below.

Functional Specificity

"Specificity of competence" and "specificity of the scope of concern" are considered under this rubric. The former refers to the expectation that the physician will practice only the techniques and areas of medicine in which he is competent, and it also involves his right not to treat patients requiring skills he does not possess.

Through expectations concerning the specificity of the scope, the physician is expected to engage in the privileges, such as the exemption from the prohibitions concerning invasion of privacy, *only for the purpose of medical care.* This expectation tends to allay anxieties on the patient's part about being exploited by the physician.

Society supports the maintenance of the functional specificity of the physician by "segregation of the context of professional practice from other contexts." Thus, information gained in the context of medical practice is expected to be privileged and confidential, and situations suggestive of sexual or aggressive encounters in other contexts are perceived differently in the medical context, for example, having members of the opposite sex undress in the same room or cutting a person's skin with a knife.

Parsons states, "the importance of functional specificity is to define, in situations where potential illegitimate involvements might develop, the limits of the 'privileges' in the 'dangerous' area which the physician might claim." Affective neutrality is considered to be the expected attitudes of the physicians within these limits.

Affective Neutrality

This refers to the expectation that physicians will maintain *objectivity* in regard to their patients and will not become "emotionally involved." Included in this are the expectations that the doctor will treat his patients equally, whether he likes them personally or not, that he will not become emotionally aroused in the course of his professional activity (such as erotic arousal), and that he will not reciprocate some patients' pull to become more "intimate" with them, such as becoming personal friends. Parsons sees a similarity between this and the affective neutrality essential in psychotherapy situations and infers that a functional significance of this aspect in medical practice might be that *there is a certain amount of "unconscious psychotherapy" in all medical practice.*

Affective neutrality does not mean that the physician should express no concern about his patient, but rather that this attitude is expected to be one of *professional* concern.

The Physician's Collectivity Orientation

This refers to the service orientation of the physician to *subordinate his own personal gain to the welfare of the patient.* The collectivity orientation is considered to be the foundation of the "trust" that the patient is expected to have in his physician. Parsons states that this orientation is found in all cases of institutionalized authority. In the doctor–patient relationship, this authority is legitimized in a reciprocal relationship—the doctor has the "obligation faithfully to accept" the implications of the fact that he is the patient's doctor.

The significance of this orientation is in allowing the development of a trusting relationship between the doctor and the patient by reducing the threat of exploitation on the doctor's part.

The collectivity orientation of the doctor is protected, according to Parsons, by a series of symbolic practices which differentiate the medical profession from other business enterprises. They include sanctions against advertising, against bargaining over fees, and against refusing patients on the grounds of being "poor credit risks."

In summary, then, the society gives the physician the mandate to use certain *privileges* in helping the patient, accompanied by the expectation that he has high *technical competence,* that he will treat his patients scientifically, using *objective criteria* for diagnoses and treatment rather than personal feelings, that he will treat patients *only in the areas in which he has professional competence* and not spread out his practice and areas of competence too thin, that he will maintain *objectivity* concerning patients by not becoming personally involved with them, and that he will always put the *welfare of the patient* before his own welfare in the practice of medicine.

Summary

Physicians and patients have the mutual expectation that the doctor will *help* the patient. The patient's priority is usually *relief* from suffering or distress. The physician's priority is generally the treatment of underlying *disease,* which is then expected to result in relief from distress. Neglect of the patient's main concern of relief from distress can result in a strained doctor–patient relationship.

In assuming the sick role, the patient expects to offer cooperation and compliance to the doctor, in return for some assurance that attempts will be made to relieve the distress. Effective doctor–patient *communication* and *information exchange* are necessary for optimal cooperation and compliance of the patient and effective treatment. Factors that can impede effective communication include differences in *social class* and *language style* (elaborated code vs. restricted code) and problems related to *medical jargon*.

Previous experiences with illness, doctors, and hospitals determine the patient's unique expectations in the consulting room. The physician's past experiences also influence his own expectations about a particular class of patients or illnesses. Many physicians have the covert expectation that distress should stem from physical causes, and patients with distress due to psychosocial events might be unfortunately viewed with negative bias.

The doctors are expected, in general, to fulfill the doctor role expectations: (1) technical competence; (2) universalism; (3) functional specificity; (4) affective neutrality; and (5) collectivity orientation.

Implications

For the Patient

When a person consults a doctor, he has certain expectations about what the doctor will do for him, how he should behave in becoming a patient, and how the doctor will behave as a professional. Some of the expectations are generally shared by most patients, while others are uniquely personal, based on "priming experiences." Some general expectations include *relief from distress,* treatment of *underlying cause of the symptom producing the distress, cooperation* and *compliance* with the physician who is *competent* and *interested* in helping the patient, and *communication* of information from the physician. The patient may feel that the doctor is uninterested in relieving his immediate distress or incompetent if he does not understand that the doctor's concern over the underlying disease is a necessary step in the ultimate relief from his distress. This danger arises especially if there is a problem in communication between the doctor and the patient.

For the Physician

The physician should be aware of the fact that the first *priority for the patient* in seeking medical help is relief from distress. The physician should effectively *communicate* to the patient his interest in relieving the distress and his *overall plans* in evaluating and managing the patient. He should recognize that the social class and language differences (related both to the social class and medical jargon) can interfere with effective communication with the patient. After imparting information to a patient, the physician should specifically *ask the patient to explain, in his own words,* what his understanding of the information is. In general, patients are interested in *receiving more information than they actually request.* The physician should *ask specific questions* about the patient's experiences with illness, doctors, and health care systems to understand the implication of individual "priming factors" for expectations. He should also understand the *effect of his own past experiences* on his expectations about patients and this particular patient. The physician should also be aware of the *doctor role,* which defines what is generally expected of physicians by the patients and by society at large.

Above all, the physician should recognize that the *expectations* and *hopes* of both the doctor and the patient are essentially the same, and he should form a *collaborative alliance* with the patient in planning evaluation and management.

For the Community and Health Care System

The health care system should recognize that the "problem" patient is often a person whose adjustment to the sick role (expectations of the health care personnel) is difficult. Recognition of its own expectations of the patient and understanding the patient's personality traits that may make it difficult for him to meet these expectations can resolve an impasse (see Chapter 15). Medical education should emphasize relief of distress as well as treatment of underlying disease in order to facilitate collaboration between physicians and patients. Hospitals and medical schools should devise methods of more effective *communication* with the patients concerning medical matters such as diagnostic and treatment procedures. Health policy planning should include considerations of the impact on the doctor role, the sick role, and the expectations on both sides and how they might change as a response to policy decisions (e.g., advertising by doctors). Attempts should be made to prevent an increase in the frustration levels of patients concerning their expectations that the physician will be interested in helping them as persons as well as in treating their disease.

Recommended Reading

Freidson E: *Profession of Medicine: A Study of the Sociology of Applied Knowledge.* New York, Dodd Mead & Co., 1970, chap 10 (Illness as social deviance) and 11 (The professional construction of concepts of illness). Freidson is a sociologist who is a leading critic of Talcott

Parsons. Although some of his writing is quite unsympathetic to the medical profession, there are very astute observations, such as that physicians are more likely to see illness than to diagnose normality, and this tendency may result in overuse of medical technologies (such as unnecessary surgery). Illness is seen as a social state, and a point is made that an idea about what is normal, desirable, and moral is essential to considering what an illness is.

Parsons T: *The Social System*. New York, The Free Press, 1951, chap X (Social structure and dynamic process: The case of modern medical practice), pp 428–479. A lucid discussion of the "doctor role" with elaboration on the five expectations. Discussion also of the sick role. A must reading.

Waitzkin H, Stoeckle JD: The communication of information about illness, in Lipowski ZJ (ed): *Advances in Psychosomatic Medicine*. Vol. 8: *Psychosocial Aspects of Physical Illness*. Basel, Karger, 1972, pp 180–215. A good discussion concerning the communication of information about illness to patients. A review article.

References

Bernstein B: Elaborated and restricted codes: Their social origins and some consequences. *Am Anthropol* **6**:55–69, 1964.

Cartwright A: *Human Relations and Hospital Care*. London, Routledge & Kegan Paul, 1964.

Chomsky N: *Aspects of the Theory of Syntax*. Cambridge, MIT Press, 1965.

Davis MS: Variations in patients' compliance with doctors' advice: An empirical analysis of patterns of communication. *Am J Public Health* **58**:274–288, 1968.

Duff RS, Hollingshead AB: *Sickness and Society*. New York, Harper & Row, 1968.

Freidson E: *Profession of Medicine: A Study of the Sociology of Applied Knowledge*. New York, Dodd Mead & Co, 1970.

Parsons T: *The Social System*. New York, The Free Press, 1951, pp 428–479.

Pratt L, Seligman A, Reader G: Physicians' views on the level of medical information among patients. *Am J Public Health* **47**:1277–1283, 1957.

Skipper JK, Leonard RC (eds): *Social Interaction and Patient Care*. Philadelphia, Lippincott, 1965.

Waitzkin H, Stoeckle JD: The communication of information about illness, in Lipowski ZJ (ed): *Advances in Psychosomatic Medicine*. Vol. 8: *Psychosocial Aspects of Physical Illness*. Basel, Karger, 1972, pp 180–215.

PART II

ON BEING A PATIENT

Psychophysiologic Considerations

CHAPTER 4

Anxiety

1. A 40-year-old white woman came to the doctor with the following complaint: "I am afraid my heart will burst and that I will drop dead." On examination, mild hypertension and rapid pulse were noted. After thorough workup and study of the patient, the physician concluded that anxiety was probably the most important factor in producing her symptoms.

2. An attractive female college student, 22 years old, told her physician that she felt she needed sex therapy. She had had difficulty achieving orgasm during intercourse for several years and now found herself withdrawing socially because of fear of getting into sexual relationships in which she would feel frustrated. She was successful and a high achiever in all other areas, for example, scholastic activity, and felt that she should achieve orgasm every time she had intercourse. The physician's impression was that her anxiety concerning sexual performance was interfering with her ability to enjoy it fully.

3. A 30-year-old housewife would develop overwhelming panic whenever she went out of the house alone, particularly in crowded places. She refused to leave her house unless her husband would go with her and stay by her side. Her physician diagnosed her condition as agoraphobia and referred her to a psychiatrist.

Some writers have labeled our present times "the age of anxiety." "Anxiety" is one of our most commonly used words, and virtually everyone is familiar with it. Like pain, everyone has experienced it, and all wish to avoid it. At the present time, antianxiety medications are the most commonly prescribed drugs in this country. Anxiety is important in medical practice because it constitutes one of the most common, but often unrecognized, reasons for seeking medical help. In addition to the familiar and easily recognizable symptoms it may produce, it may also contribute to the development of a myriad of physical symptoms that patients may not attribute to it.

While a great deal is known about this ubiquitous and highly important phenomenon of anxiety, we still have not achieved a fully and satisfactorily integrated understanding of its nature or of the pathophysiologic mechanisms whereby it may both induce and influence as well as arise out of physical dysfunction (disease). In this chapter, we will first discuss some relevant theories and various aspects of anxiety—that is, its phenomenology, central neurophysiology and neurochemistry, peripheral physiology, function, and regulation (and disregulation)—and will then turn to its clinical evaluation, diagnosis, and management. To discuss so many aspects of such a complex phenomenon presents a problem similar to that presented in the fable of the blind men and the elephant—the very same thing can seem so different depending upon which aspect one apprehends and upon the amount and kind of detail that various approaches can elucidate (i.e., upon the relative technical and theoretical sophistication of different disciplines). In discussing the various aspects of anxiety in the sections that follow, we have attempted to balance presentation of detail in relation to sketching overall patterns in such a way as to achieve maximum relevance for the physician. We ask the readers to bear in mind (as a matter of faith?) that these disparate renderings all do, in fact, pertain to the same thing.

Phenomenology of Anxiety

As in the first vignette, the most prominent subjective feature of anxiety is identical to what is experienced in the *emotion* of *fear*—namely, a sense of dread and apprehension. This fearful feeling is usually vague and diffuse, but it may also focus on a specific idea, such as fear of dying, or of cardiac arrest, or of having a dreadful disease such as cancer. When the patient is questioned carefully, one can often determine that the vague feeling of dread came first and was later followed by more specific thoughts and ideas such as those mentioned above. *Physiologic changes* are part of anxiety. They are mediated by activation of the central and autonomic nervous systems and of neuroendocrine mechanisms. In a fully developed reaction, all structures influenced by these systems may show functional changes. Thus, the symptoms and signs may include rapid pulse, increased blood pressure, excessive sweating, change in bowel function, changes in appetite, trouble sleeping, and difficulty breathing. In essence, then, *subjective feelings* of *dread and fear* accompanied by *symptoms* and objective *signs* of appropriate physiologic changes indicate the presence of anxiety.

Theories of Anxiety and Emotions

Since anxiety is an emotion, we should first take up some general considerations about emotions. *Emotions,* or *affects,* as they are sometimes otherwise called, include three main components: (1) a subjective state of mind or feeling tone (e.g., dysphoria–dread–awe); (2) a neurovegetative motor discharge (e.g., increased heart rate); and (3) perception by the person of the bodily sensations caused by the motor discharge (e.g., palpitation of the heart). Various theories relate these three components to one another in different ways.

The James–Lange theory of emotions, proposed in late 19th century by the famous psychologist William James and the Danish physician Carl Lange postulated that bodily changes (motor component) follow directly the perception of an exciting event and that the person's perception of the bodily changes (sensory component) was what we call "emotion" (James and Lange, 1922). According to this theory, changes in the viscera and/or skeletal muscles were essential for the occurrence of emotions. The subjective component was omitted or assumed to be part of the sensory component. These assumptions were later put to test and disproved by Walter Cannon, the famous American physiologist and also William James' son-in-law. He showed that emotions were felt in persons who had had upper cervical spinal cord transections (thus effectively cutting off all the afferents from the viscera and skeletal muscles) and that in normal individuals, the latent periods for the bodily changes were much longer than the felt emotions (i.e., emotions occurred before bodily changes, not after). This led Cannon to believe that perceptions of noxious stimuli at the level of the *thalamus* (see Figures 2 and 3) in the brain led to two distinct pathways of excitation, one upward to the cortex, adding affective quality to the experience through associations with memory traces, etc., and a downward discharge from the thalamus effecting redistribution of blood to viscera and skeletal muscles and changes in metabolism (e.g., rise in blood sugar)—all of such a nature as to prepare the animal for the vigorous muscular work involved in attacking *(fight)* or getting away from *(flight)* the danger. Cannon made extensive investigations into the fight–flight responses, which he felt were related to the basic emotions of displeasure, anger, and fear (anxiety) (Cannon, 1932). Cannon's theory concerning emotions was later modified by Papez (1949) and MacLean (1949), placing more emphasis on the limbic brain structures than on the thalamus (see Figure 4, below). This *limbic system model* forms the basis of modern neurophysiological theories concerning emotions (see section on the brain mechanisms of anxiety, below).

The two major theories that address the psychological mechanism (higher cortical function of the brain) by which situations may be *perceived* and

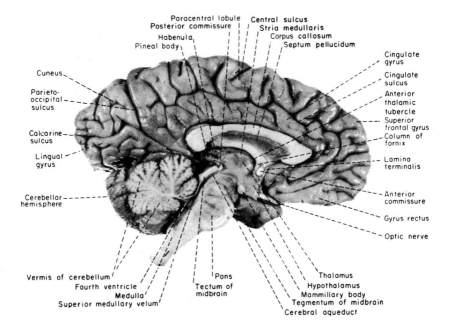

Figure 2. Photograph of the medial surface of the adult brain cut in sagittal section. (From Everett *et al.*, 1971. Copyright 1971 by Lea & Febiger. Reproduced with permission from the publisher and author's estate.)

appraised as dangerous, leading to the generation of anxiety as an emotion, are (1) the *learning theory or conditioning model* of anxiety based upon the studies of Pavlov (1927) and (2) the modern *psychoanalytic theory* of anxiety ("signal theory") first articulated by Freud in 1926 (Freud, 1926/1953).

Learning Theory Model

When a stimulus is inherently dangerous, such as the sight of a growling tiger, a fear response occurs naturally. A stimulus that is neutral and not inherently dangerous, such as open spaces or elevators, can become associated with a dangerous situation through a process called "conditioning." According to the learning theory model, then, anxiety is a *conditioned fear response.*

The *conditioning process* by which a neutral stimulus becomes aversive, creating a fear response, may be stated as follows: A neutral stimulus (the sound of a bell) that occurs in close *proximity* to an inherently noxious stimulus (e.g., electric shock) becomes *associated* with the noxious stimulus so that,

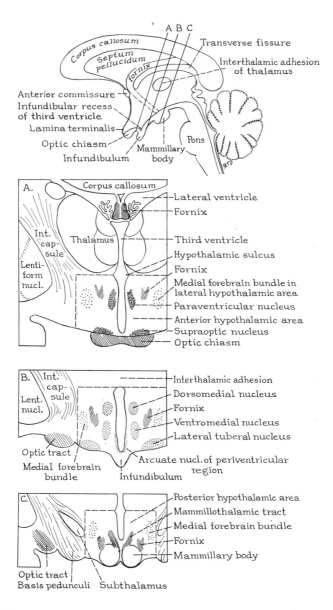

Figure 3. Schematic drawing of a sagittal section of the brain stem showing the relations of the hypothalamus to surrounding brain structures. Lines A, B, and C correspond to the levels at which the three lower drawings were made. Section A is through the supraoptic area, B is through the tuberal area, and C is through the mammillary area of the hypothalamus. (From Everett et al., 1971. Copyright 1971 by Lea & Febiger. Reproduced with permission from the publisher and author's estate.)

even in the absence of the noxious stimulus, it acquires the power to *elicit response* in the organism *as if it were the noxious stimulus.*

For example:

1. Electric shock (inherently noxious, and thus called the *unconditioned stimulus,* or US, meaning that no "conditioning process" is necessary to produce the response in question) → fear response (called the *unconditioned response,* or UR, e.g., increase in pulse rate or dilated pupils).
2. Light (usually "neutral" to animals) → no fear response.
3. Light plus electric shock → fear response. In this *pairing* of light and shock, the neutral stimulus is called the *conditioned stimulus,* or CS. If this pairing within a set time interval occurs repeatedly, then . . .
4. Light (CS) alone → fear response. The fear response occurring in response to the CS is called the *conditioned response,* or CR.

Conditioning, of course, occurs to various stimuli, including both pleasant and aversive stimuli. For example, Pavlov's famous experiments involved training dogs to salivate at the sound of a bell using the above paradigm.

Ordinarily, conditioned responses will disappear *(extinguish)* if the conditioned stimulus is repetitively experienced without any further pairing with the unconditioned stimulus (reinforcement).* This phenomenon is the basis for a form of behavioral therapy (desensitization) which is particularly useful in treating phobias, where an ordinarily neutral stimulus (e.g., elevator) has acquired the capacity to elicit the anxiety response. In phobias, the patient will go to any length to avoid the phobic object or situation in order to avoid experiencing the anxiety reaction. A patient with a phobia for crowds [and open spaces (agoraphobia)] may ultimately become a virtual recluse (vignette 3). This illustrates an aspect of anxiety with highly important clinical implications, namely, that human beings have little tolerance for free anxiety and that individuals develop behaviors (coping mechanisms, defense mechanisms) to avert or avoid it. In classical learning theory, this is conceptualized as follows: *Anxiety is so unpleasant that a person will repeat behaviors or seek situations that have been associated with its diminution.* Behaviors that lessen anxiety can be learned through instrumental conditioning; that is, relief from anxiety can be regarded as motivation for behavior (see Chapter 17).

---

*If the unconditioned stimulus has been strong enough, the conditioned response may resist extinction permanently (Solomon and Wynne, 1954; Wynne and Solomon, 1955). Sailors who had served during World War II, when a bell was used to signal air attacks ("battle stations"), still showed an increased galvanic skin response to the same gong tone 20 years later (Edwards and Acker, 1962).

Psychoanalytic Signal Theory of Anxiety

As we will see below, psychoanalytic theory assigns central clinical importance to this noxious aversive quality of anxiety and labels the psychological mechanisms that are developed for averting anxiety "ego defenses" (*see* Chapter 5).

In making a distinction between fear, where the danger stimulus is external and recognized (e.g., an escaped grizzly bear), and anxiety, where the danger stimulus is internal and unrecognized (e.g., an unconscious conflicted impulse such as a murderous wish), psychoanalytic theory turns our attention to a careful and close consideration of "intrapsychic" phenomena. This signal theory of anxiety* starts with the idea that every human being is endowed with an inborn capacity for experiencing the combined physiological–psychological reaction that we call anxiety. Freud's theory of anxiety, however, concentrates on the importance and role of anxiety in mental life rather than on providing a fundamental explanation of its nature and basic origin (Brenner, 1955). It assigns to anxiety the central role in the neuroses by asserting that it occurs when there is *conflict* between unconscious wishes for pleasurable gratification and the person's opposing mature goals and moral standards.

The theory further specifies that the form of anxiety with which we are most familiar, that is, the response associated with subjective feelings and motor and conscious sensory components, is but one of two forms of anxiety—a clinical form *(free anxiety)*. Free anxiety occurs *when psychological defense mechanisms have failed.* It may vary in intensity from relatively mild apprehension to intense disorganizing panic. The *second* form, which Freud called *signal anxiety,* is conceptualized to be so mild and attenuated as to go unnoticed (or perhaps barely noticed) in consciousness. Nonetheless, it is perceived in the mind and reacted to as a signal of an *impending* danger situation.

The theory specifies a stepwise series of events: (1) When an unconscious wish (that would lead to unacceptable thoughts and/or behavior) is about to attain conscious recognition, an attenuated form of anxiety is generated; (2) this attenuated anxiety reaction then serves as a signal (signal anxiety) indicating that a dangerous situation will develop if the conflictual impulse becomes conscious and gains access to the motor systems that could carry it out in action; (3) in response to the signal anxiety, psychological defense mechanisms come into motion that prevent the dangerous situation from developing by barring access of the threatening impulse to consciousness and the motor systems of the body (see Chapter 5). In other words, the person reacts to the

*Freud replaced with this theory the older "toxic" theory, which is now of historical interest only.

impending emergence into consciousness of a conflictual impulse as to an impending danger and so experiences attenuated anxiety. In response to this attenuated (signal) anxiety, psychological defense mechanisms are mobilized to deal with the offending impulse. In summary, the *attenuated anxiety signals a state of tension within the personality system* —that is, conflict between basic primitive organismic demands *(id)* and demands of the individual's social environment and conscience *(superego)*. It is the function of a part of the personality system called the *ego* to appraise and mediate between those opposing forces and to defend against the forbidden impulses (see Chapter 5).

Success of the personality system, more specifically, the ego, is reflected in satisfactory adaptation without experience of noticeable anxiety; partial success results in experience of somewhat attenuated, but felt anxiety (clinical anxiety states) and/or adaptive states marred by neurotic symptoms and/or behavior. Failure is regarded as resulting in panic states (unattenuated anxiety) and perhaps psychotic experience and behavior.

The psychoanalytic theory of anxiety as summarized has been incorporated into clinical psychiatric theory and is regarded as basic and essential for understanding clinical disorders involving the personality system.

Anxiety is considered also to function as a stimulus to growth and to development of adaptive behaviors. This aspect will be discussed in a later section of this chapter. More detailed aspects of the theory dealing with the ontogenetic developmental aspects and metapsychology of anxiety are more controversial but perhaps of less general importance to those working outside of psychiatry.*

While the learning theory model and the psychoanalytic theory of anxiety are quite different with respect to formulations concerning the nature and origin of anxiety and of danger situations, there are many aspects of both theories that are congruous with each other, even though they may differ in emphasis. For example, both theories recognize that anxiety is associated with potential danger situations. The emphasis in learning theory is on external danger situations and how neutral stimuli might have become deliberately or accidentally associated with them; psychoanalytic theory emphasizes intrapsychic danger situations arising from psychological conflicts.

Psychological defense mechanisms are mobilized to reduce the unpleasant affect of anxiety in potentially dangerous situations (including being ill and being in the hospital) that threaten the individual's personality system.

*Recommended readings by Freud and Brenner at the end of this chapter should be consulted for acquaintance with these more specialized features. Brenner is particularly recommended as an introduction for those without a fair amount of previous reading in the literature of psychoanalysis.

Physiology of Anxiety

As already noted, when a stressful event is perceived, the cerebral cortex and its efferent pathways are activated, including the reticular activating system. This increases the arousal level and the motor outflow through the pyramidal and extrapyramidal systems, thereby increasing general muscle tension and causing specific changes in the tone of the facial muscles, giving rise to the tense expression seen in anxiety states. Tension of vocal cords may sometimes seriously interfere with speech. In general, these changes are demonstrable by the use of electroencephalogram (EEG) and electromyogram (EMG), the EEG showing fast, low-voltage waves typical of arousal and the EMG showing increased electrical activity of muscles involved in the response.

At the same time, activation of the limbic system (see Figure 4, below) results in activation of the *hypothalamus* and *autonomic nervous system* (predominantly, but not exclusively, the sympathetic division) and of the hypothalamic nuclei that secrete the *releasing factors* (hypophysiotropic hormones). The hypothalamic releasing (or inhibiting) factors influence the *pituitary gland* and lead to the stimulation or inhibition of the release of various tropic hormones. Autonomic nervous system arousal leads to an increase in circulating *epinephrine* and *norepinephrine* by sympathetic stimulation of the adrenal medulla.

Direct effects of the autonomic arousal in acute anxiety include (1) *circulatory changes*—increase in systolic blood pressure and pulse pressure (diastolic pressure and peripheral resistance may remain the same or fall); increase in stroke volume, heart rate, and cardiac output; increased blood flow to skeletal muscle, heart, lungs, and brain and decreased blood flow to the splanchnic vascular bed and skin; (2) exocrine *changes in skin*—increased sweating and skin conductance (cold clammy hands); (3) dilation of the pupils; (4) changes in rate and depth of respiration; (5) changes in gastrointestinal function—secretion, motility, and mucosal vascularity; and (6) some metabolic changes such as increase in levels of sugar, free fatty acids, and lactic acid in the blood. Imbalance of sympathetic and parasympathetic components may contribute to untoward reactions such as development of disturbances in cardiac rate and rhythm and even fainting, as will be discussed in a later section of this chapter.

Indirect effects of anxiety (via effects of released hypothalamic factors on pituitary tropic function) include increase in the secretion of adrenal cortical hormones, which gives rise to profound metabolic changes (in water and electrolyte balance, in suppression of immune mechanisms, and in catabolic carbohydrate and protein metabolism), and other widespread hormonal changes, for example, in secretion of growth hormone, prolactin, and thyrotropic, gonadotropic, and antidiuretic hormones.

In general, the longer-lasting endocrine systems are called into play when response to danger is intense and sustained. Then, more profound metabolic effects are added to the more acute autonomically innervated reactions. Selye's now classic studies of stress call attention to the role of the pituitary–adrenal cortical system and the adrenal cortical hormones in the *adaptation syndrome* and point to their importance as probable contributors to pathogenesis of a variety of clinical disorders of (unknown) multiple-factor etiology such as rheumatoid arthritis and essential hypertension (Selye, 1950).

As the preceding discussion shows, consideration of the psychophysiology of anxiety leads quite naturally to a more general look at the psychophysiology of stress and to contemplation of some clinical implications. For the student of medicine, there are two highly important points to emphasize here. The first concerns the distinction between stress and strain. *Stress* consists of an *external* and/or internal *challenge* to the integrity of a structure requiring adaptation or adjustment, whereas *strain* is a measure of the tension or imbalance endured *within* the responding (stressed) structure. A physical analogy would be that of a heavy truck crossing a bridge, the weight of the truck constituting the stress and the disturbance in molecular alignment of the bridge structure constituting the strain. In psychophysiologic systems, the stress might be a psychosocial crisis (e.g., death of a close relative); strain would be measured by the degree to which balance of psychophysiologic systems is upset and required to adjust in order to restore a previously steady state.

The second point to emphasize is that there is in the human an *inverse relationship between the effectiveness of psychological defenses and the degree of physiologic activation* (reviewed by Mason, 1975). When defenses break down or are ineffective, physiologic changes are intense; when defenses are highly effective, physiologic changes, if any, are minimal. Thus, the effectiveness of psychological defenses is a crucial variable in determining the degree of strain in the individual. For further discussion of defense mechanisms, see Chapter 5.

Psychosocial stress, then, carries the potential for inducing profound and widespread physiologic, metabolic, and chemical effects in virtually all systems, organs, and tissues of the body—effects that may influence the balance between health and disease—but the extent and intensity (potential seriousness) of such effects depend upon the efficiency of psychological defenses. The physiologic, metabolic, and chemical effects referred to above probably influence the health–disease balance in a nonspecific fashion, that is, by affecting the resistance or receptivity of tissues to pathogenic vectors of any type (e.g., bacteria, viruses, metastatic neoplastic cells, and allergens). These are the mechanisms and relationships that account for the profound effects of life change upon morbidity and mortality as well as upon illness and help-seeking behavior (see Chapters 1 and 11).

Brain Mechanisms of Anxiety

We mentioned earlier that the modern concept of emotion is based on the neuroanatomical model proposed by Papez and MacLean. According to this model, the structures of the limbic system, the inner core of the brain, play a major role in the brain mechanisms of emotions, including anxiety. The word "limbic" refers to a border or a hem. This term was coined by Broca in 1878 to denote the inner brain tissue surrounding the brain stem and lying under the neocortical mantle (Figure 4). The microscopic structures of the limbic brain are presumed to be organized into two layers. The phylogenetically oldest tissue (allocortex) makes up the inner ring, and the outer ring (called the transitional cortex) consists of a peculiar cellular structure, not resembling either the neocortex or the allocortex (Isaacson, 1974). Some portions of the inner aspects of the neocortex and thalamus, although not part of the original "limbic lobe" described by Broca, are often considered as being part of the functional unit, the limbic system. Thus, the structures involved with this system include the *hypothalamus,* the *amygdala,* the *hippocampus,* the *septum,* and the

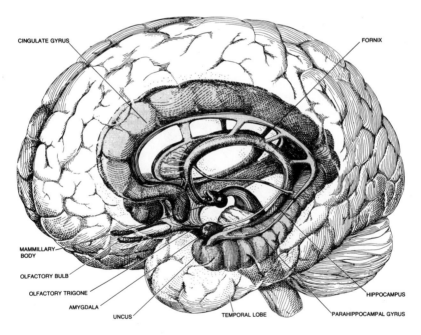

CINGULATE GYRUS

FORNIX

MAMMILLARY BODY

OLFACTORY BULB

OLFACTORY TRIGONE

AMYGDALA

UNCUS

TEMPORAL LOBE

HIPPOCAMPUS

PARAHIPPOCAMPAL GYRUS

Figure 4. The limbic system (shaded area): a series of evolutionarily primitive regions at the core of the brain that are primarily involved with smelling in lower vertebrates and with the arousal of emotions in humans. (From Synder, 1977. Copyright 1977 by Scientific American, Inc. Reproduced with permission.)

cingulate gyrus. These structures are closely related to the *anterior thalamus* and the *reticular activating system,* which runs through the limbic system and the brain stem and extends into the spinal cord (see Figures 2– 7).

Various studies, including direct electrical stimulation and surgical ablation of structures of the limbic system, indicate that basic emotions and drives manifested by eating, sexual behavior, drinking, "sham rage," and attacks are controlled by these structures.

In general, pleasurable feelings are produced by stimulation of certain areas of the limbic system and related structures, such as the lateral hypothalamus and the medial forebrain bundle, a neuron system arising from the noradrenergic, serotonergic, and dopaminergic neurons of the brain stem and distributing widely through the limbic system and to the forebrain (see Figures 3 and 6). Lesions of the medial forebrain bundle produce a drop of 90% or more of the norepinephrine levels in the forebrain, which may be of significance in disorders of mood, such as manic or depressive disorders (see Chapter 6). Stimulation of other areas of the limbic brain, such as the medial hypothalamus or the medial portion of the amygdala, the almond-shaped structure lying at the top of the hippocampus, produces aggressive and angry responses.

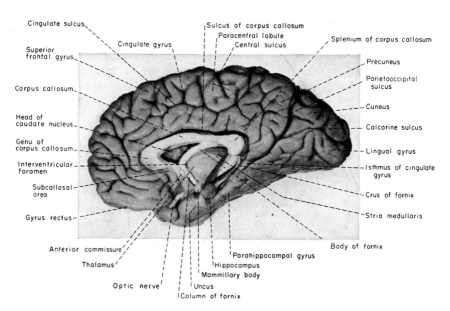

Figure 5. Photograph of the medial surface of the adult brain cut in sagittal section and partially dissected to show the hippocampus and fornix. (From Everett *et al.,* 1971. Copyright 1971 by Lea & Febiger. Reproduced with permission from the publisher and author's estate.)

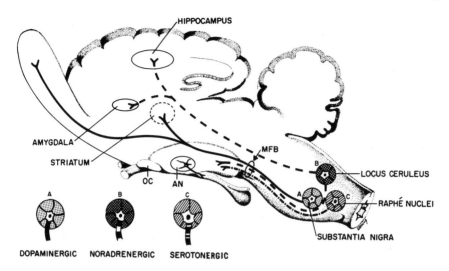

Figure 6. Monoaminergic pathways in mammalian brain. The principal localization of the neurons containing norepinephrine, dopamine, and serotonin is in the mesencephalon and pons. Axons of these cells are distributed to widespread areas of the cortex, limbic system, and striatum. The dopaminergic system of the arcuate is an exception to this general scheme of distribution. Abbreviations: MFB, medial forebrain bundle; AN, arcuate nucleus; OC, optic chiasm. (From Martin *et al.*, 1977. Copyright 1977 by F.A. Davis Co. Reproduced with permission from the publisher and authors.)

If an internal or external stimulus is processed by the neocortex and the stimulus is found to be associated with unpleasant or painful memories, then the signal of anxiety would be generated. That is, the neocortex would play a major role in the processing and integration of perception and the activation of associative pathways. The result of such activation may be stimulation of certain parts of the limbic system concerned with the feeling of anxiety. In fact, there are extensive connecting pathways between many parts of the neocortex, especially between and among the prefrontal cortex concerned with intention and plans, the temporal cortex concerned with verbal memory, and the amygdala and hippocampus of the limbic system. The limbic system and the neocortex have extensive connections with the brain stem. Nuclei in the brain stem, especially the noradrenergic locus ceruleus (see Figure 6), may have important functions in anxiety– fear mechanisms, as we will discuss in the next section.

The amygdala, hippocampus, and septum all have modifying influences on the functions of the *hypothalamus*, which is the *final common pathway* of limbic system functions. Different areas of the *amygdala* are concerned with searching, curiosity, and aggressive reactions. Complete ablation of both amygdalae in animals tends to produce placidity and lack of fear. This is a part

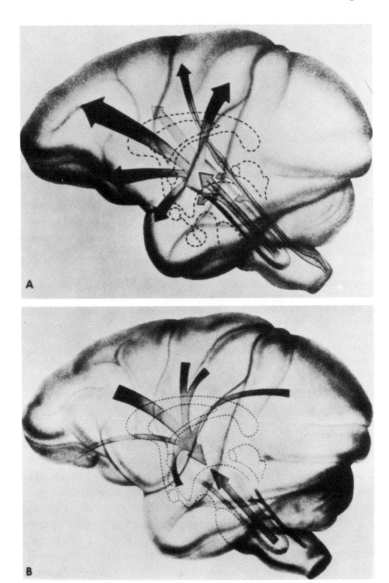

Figure 7. The reticular activating system. A: The ascending reticular activating system schematically projected on a monkey brain. (Originally published in Lindsley; *Reticular Formation of the Brain.* Boston, Little, Brown & Co.) B: Convergence of pathways from the cerebral cortex and from the spinal afferent systems on the reticular activating system. (Originally published in French, Hernandez-Peon, and Livingston; *J. Neurophysiol.* **18:**74, 1955.) (From Guyton, 1976. Copyright 1976 by W.B. Saunders Co. Reproduced with permission from the publisher and author.)

of the *Klüver–Bucy syndrome,* produced by bitemporal lobectomies. Other features of the Klüver–Bucy syndrome include visual agnosia, a compulsiveness to contact and examine objects, a strong oral tendency, and hypersexuality.

The *hippocampus* is connected to the septum via the fornix, which terminates in the mammillary body of the hypothalamus (Figures 3, 4, and 5). Destruction of the hippocampus in animals usually results in a greater willingness to undertake new actions and decreased fear reactions. The hippocampus, together with the septum, forms an inhibitory system, the excitation of which causes behavioral inhibition. The hippocampus is also intimately involved in the conversion of *recent memory* into long-term memory and in the association of stimulus with painful experience in avoidance conditioning (Isaacson, 1974; Gray, 1972). Parenthetically, *psychomotor epilepsy* (also known as temporal lobe epilepsy) is often associated with extensive scarring of the hippocampus and neighboring structures and with many behavioral and emotional problems.

The *amygdala* and the *septohippocampal system* are considered by many to act as a push–pull balanced control system with regard to anxiety. The hippocampus is thought to be primarily responsible for recognition of a "mismatch" between the incoming stimulus and an expected stimulus. Together with the amygdala, the septohippocampal system determines the degree of *uncertainty* in a given situation and determines the overall reaction of the organism via the final common pathway of the hypothalamus.

The *hypothalamus* is the final common pathway and effector organ of the limbic system. The hypothalamus may be divided loosely into an *anterior, parasympathetic* part and a *posterior, sympathetic* part. The anterior hypothalamus is considered to be "trophotropic," that is, related to energy conservation and pleasurable states. The posterior hypothalamus is "ergotropic," having to do with the interaction between the organism and the environment. Stimulation of the posterior hypothalamus results in sympathetic nervous system activation and anxiety–fear responses as well as anger. Stimulation of the anterior hypothalamus can result in either relaxation or acute distress.

The hypothalamus is sometimes called the *"homeostat"* of the body, since it controls most of the homeostatic mechanism through its outflow into the autonomic nervous system and the endocrine system via the pituitary gland. When the outcome of the excitation of the neocortex and the limbic system structures of the amygdalo-septo-hippocampal system is excitation of the posterior, sympathetic part of the hypothalamus, a *fight–flight reaction* may be elicited with concomitant emotions of anxiety, fear, and anger. If the outcome is stimulation of the anterior, trophotropic part of the hypothalamus, a *relaxation* response might be elicited. Various gradations of simultaneous stimulations also occur, thus eliciting mixtures of ergotropic and trophotropic responses. Also, in situations of acute fear and distress, the stimulation of the trophotropic, parasympathetic system may be considerable, and sometimes predominant (such as decreased blood pressure, decreased heart rate, and immobilization with depressive or apathetic affect).

In addition to the brain structures described above, the *reticular activating system* plays an important role in anxiety mechanisms (see Figure 7). The diffuse network of nerve cells extending from the neocortex through the limbic system into the spinal cord (called the reticular formation) has both ascending and decending pathways. The major function of this system is the control of the *tone* of the central nervous system *(arousal)*. The perception of a potentially dangerous situation results in an *activation of the reticular activating system,* thus preparing the brain and the central nervous system for the fight–flight response, and contributes to the emotional experiences of anxiety, fear, and anger.

With the anxiety–fear response, the hypothalamus facilitates the release of certain *"stress" hormones* through its control of the pituitary gland by means of the *hypothalamic releasing and inhibiting factors* (hypophysiotropic hormones).

Central Neurochemistry of Anxiety

At present, data concerning the roles of various neurotransmitter substances in the brain during anxiety states are confusing and often contradictory. Suffice it to say that all the known central nervous system neurotransmitters seem to be involved in the functioning of the various structures involved. The substances include catecholamines (including norepinephrine, epinephrine, and dopamine); the indoleamine serotonin; acetylcholine; γ-aminobutyric acid (GABA); glycine; substance P; and endorphins (enkephalins). Recent evidence tends to indicate that the noradrenergic system is involved in the pleasure–reward system as well as in anxiety–fear, the serotonergic pathways in sedation and sleep mechanisms, the cholinergic pathways in arousal determined by the reticular activating system as well as in functions of the neocortex and movement, and the dopaminergic pathways in attention and modification of movement; GABA seems to exert a generalized inhibitory effect within the central nervous system.

Endorphins are also implicated in analgesia, euphoria, and, perhaps, anxiety (see Chapter 7). There is some recent evidence that there may be specific receptors in the brain that bind a class of antianxiety drugs, the benzodiazepines (Squires and Braestrup, 1977). An implication of this finding is that, as in the case of opiate receptors in the brain, there might be as yet unidentified endogenous substances that regulate anxiety levels in the brain analogous to the endorphins in relation to pain perception.

Stimulation of the *locus ceruleus* in the brain stem (pons) in monkeys results in typical anxiety–fear behaviors, and most antianxiety agents appear to inhibit the locus ceruleus or its synaptic projections (Redmond *et al.,* 1977). The locus ceruleus seems to provide more than 90% of the noradrenergic input into the brain. Thus, this nucleus might serve as an "anxiostat," contributing important modifying effects on the limbic system, neocortical, and brain stem structures in their mediation of anxiety and fear responses.

Once the anxiety–fear response has been elicited by specific activation of the hypothalamus and the pituitary gland, the effect on the brain of the sensory input from the bodily changes due to sympathetic activation, such as increased heart rate and blood pressure, and the direct effect on the brain of the hormones released by the pituitary may form a *secondary component* of the experience of anxiety and fear. This component (the effect on the brain of the bodily changes accompanying stimulus) of emotion had been equated with emotion itself in the *James–Lange theory of emotions.* Although Cannon disproved the equation, further studies have shown that some bodily changes accompanying emotion, such as levels of epinephrine in the blood, can influence the *readiness of individuals* to experience specific emotions, although this reactivity is modified a great deal by cognitive factors, such as what the subject had been told prior to an intravenous infusion of epinephrine (Schachter and Singer, 1962). For example, intravenous infusion of norepinephrine and epinephrine simulates the bodily changes observable in anxiety–fear or rage reactions, and the subject will experience these emotions at the slightest provocation. However, if the subject has had explained exactly what bodily changes to expect, he will not be as ready to react emotionally.

Studies on the direct effects of "stress hormones" on the brain indicate that adrenocorticotropic hormone (ACTH) increases the anxiety–fear response in animals. For example, ACTH injection increased the latency period for animals to enter a cage where they had been shocked previously. Adrenocortical steroids such as cortisol seem to improve avoidance learning in animals, suggesting an increased anxiety–fear response. On the other hand, in humans, exogenous corticosteroids tend to cause euphoria, although anxiety symptoms also occur in some subjects. Some studies indicate that ACTH enhances, while cortisol tends to inhibit, the dorsal area of the hippocampus.

Function of Anxiety

Anxiety is an unpleasant emotion and certainly a major cause of suffering. One might wonder, then, why we have anxiety at all; that is, why have we not discarded anxiety eons ego in the evolutionary process? The obvious reason is that anxiety serves highly important *adaptive functions.* We have already seen that anxiety prepares the organism physiologically for fight–flight reactions essential for survival, and we have discussed the role of anxiety in learning; that is, it *facilitates avoidance learning,* thus preventing repeated exposure of the organism to dangerous situations. Another highly important function of anxiety that we have discussed is its signal function and role in initiating the *mobilization of psychological defense mechanisms.*

But beyond these more immediate and obvious survival values, anxiety serves broader and more far-reaching functions—it is an important force in stimulating and supporting *personality development,* particularly maturational processes responsible for acquisition and effective performance of *socially valued skills.* Perhaps the easiest way to open discussion of the productive, constructive, or generative function of anxiety is to look at its immediate or short-term role as an influence on skilled performance. Anyone who has had to face the challenge of an important academic examination, or athletic competition, or public speaking knows very well that there is an optimal level of "tension" or anxiety for realizing the best of one's capabilities. With too little anxiety (and insufficient motivation), performance is likely to be lackluster and below par. We all have our own ways of getting "psyched up" for such challenges. On the other hand, if the level of anxiety becomes too high, performance suffers because of the disorganizing effects on finely tuned cognitive and sensorimotor mechanisms—increased incidence of forgetting and of errors, loss of fine motor coordination, loss of confidence, feeling "clutched up," panic, and so on. In vignette 2, it seems likely that excessive anxiety in relation to success in sex may have played a disruptive role in the patient's experience of sexual activities and contributed to her eventual aversive response. The *inverted U relationship* between *level of drive and performance* (Yerkes–Dodson law) in this way can be seen to apply to anxiety, again calling attention to its "drive" or motivational quality.

Many theories of personality development postulate a similar motivational, generative, and facilitating–inhibiting function for anxiety in cognitive and social development. Psychoanalytic theory (particularly developmental ego psychology) details how frustration generates anxiety and motivates development of the requisite cognitive and defensive ego functions and related social skills upon which mature adult adaptive behavior depends (Freud, 1926/1953; Hartmann, 1958, 1964).

Disregulation of Anxiety

As is the case with other primarily adaptive mechanisms (e.g., immune responses, fever, and inflammation), anxiety is subject to disregulation. Major disruptions in its regulation not infrequently contribute to clinical morbidity—and sometimes even to fatal reactions. Walter Cannon, fascinated by the phenomenon of voodoo death, reviewed the world literature on it and wrote a now classic paper on the subject (Cannon, 1942). In Africa, some superstitious primitive tribes believed that certain powerful medicine men or witch doctors had the power to kill through the magical ritual of "bone pointing." There were numerous accounts describing how vigorous, healthy individuals, after having had the bone pointed at them and being convinced they were going to die, would leave the tribe and within a few days be dead—of no apparent or usual natural cause.

Cannon speculated that the mechanism might be excessive sympathetic adrenal stimulation. Richter studied an experimental model of sudden functional death in captured wild Norway rats and demonstrated (1) that the pathogenic mechanism was vagal inhibition of the heart and (2) that the phenomenon was influenced by sensory and psychological factors. There are, in fact, quite a number of examples of behaviorally induced or associated sudden death or feigned death in animals (Richter, 1957). Sudden death due to fatal arrhythmia is not an unusual occurrence in humans (400,000 deaths each year are attributed to it in the United States) (DeSilva and Lown, 1976). Most studies of this phenomenon implicate the effects of abrupt autonomic imbalance upon the cardiac rate-setting and impulse-conducting tissues (Lown et al., 1977). This effect is probably most apt to occur in individuals with structural damage to these tissues (e.g., due to arteriosclerosis), but it is not really known whether or not the phenomenon can occur in individuals with entirely healthy hearts.

Two other common and clinically important examples of anxiety disregulation are fainting (syncope) and hyperventilation.

Fainting

In the common form of fainting *(vasodepressor syncope)*, the mechanism involves primarily the cardiovascular aspects of the anxiety reaction, specifically as it affects distribution of blood throughout the body. The *loss of consciousness* is caused by inadequate blood supply to the brain despite the fact that the anxiety response normally increases cardiac output and redistributes blood so as to increase blood flow to the brain as well as the skeletal muscle, heart, and lungs. In vasodepressor syncope, blood pools in the periphery, particularly in the extensive vasculature of the skeletal muscle of the lower extremities. This results in decreased venous return to the right side of the heart, decreased cardiac filling, and fall in cardiac output—sufficient to result in inadequate blood supply to the brain. Engel (1962) postulates that the circulatory changes of anxiety prepare for fight or flight, both of which require vigorous muscle activity, which, in turn, keeps the increased blood supply to muscle circulating and literally massages it out of the muscle bed back toward the heart, ensuring adequate cardiac filling and output. If, however, the danger situation is abrupt, overwhelming, and one which the individual is powerless to influence, and if the person would be ashamed to flee (retreat) and does not act, that is, does not move, the large amount of blood sent to the muscles stays there instead of being pumped back to the heart by muscle contraction. Epidemics of vasodepressor syncope commonly occur among army recruits when the young men are lined up for blood tests by venipuncture. If one recruit faints, it is common for several more to follow suit in short order, illustrating another interesting aspect, namely, social contagion. The issue of pride (shame) preventing retreat in this situation is clear. Another aggravating circumstance is that the subjects are standing up, so that gravity aggravates or accentuates the pooling of blood in the legs.*

Hyperventilation Syndrome

The second clinically important acute disregulation syndrome is the "hyperventilation syndrome." In this condition, an exaggeration of the respiratory aspect of the anxiety response leads to difficulty, that is, excessive increase in rate and/or depth of breathing. This is easily observed by the physician, although the patient most often is not aware of it. With the overbreathing there is excessive loss of carbon dioxide, leading to *respiratory alkalosis* (reduced pCO_2). The increased blood pH leads to decreased ionization of calcium, which may produce clinical signs of tetany (in which painful muscle contractions occur). In addition to the usual symptom of anxiety, the hyperventilating patient experiences light-headedness (altered blood gases), headache, nausea, tingling around the mouth, tingling of the fingers and toes (hypocalcemia), and, if the overbreathing lasts long enough, even cramping or spasm of muscles in the extremities. All of this is enough to make the person even more anxious, resulting in a vicious circle. A patient who has such attacks is usually terrified by the experience. Dramatic reassurance can be given by demonstrating that the attacks can be reproduced at will by deliberate overbreathing. Then the symptoms can be reversed by having the patient breathe into a paper bag and rebreathe the exhaled air which has a higher concentration of carbon dioxide. Confirming this diagnosis through the above technique can be dramatic and highly gratifying to both patient and physician. Most doctors remember with great pleasure the first time they had the opportunity to use this treatment for hyperventilation. Further evaluation should then be done

---

*For a thorough description and discussion of mechanisms of all forms of syncope, readers are referred to Engel (1962) and medical textbooks.

to understand the underlying cause of anxiety in the patient which leads to hyperventilation.

Stress-Related Disorders

As noted in the section on the physiology of anxiety, when stress (and strain) is prolonged, anxiety responses merge into states in which additional systems, for example, neuroendocrine systems, are mobilized, and extensive metabolic chemical changes eventuate in the central nervous system and throughout the entire body. These changes in interaction with other factors (constitutional, specific tissue vulnerabilities, specific pathogens, etc.) may contribute to or aggravate many clinical disorders such as hypertension and peptic duodenal ulcer. Although there is growing experimental literature on stress-related disorders, the mechanism of interaction between stress and disease is far from completely understood. We are only beginning to appreciate the multiple interacting and intervening variables that can influence the response of somatic systems to psychological–social stress. For example, let us look at just two (somewhat contradictory) experiments in the vast experimental literature on production of gastric ulcers in animals by exposure to stress.

When monkeys were trained to press bars constantly to avoid electric shock in a complex and highly demanding operant conditioning program with many contingencies, they developed bleeding gastric ulcers and died ("executive" monkeys). On the other hand, yoked control monkeys who were shocked the same amount but did not have to press bars to avoid shock did not develop bleeding ulcers (Brady, 1958). In another experiment, rats who were trained to avoid shock by bar-pressing did not develop bleeding ulcers, while yoked *control* rats who were exposed to inescapable shock developed bleeding ulcers (Weiss, 1968). In the latter experiment, however, the rats trained to press bars to avoid shock had *feedback* in the form of light; that is, the light indicating impending shock was turned off as the bar was pressed, unlike the "executive" monkey situation where there was no direct feedback concerning adequate performance.

One might speculate that the *"executive" rats* had a *sense of control* with performance of bar-pressing, while the monkeys had to perform without this sense of control. In any case, it seems that a sense of control and feedback of success from coping strategies in anxiety states may be one important factor in buffering the physiologic strain resulting from the stress and in influencing whether or not a "stress disorder" will result.

Disregulation of anxiety and stress reactions may occur due to *uncontrollable* and *sustained external or internal anxiety-provoking situations* (e.g., as in battle fatigue or unresolved conflict), or it may occur due to *inherent instability, defect, or malfunction* in *any of the many structures and systems* involved, *including the target organs of physiologic arousal.*

A somewhat unique side effect of modern medicine is the increase in *iatrogenic disregulations* of anxiety. This often results when physicians, overlooking the psychosocial origins of the reactions or, in some cases, the adaptive significance of mild to moderate levels of anxiety, prescribe *antianxiety medications at times* and *in dosages* that are *not indicated.* Since antianxiety medications, especially minor tranquilizers such as the benzodiazepines, are habit-forming, a person would have to take increasing doses in order to maintain anxiety at an imperceptible level. This would be especially marked when the psychological and/or social roots of the anxiety are ignored and allowed to continue operating unabated. As a further complication, the patient will eventually experience exacerbation of the anxiety when the dose of the medication is lowered due to the effects of withdrawal. This is *not* to say that antianxiety medications should not be used—there are many situations in which they are indicated. The physician should, however, have a clear idea as to why, and for how long, the medication is to be prescribed.

Classification of Anxiety Disregulation Syndromes

While it is not within the scope of this book to discuss all stress disorders, a brief discussion about the classification of anxiety disregulation syndromes is in order. Essentially, anxiety disregulation syndromes can be categorized according to whether they involve (1) dysfunction in the experience of anxiety (excessive or insufficient); (2) dysfunction in psychophysiologic systems; or (3) dysfunction in behavior.

Disorders in the Experience of Anxiety. The *locus* of the problem in this category is often the *brain* and the *personality system.*

Excessive Experience of Anxiety. Anxiety disorders (neurosis), anxious personality traits, impulsiveness, tendency to become paralyzed with anxiety in the face of moderately stressful situations, etc., fall within this category. Drug abuse, including alcoholism, may be secondary to this type of anxiety disregulation.

Insufficient Experience of Anxiety. Persons who chronically experience little or no anxiety tend to lack motivation and become underachievers. Some individuals, on the other hand, tend to seek extremely dangerous situations to experience arousal (excessive risk-seeking behavior). Inability to learn from unpleasant experiences may be one factor contributing to development of antisocial personality disorders.

Psychophysiologic Disorders. Stress disorders in the form of tissue damage and/or organ dysfunction may occur following *sustained physiologic* *arousal* in anxiety. The *locus* of the problem may be in the perceptual apparatus, cerebral cortical structures, and the *personality system* (excessive generation of anxiety); and/or in the *neuroendocrine* and *autonomic nervous systems* (instability or excessive excitation); and/or in the *target organs* (vulnerability). Psychophysiologic disorders may occur in relatively healthy and disease-resistant individuals with intact personality systems and central nervous and endocrine systems if the organism—environment interaction is such that the physiologic component of anxiety is activated for prolonged periods in an uncontrollable way. If disease (such as essential hypertension, peptic ulcer, migraine, the depressive syndrome, schizophrenia) eventuates, the selection of the affected system probably rests upon *constitutional* (genetic and developmental) *predisposing* factors related to the organ system involved.

Dysfunction in Behavior. *Heterothetic Behaviors.* As we discussed in Chapter 1, some individuals who find themselves in anxiety-provoking situations seek medical help for minor physical symptoms without recognizing that the help-seeking behavior is motivated by anxiety. An example is the woman who, when family problems arose, came to see her physician for varicose veins she had had for 20 years. Prompt recognition of the presence of heterothetic behaviors is important for the physician to prevent "addiction to sick role behavior" and/or unnecessary and potentially dangerous medical procedures (see Chapters 2 and 15).

Cognition—Action Dissonance. This occurs when an individual takes no action to alleviate an anxiety-generating situation, even when the situation is readily identifiable and the means of avoiding danger is readily available. The *locus* of the problem in this case is obviously in the personality system and, secondarily, in the organism—environment interaction. This syndrome can eventually, of course, contribute to development of any of the disorders discussed above. "Learned helplessness" may be one possible explanation for this disorder (Seligman and Maier, 1967). Animal and human experiments show that repeated prior exposure to situations in which behavior has no effect (learning helplessness) may influence individuals' behavior in future situations. They may tend to "give up" the quest for ways of coping, even in new situations in which their behavior could have an effect. Such learned helplessness is often encountered in depression (see Chapter 6).

Evaluation of Anxiety

The diagnosis of anxiety is based upon the signs, symptoms, and behavioral changes that have been discussed in previous sections of this chapter.

Once having established the presence of anxiety, the evaluation should proceed to the contexts of its occurrence, that is, the questions of the meaning and significance of anxiety (What is the danger situation?); the kind of individual (prone to anxiety? tending to deny anxiety? etc.); the cultural–social matrix (What is the method of expressing anxiety the patient is accustomed to? by complaining of physical symptoms? by taking medications?); and the reasons the patient is seeking help now (limit of tolerance? heterothetic? occurrence of psychophysiologic disorder?). The contexts should be considered in terms of current, recent, and background contexts.

Contexts of Anxiety

Current Context. Presenting symptoms. What are the immediate circumstances (and accompanying thoughts) under which the anxiety is experienced? Include considerations of patient's antianxiety medications or withdrawal therefrom. How effective are the psychological defenses?

Recent Context. What is the danger situation? Why is the situation seen to be dangerous in the light of the patient's experience? Any cumulative effect of stressful events in the recent past? Has the body been weakened by physical illness (e.g., recovering from an infection, presence of chronic disease)? Are there any physical illnesses or vulnerabilities that may tend to disregulate anxiety at central nervous system, neuroendocrine, or target organ levels?

Background Context. Is the patient habitually prone to experience anxiety? What psychological defenses does he ordinarily use? How is anxiety handled in the patient's cultural and social class matrix (by somatization, suppression, etc.)? If a physical symptom related to anxiety is present, what is the patient's early experience concerning such symptoms either in himself or in a relative?

A fuller discussion on the systematic evaluation of patients will be presented in Chapter 9.

Differential Diagnosis of Anxiety States

Any *disease* of any part of the brain, autonomic nervous system, and neuroendocrine system associated with the anxiety mechanism can mimic anxiety states, as can some diseases of target organs. It is important to *rule out* such diseases. Physical examination and psychiatric evaluation, including mental status examination and appropriate laboratory tests, will usually clarify the diagnosis. To establish the psychiatric diagnosis of anxiety disorder (neurosis), it is not sufficient to "rule out organic disease" by negative physical examination and laboratory findings. It is necessary also by psychiatric evaluation to adduce evidence for a positive psychiatric diagnosis, such as clarification of the psychosocial context or the danger situation. Some diseases capable of mimicking anxiety states are thyrotoxicosis, pheochromocytoma, carcinoid syndrome, hypoglycemia, seizure disorders, drug withdrawal states, brain tumors, and Cushing's syndrome. Some major psychiatric disorders such as schizophrenia and affective disorders are often accompanied by anxiety, but, in addition, one would find evidence of other psychiatric difficulties such as a thought disorder in patients with schizophrenia and altered neurovegetative function and sleep disorders in patients with the depressive syndrome.

Management of Anxiety

Careful evaluation and appraisal of the patient with anxiety should lead naturally to formulation of a rational management plan. The first order of business is to determine whether or not the experienced anxiety is excessive, that is, whether it threatens to paralyze or decrease *coping* and adaptive *abilities* of the patient or to cause other disregulation syndromes such as psychophysiologic disorders. If excessive anxiety is present, then prompt reduction of such anxiety by means of appropriate reassurance and antianxiety medications is indicated. (Sometimes even hospitalization is desirable as a way of getting the patient away from a stressful life situation and providing a supportive setting.) In prescribing antianxiety agents such as diazepam (Valium) or chlordiazepoxide (Librium), the physician, being aware of the habit-forming qualities of the medications, should take care that they are used only *temporarily,* almost as an emergency measure. Major tranquilizers such as perphenazine (Trilafon) or haloperidol (Haldol) in small doses (e.g., 2 mg Trilafon b.i.d. or t.i.d. p.r.n.) may be equally effective in reducing anxiety without addictive qualities, but they can also produce serious and irreversible side effects in some individuals if used excessively and over prolonged periods. (A more comprehensive discussion of these and other medications will be found in Chapter 18).

Having determined the severity of anxiety present, and having made a decision as to whether or not to *treat the manifest anxiety per se,* the physician should next attempt to define the *causes* and *contexts* of the anxiety and, having done so, to institute appropriate treatment modalities. A few examples follow.

Careful evaluation of the contexts of anxiety may reveal that the main danger situation is an *intrapsychic* one (intensification of psychological conflicts, e.g., between basic drives and learned inhibitions). In this instance, *psychotherapy* is indicated. The danger situation may be an external one, such as threats to health or occupation. *Medical treatment* or *counseling* may be necessary in these situations. On occasion, it may be necessary to advise *environmental change* or suggest *new coping strategies* (especially in the presence of action– cognition dissonance). If the anxiety-provoking situation is pervasive and seems to be a result of *faulty learning, behavioral treatment modalities,* such as desensitization or learning of relaxation techniques, may be helpful.

If a target organ disorder, such as hypertension, is present, *it should be treated medically in parallel with the management of the psychological and social factors* that might have contributed to it. Excessive anxiety determined predominantly by *intrinsically unstable brain structures* (acute toxic or structural brain damage) may be managed successfully by teaching the patient new coping strategies and relaxation techniques.

Summary

Anxiety, together with pain, is one of the most common major causes of help-seeking behavior. The experience of anxiety involves *subjective* feelings of fear and dread which are usually vague, although on occasion the patient may complain of specific fears such as fear of dropping dead. *Physical examination* will usually reveal signs of sympathetic nervous system activation, including rapid pulse rate, elevated blood pressure, and excessive sweating.

Anxiety can be regarded as a *warning response* to impending danger which may be external or intrapsychic. The term "signal anxiety" in psychoanalytic theory refers to the special case in which we are not aware of the nature of the danger situation (i.e., the impending situation is internal, psychological, and "unconscious"). Anxiety may develop as a conditioned response to previous exposure to unpleasant or dangerous situations. Anxiety serves the adaptive *functions* of preparing the organism for fight or flight, of mobilizing psychological defense mechanisms, and of facilitating performance.

All parts of the *brain* participate in the anxiety mechanism. The most important parts of the brain include the neocortex for processing of information, the limbic system for the emotional reactions leading to the neural and endocrine discharge via the hypothalamus, the brain stem nuclei, especially the locus ceruleus, which may play a major role in the generation and suppppression of the anxiety– fear response, and the reticular activating system for the arousal levels of the central nervous system accompanying anxiety.

Activation of specific parts of the hypothalamus in anxiety– fear reactions results in specific patterns of excitation of autonomic and endocrine systems. Anxiety is usually associated with excitation of the autonomic nervous system and altered function of neuroendocrine systems.

Although anxiety serves a useful function in moderate levels, it may, so to speak, go out of kilter, resulting in "anxiety disregulation syndromes." The cause of disregulation may be multiple, and any combination of the following may be involved: the perceptual apparatus, the brain and personality system, the neuroendocrine and autonomic nervous systems, target organs, organism–environment interaction, and iatrogenic factors.

Anxiety disregulation syndromes may be classified broadly into (1) disorders in the experience of anxiety (excessive or insufficient), (2) psychophysiologic disorders, and (3) dysfunction in behavior, including heterothetic behaviors and cognition–action dissonance.

Evaluation of anxiety should include the determination of the presence of the *state* of anxiety by means of indicators including subjective reports and an evaluation of the *contexts* of anxiety, which include current, recent, and background contexts. The recent context includes determination of the possible danger situation generating the anxiety, recent life events, and stresses. The background context includes the cultural factors, early learning factors, and the *trait* of the patient in experiencing anxiety.

The *management* of anxiety should naturally follow the information obtained in the evaluation phase. Excessive anxiety may be successfully treated by medication, behavioral treatment modalities, and reassurance. The danger situation should be identified and coped with, for which psychotherapy or counseling is often indicated. Target organ disorders may need specific medical treatment.

In general, antianxiety medications should be used only temporarily to alleviate massive and paralyzing anxiety while evaluation and treatment continue to deal with situational and psychological factors generating anxiety.

Implications

For the Patient

As anxiety is an unpleasant and vague feeling whose cause is usually not obvious, some patients may tend to *attribute the cause of dysphoria to a physical illness* or may displace their concern onto physical sensations associated with minor disorders. Thus, the presence of anxiety is one of the most common reasons for help-seeking behavior, *ostensibly for other physical symptoms* (heterothetic, or problems of living presenting as a symptom). In such instances, the fact that physical examination and laboratory tests reveal no serious medical condition will not completely reassure the patient, since the cause of the anxiety was not related to the physical symptoms in the first place. If the situation (usually interpersonal and/or intrapsychic) generating anxiety is not explored by the physician, the patient often interprets continuing high levels of anxiety as evidence that the physician either lacks competence or "does not care."

For the Physician

The physician should be aware that the patient is *suffering* when anxiety is present. Alleviation of this suffering can only be achieved by a comprehensive evaluation and management of the patient. Although anxiety often results in heterothetic behaviors, the physician should also be aware that (1) actual physical illness, especially chronic illnesses, may increase the patient's propensity to experience anxiety and that (2) on occasion, some medical illnesses *simulate* anxiety states. Any disease affecting the brain and peripheral structures concerned with anxiety mechanisms can mimic anxiety states. A rational management plan can only be obtained after a thorough evaluation of the patient according to the principles outlined in this chapter. Emphasis should be placed on understanding the recent context, or the danger situation to which the patient may be responding with anxiety. In order to elicit this information, the physician has to ask *specific questions* about recent events, such as the patient's *relationships* with spouse, relatives, and friends, the financial situation, and the health status of close people. Questions should be asked about the patient's *demographic data* and early experiences, especially in relation to anyone who had a disease or symptom similar to the one the patient is complaining of now, in order to elicit information concerning the background context. The patient should also be asked whether or not he has a tendency to feel anxious or to get upset easily, whether he has had many physical illnesses and complaints in the past, etc. (the "trait" of the patient). An evaluation of the current context should include the question, "What do you think, or theorize, is causing your present symptoms?" (e.g., palpitations, dizziness, or whatever). Often the patient may tell you, "I think it's because I have cancer" (or heart disease, or leukemia, etc.). This should be followed by the questions, "Why do you think that?" or "Do you know of anyone who had cancer?" (or heart disease, or leukemia, etc.). This will often give the physician information concerning what the *meaning* of the symptom might be for the patient and, sometimes, what the danger situation might be, given the patient's unique experiences and exposures ("priming factors").

For the Community and Health Care System

We are often told that we live in an age of anxiety. We have seen that one of the important elements in reducing undesirable effects of anxiety (or perhaps anxiety itself) in animals and humans is a *sense of control or mastery* and *feedback* indicating that the attempt to control or master the situation generating anxiety has been successful. At the level of social systems, it seems imperative to facilitate, as much as possible, the sense of mastery available to the individual members and to provide feedback of such mastery. More responsive decision-making and administrative structures with a minimum of bureaucratic red tape (an excellent device to reduce or delay feedback) at all levels of the social system would be highly desirable. This would apply particularly to the health care system, including the hospital, the ward, and the treatment team.

Patients with anxiety disorders can become more anxious, frustrated, and sick when their requests for p.r.n. ("when necessary") medications (or bedpan or whatever) remain unanswered or ignored for hours.

Medical curricula should include the evaluation and management of anxiety and anxiety disregulation disorders. Special emphasis should be placed on the role of anxiety in facilitating heterothetic help-seeking behaviors and in the treatment of target organ disorders, as well as on the psychopharmacologic management of acute anxiety. Drug treatment of anxiety should always be accompanied by an attempt to understand and cope with the danger situation and underlying factors generating the anxiety.

Recommended Reading

Brenner C: An Elementary Textbook of Psychoanalysis. New York, International Universities Press, 1955, pp 81–92. An exceptionally lucid, accurate, and detailed synopsis of the theory of signal anxiety. The entire volume is recommended as an excellent and authoritative introduction to psychoanalytic theory.

Freud S: Inhibitions, symptoms, and anxiety, in Strachey J (ed): *The Standard Edition of the Complete Psychological Works of Sigmund Freud.* London, Hogarth Press, 1953, vol 20, pp 71–175. (Originally published, 1926.) A classical psychoanalytic view of the mechanisms of anxiety and symptom formation.

Hilgard ER, Bower GH: *Theories of Learning.* Englewood Cliffs, NJ, Prentice-Hall, 1975. This is comprehensive textbooks on various learning theories and theoreticians. The chapters on Pavlov's classical conditioning and Skinner's operant conditioning are well worth reading if you have not already read them in a psychology course. A good reference concerning any questions about learning theory and conditioning.

Isaacson RL: *The Limbic System.* New York, Plenum Press, 1974. A review of the structure, functions, and experiments concerning the limbic system. Recommended for those interested in the specific structures.

Izard C: *Patterns of Emotions.* New York, Academic Press, 1972. A comprehensive psychological analysis of anxiety and depression. The author believes that anxiety is a complex emotion consisting of fear, distress, and anger.

Kollar EJ, Alcalay M: The physiological basis for psychosomatic medicine: A historical view. *Ann Intern Med* **67**:883–895, 1967. A nice and reasonably comprehensive review of psychophysiology of emotions.

Levi L: *Emotions: Their Parameters and Measurement.* New York, Raven Press, 1975. This is a multiauthored comprehensive volume on the biological and psychophysiological aspects of emotion, including anxiety. Quantification of emotion is also discussed extensively. An excellent reference.

Spielberger CD (ed): *Anxiety: Current Trends in Theory and Research.* New York, Academic Press, 1972. This two-volume multiauthored book deals more specifically with anxiety, its nature, measurement, biological aspects, and relationship to stress.

Warburton DM: *Brain, Behavior and Drugs.* London, John Wiley & Sons, 1975. A comprehensive review of the neurochemistry of behavior, including mood, homeostasis, sleep and dreams, and memory.

References

Brady JV: Ulcers in "executive" monkeys. *Sci Am* **199:**95–100, 1958.

Brenner C: *An Elementary Textbook of Psychoanalysis.* New York, International Universities Press, 1955.

Cannon WB: *The Wisdom of the Body.* New York, WW Norton & Co, 1932.

Cannon WB: "Voodoo" death. *Am Anthropol* **44:**169–181, 1942.

DeSilva RA, Lown B: Ventricular premature beats, stress, and sudden death. *Psychosomatics* **19**(11):649, 1978.

Edwards AB, Acker LE: A demonstration of the long-term retention of a conditioned GSR. *Psychosom Med* **24:**459–463, 1962.

Engel GL: *Fainting,* ed 2. Springfield, Ill, Charles C Thomas, 1962.

Everett NB, Sundsten JW, Lund RD: *Functional Neuroanatomy,* ed 6. Philadelphia, Lea & Febiger, 1971.

Freud S: Inhibition, symptoms, and anxiety, in Strachey J (ed): *The Standard Edition of the Complete Psychological Works of Sigmund Freud.* London, Hogarth Press, 1953, vol 20, pp 77–175. (Originally published 1926.)

Gray JA: The structure and emotions of the limbic system, in *Physiology, Emotion and Psychosomatic Illness.* Ciba Foundation Symposium 8 (NEW series), New York, Ciba Foundation, 1972, pp 87–130.

Guyton AC: *Textbook of Medical Physiology.* Philadelphia, WB Saunders Co, 1976.

Hartmann, H: *Ego Psychology and the Problem of Adaptation.* New York, International Universities Press, 1958.

Hartmann H: The mutual influences in the development of ego and id in *Essays of Ego Psychology: Selected Problems in Psychoanalytic Theory.* New York, International Universities Press, 1964.

Isaacson, RL: *The Limbic System.* New York, Plenum Press, 1974.

Izard C: *Patterns of Emotions.* New York, Academic Press, 1972.

James W, Lange CG: *The Emotions.* Baltimore, Williams & Wilkins, 1922.

Lown B, Vernier RL, Rabinowitz SH: Neurologic and physiologic mechansims and the problems of sudden cardiac death. *Am J Cardiol* **39:**890–902, 1977.

MacLean P: Psychosomatic disease and the "visceral brain." *Psychosom Med* **11:**338–353, 1949.

Martin, JB, Reichlin S, Brown G: *Clinical Neuroendocrinology.* Philadelphia, FA Davis, 1977.

Mason JW: Clinical psychophysiology: Psychoendocrine mechanism, in Reiser MF (ed): *American Handbook of Psychiatry,* ed 2. Vol 4: *Organic Disorders and Psychosomatic Medicine.* New York, Basic Books, 1975, pp 553–582.

Papez JW: A proposed mechanism of emotion. *Arch Neurol Psychiatry* **38**:725–743, 1949.

Pavlov IP: *Conditioned Reflexes*. London, Oxford University Press, 1927.

Redmond DE, Maas JW, Huang YH, *et al.*: Does the locus ceruleus mediate anxiety and fear? Presented at the meeting of the American Psychiatric Assocation, Toronto, 1977.

Richter CP: On the phenomenon of sudden death in animals and man. *Psychosom Med* **19**:191–198, 1957.

Schachter S, Singer JE: Cognitive, social, and physiological determinants of emotional state. *Psychol Rev* **69**:379–399, 1962.

Seligman ME, Maier SF: Failure to escape traumatic shock. *J Exp Psychol* **74**:1–9, 1967.

Selye H: *The Physiology and Pathology of Exposure to Stress*. Montreal, Acta, 1950.

Solomon RL, Wynne LC: Traumatic avoidance learning: The principles of anxiety conservation and partial irreversibility. *Psychol Rev* **61**:353–365, 1954.

Synder SH: Opiate receptors and internal opiates. *Sci Am* **236**:45, 1977.

Squires RF, Braestrup C: Benzodiazepine receptors in rat brain. *Nature* **266**:732–734, 1977.

Weiss JM: Effects of coping responses on stress. *J Comp Physiol Psychol* **65**:251–260, 1968.

Wynne LC, Solomon RL: Traumatic avoidance learning: Acquisition and extinction in dogs deprived of normal peripheral autonomic functioning. *Genet Psychol Monogr* **52**:241–284, 1955.

CHAPTER 5

Psychological Defense Mechanisms

1. A 45-year-old man was quite surprised to discover that he had completely forgotten his doctor's appointment one Monday until his wife asked him about it that same evening. He had suffered severe chest pain a week before, but after it subsided, he decided not to call the doctor because his routine checkup appointment already had been scheduled for that Monday.

2. The young physician admitted a 29-year-old woman to the surgical service but could not understand his patient. Earlier the same day, she had gone to her family doctor's office complaining of a sore throat. When her doctor examined her, he found an area of ulceration on her breast and a hard lump under the ulcerated area. Upon admission to the surgical service, she told the admitting physician that she entered the hospital because of a sore throat—completely ignoring the breast condition. When asked about it, she said that she had noticed it three months ago but had not paid any attention to it.

3. A respected surgeon specializing in the surgical treatment of cancer always appears cheerful and optimistic. When a colleague commented to him that it must be difficult to maintain such cheerfulness while treating cancer patients, he said, "All cancer patients want to be cheerful and optimistic. So, I am cheerful, and they are cheerful." One of his patients, however, was not always cheerful and was referred to the psychiatrist. She told the psychiatrist, "I feel like a failure. I cannot keep up a cheerful front for my doctor."

4. A patient in the coronary care unit who had witnessed the death of the patient in the next bed was asked what had happened. He said, "The guy in the next bed improved and was transferred to the medical floor, since he doesn't need to be on intensive care any more."

5. An intern proposed a crippling radical operation for a patient, despite the fact that cancer was widespread throughout the body and could not be ameliorated by the proposed surgery.

6. A 45-year-old man underwent open-heart surgery for replacement of the mitral valve. He was recuperating satisfactorily in the recovery room until the second postoperative day. At noon, the nurses noted that he was becoming confused and restless. Shortly thereafter, he was openly agitated and attempted to pull out his intravenous tubing. He insisted that the women in the room (nurses) were plotting to kill him by injecting poison through the intravenous apparatus. On mental-status examination, he was noted to be grossly disoriented as to time and place and unable to remember even simple things such as a three-digit number.

In the first five cases presented above, either the patient or the doctor avoided or minimized a potentially unpleasant situation and feelings, for example, finding out that he or she might have a serious disease (vignettes 1 and 2), having to discuss the gravity of illness with the patient, or recognizing that patients may sometimes feel discouraged (vignette 3). This kind of avoidance or minimization is effective only temporarily and, in the long run, is often *detrimental*—unduly delaying help-seeking behavior and prompt medical treatment. On the other hand, as a short-term reaction, it can be *beneficial* when the *danger situation abates spontaneously* or in situations when *everything that can be done to deal with the danger is already being done* and when the *physiologic change of anxiety could be harmful.* For example, patients who deny feeling frightened or apprehensive in the coronary care unit for the first few days after suffering from a heart attack have been shown to have better survival rates as compared to those patients who admit feeling frightened or apprehensive (Hackett et al., 1968). Understanding the psychology of defense mechanisms can help in developing an appreciation for some of the (sometimes inscrutable) adaptive and maladaptive ways that patients and doctors behave when exposed to the myriad of unpleasant situations and emotions connected with illness and death.

Distress, Anxiety, and Defense Mechanisms

As we discussed earlier, help-seeking behavior occurs when a person has reached his limit of tolerance of anxiety because of a symptom or disability. Anxiety arising from problems of living may also result in help-seeking behavior by lowering the individual's threshold for tolerance (e.g., of pain), increasing his awareness of discomfort associated with the symptom, or motivating him to seek comfort through interpersonal contact with the doctor. In each of these situations, the common denominator is a *felt distress* by the individual (or, in some instances, by other persons involved with the patient) that moves him to seek help.

When perceptual and psychological stimuli activate *memories* associated with dangerous situations or are themselves perceived and evaluated as being *directly threatening,* then *anxiety* results. The brain structures as well as the physiological and psychological mechanisms involved in the generation of anxiety and the anxiety response have been discussed in Chapter 4. We have seen that anxiety serves as a signal to the organism that it has to somehow cope with a potentially dangerous situation. Human beings may deal with anxiety (and thus the danger situation in two ways: (1) by fleeing from or eliminating the source of the stimuli, that is, *fight or flight,* or (2) by internal adjustments in the central nervous and psychological systems whereby the anxiety sensation is reduced and the potential danger situation "avoided," although the stimuli may be still present. This is always the case when the stimuli are internal rather than external—since we cannot flee from internal psychological– motivational sources of potential danger. The internal adjustment mechanisms are what are called the *"psychological defense mechanisms."*

When the stimuli associated with danger come from outside of the person, elimination of the source would be most desirable, but it is not always possible. Sometimes we have to make *inner adjustments to ignore unpleasant events* outside because we are not powerful enough or are otherwise unable to change them. If the danger situation exists internally, that is, a psychological conflict has been activated, which, if allowed to run its course, threatens to overwhelm the person emotionally—the only recourse lies in the use of *internal adjustments.* For example, certain past memories and/or mental representation of forbidden conflictual drives may be rendered inaccessible to consciousness; this is called "repression" in psychological terms. Of course, there must be changes in the central nervous system that subserve these phenomena, such as, perhaps, attenuation of associative pathways in parts of the brain involved in memory storage and retrieval. We do not yet have the technology which permits study and description of these different aspects in a unified way. The best we can do, then, is to refer to states and changes in the brain that manifest themselves in both the physiological and psychological realms and to describe the changes in the two realms insofar as they are known separately and in parallel.

We should emphasize that the defense mechanisms come into being *automatically* ("unconsciously"), that is, without conscious "willing" on our part. According to psychoanalytic theory, the generation of a small amount of anxiety as a signal is considered to usher in the defense mechanisms, which, in turn, avoid the development of clinical anxiety. There are individual variations in the kind of defense mechanisms habitually used in the face of potential danger. Some individuals usually or preferentially cope with danger situations by using internal adjustment processes (defense mechanisms), others use mainly outer-directed defensive activity, and some use both.

During the course of development, each individual develops a repertoire of defenses, some of which are called into play (separately or in combinations) so habitually that, in effect, they become part of the person's character style. For example, if someone habitually attributes inner unacceptable feelings to others (this defense is called projection; see below), we may speak of him as a paranoid character. Since habitual defense mechanisms can be expected to be utilized when an individual encounters threatening events, including discovery of symptoms or signs of disease, these character styles have special implications for medical management, as we will see in Chapter 15.

It seems likely that developmental environmental influences, especially learning experiences within the family, contribute to the development of defenses and defensive repertoires, but there is still a great deal to be learned about the ontogeny of defenses.

As the term "defense" implies, these mechanisms are usually quite adaptive and are necessary in daily life, serving useful functions, just as inflammation serves useful physiologic defense functions. On the other hand, exaggerated and/or persistent use of certain defensive maneuvers may lead to psychopathology, just as persistent inflammation may itself contribute to certain diseases.

When defenses break down, increasing conscious experiences of free anxiety and awareness of danger develop and may lead to help-seeking behavior. In addition, as we saw in Chapter 4, when the physiologic activation is severe and prolonged, the stage may be set for precipitation or exacerbation of stress-related illnesses (Sachar et al., 1970). The variety of effective defenses and combinations of defenses that are available for flexible and appropriate mobilization when needed serve as one highly important measure of an individual's capacity to adapt successfully and maintain health in a dynamically stressful environment. This assessment is a major consideration which a psychiatrist takes into account in appraising the strength ("ego strength") of the personality.

Our discussion of defenses is oriented toward the medical reader; we have tried whenever it is appropriate to emphasize the ways in which defenses manifest themselves so as to influence the sick role, illness, and professional behaviors. Our main concern is their relevance to medical practice in all its aspects—diagnosis, treatment, research, and prevention.

Classification of Defense Mechanisms

Despite the importance of their functions, there is, unfortunately, no standard system for classifying defenses—or, for that matter, a standard com-

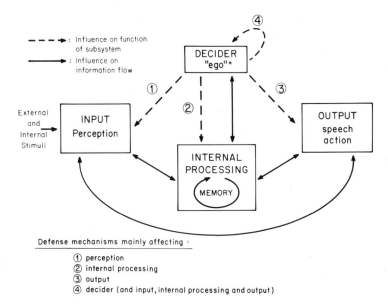

Figure 8. General systems diagram for defense mechanisms. *The executive and defensive functions of the "ego."

prehensive list of them. The classification systems that are offered differ from one another. Anna Freud (1966) proposed that repression be regarded as the primary defense, with the others then to be regarded as reinforcing it. Meissner *et al.* (1975) (following Vaillant) classify defense mechanisms into narcissistic, immature, neurotic, and mature defenses. Others classify them as successful or unsuccessful, still others into defenses that are directed primarily toward outer dangers and those that are primarily inwardly oriented. In the discussion of the defenses that follow, we have grouped them according to a scheme that is compatible or syntonic with the general systems approach that we have used in the rest of the book.*

The personality system can be seen as consisting of *input, internal processing–decider,* and *output* apparatuses or subsystems for handling information. General system concepts can be applied to classify the defense mechanisms on the basis of the subsystem most affected by the defensive process (see Figure 8). "Input" refers to the perceptual apparatus; "internal processing" refers to the associative and memory connections; "decider" refers to the hypothetical "executive" apparatus (of the ego); and "output" refers to the devices subserving motor (including verbal) function. Obviously,

*This is for the sake of consistency and continuity and to facilitate transfer of concepts and understanding between different sections of the book and permit extrapolations from one section to another.

for any defense mechanism to be mobilized, some perception of a danger situation has to occur, and the decider, through input from the internal processing apparatuses, mobilizes defense mechanisms, which, in turn, act on the functions and channels leading to any of the subsystems. As the personal system is an open system, and all of the subsystems have mutual feedback, any change in one subsystem usually affects all other systems more or less, and so, to some degree, all are involved (see Figure 8). The scheme we are using here classifies or groups defenses according to which subsystem—input, internal processing, output, or decider itself—is the one whose altered function constitutes the presenting or most obvious manifestation of the defensive operation. Thus *denial* of an external danger manifests itself mainly in the input (perceptual) subsystem. *Acting out* manifests itself mainly in the output subsystem. *Rationalization* manifests itself mainly in the internal processing subsystem. This scheme, then, simply highlights the subsystem manifestly most affected when the defense mechanism is in operation. A subsystem's function can be either increased, decreased, or altered, for example, by a reversal process in which an output device may send out a message that is opposite in character from the information contained in the internal processing subsystem. (As a result, a person may express hate in place of love or suspicion instead of trust.)

Defenses Listed According to Their Main Subsystem Effects*

1. Defense mechanisms that manifest their main effects in the input subsystem. These mechanisms reduce anxiety by changing the perception of a stimulus field that heralds the development of a potential danger situation by:
   a. Diminution or negation of its perception *(denial);* this may even occasionally take the extreme form of negative hallucinations.
   b. Switching the direction of feelings toward and/or thoughts about a highly important and meaningful person onto another, less meaningful, one *(displacement),* thereby enabling the individual to feel comfortable and safe with the negative thoughts and/or emotions.†
   c. Perceiving certain feelings, characteristics, or thoughts as belonging

---

*Illustrative examples of each of the defense mechanisms will be given in a later section of this chapter.

†This mechanism, which may also involve considerable alterations in output and internal processing mechanisms, is grouped here with those involving perception as their primary mode of presentation, since the object of the negative thought or feeling is *perceived* to be different from the original object.

to someone other than oneself *(projection)* or as being located within the self rather than in another person *(introjection)*.

  d. Reducing the perceptual sphere in a massive fashion *(constriction of awareness)*.

2. Defense mechanisms that manifest their main effects in the internal processing subsystem. (Those affecting mainly the executive or decider subsystem are discussed separately below.) The mechanisms we have included in this category involve mainly changes in cognitive, associative, and integrative functions of the brain:

  a. A stimulus or percept that reactivates and would ordinarily stimulate conscious recall of an old forgotten memory may fail to do so because of *repression,* a defense that attenuates association such that stored memories do not reach conscious awareness.

  b. If the meaning of the motives underlying a particular action has been repressed, another reasonable but more socially and personally acceptable meaning may be substituted and considered by the person to constitute the motivation for that action *(rationalization)*.

  c. *Intellectualization* refers to use of intellectual activity in an intense effort to master feelings through objective understanding.

  d. When conflictual memories and ideas enter conscious thought and/or are verbalized without activation of appropriate affects, the defense of *isolation* is being utilized.

  e. *Fantasy and daydreaming* involve associative processes that evoke pleasant feelings and may aid or reinforce denial by diverting attention away from anxiety-provoking stimuli in the environment.

  f. The affective quality associated with a particular idea or action may be turned into its opposite *(reaction formation)*; for example, a craving may be reversed and perceived as a revulsion.

3. Defense mechanisms that manifest their main effects in the output (action) subsystem. These mechanisms reduce anxiety by

  a. Concealing meanings from recognition by expressing them as actions rather than as thoughts *(acting out)*.

  b. Attempting to achieve mastery of a danger by direct active confrontation; for example, the lion tamer exposes himself to the very situation he fears and achieves a sense of security through mastery *(counterphobic maneuvers)*.

  c. Doing something that is considered to negate or "cancel out" a dangerous or guilt-producing action already performed *(undoing)*.

  d. Engaging in an activity that is socially acceptable and worthwhile in its own right but that at the same time may covertly gratify a conflictual forbidden desire *(sublimation)*.

Finally, *activity* of any sort may serve in a nonspecific way to distract one's attention from the anxiety-producing situation and thus provide some relief.

4. Defense mechanisms whose main effects are more evenly distributed in the subsystems. The effects of regression and identification uniformly pervade all of the functional subsystems through the *decider* or executive functions.

  a. In the face of anxiety, we may have tendency to revert to earlier modes of thinking, feeling, and acting in an effort to feel as we did at an earlier epoch of life when we were free of the kinds of anxiety-producing situations that presently confront us or when earlier developmentally age-appropriate modes of behavior were successful in dealing with the kind of situation that is producing anxiety at present *(regression)*. When this mechanism is manifest, we may, at least in part, perceive things as if we were a young child, concern ourselves increasingly with issues that were important in childhood, and behave and act in less mature ways. Regression may, of course, be maladaptive. In many situations, however, it serves adaptive purposes, especially when regulated and controlled, as, for example, in psychotherapy and creative activity. In hospitalized patients, it can facilitate the patient's adaptation to the sick role. When regression is execessive and uncontrolled, it can seriously impair the capacity for rational, mature adaptive behavior.

  b. Another mechanism that affects all of the input, internal processing, and output apparatuses is *identification*. By modeling much of one's own behavior and self-image upon another person's ways of perceiving, thinking, acting, dressing, speaking, and so forth, one may unconsciously feel as if he or she *is* the other person. This mechanism may protect against the anxiety over loss of, or fear of separation from, a loved person. It also is extensively involved in healthy growth, maturation, and learning.

Illustrations of Defense Mechanisms as They May Be Encountered in Medical Practice

Defense Mechanisms That Manifest Their Main Effects in the Input Subsystem

Denial. This is a mechanism by which a person manages to remain unaware of potentially anxiety-provoking external situations, perceptions, or emotional states. Some patients who have suffered heart attacks can in this way minimize the anxiety-provoking aspects of the situation and remain calm.

As noted earlier, this may have a salutary effect on the patient's clinical course during the early acute phase in the coronary care unit—probably by sparing the damaged heart muscle from physiologic burdens that may accompany anxiety, such as increased demand for cardiac work or stimulation of irritable injured ventricular muscles by circulating epinephrine. It can be overdone, though; for example, some patients, as soon as the pain subsides, refuse to believe that they have suffered a heart attack and sign out of the hospital against medical advice—only to be brought back a few hours later pronounced "dead on arrival." Similarly, too much denial during the recovery and rehabilitation phase of illness may interfere with a patient's ability to follow a prescribed regimen of carefully graded return to activity.

Some women who have found lumps on the breast may, through the use of this mechanism, delay consulting a physician (see vignettes 2 and 4).

Physicians may also use denial both adaptively and maladaptively. In dealing with a patient who is terminally ill, a certain amount of denial (of the seriousness of the illness) may be manifested as optimism in the physician's attitude, and this may help the patient to sustain the hope which is so essential in coping with his condition. Excessive denial, however, may strain the patient's credulity or capacity to respond (vignette 3) or may lead to unrealistic planning (vignette 5). Denial is one of the most common and important defense mechanisms encountered in medical practice, both in patients and physicians. It may be reflected in help-seeking behavior and in physicians' behavior and may affect the course, treatment, and outcome of disease.

Displacement. In this process, conflictual feelings, thoughts, or impulses are directed away from an emotionally significant person and instead perceived as belonging to another person. For example, a patient who was actually insulted by the doctor felt offended by the nurse and was abusive toward her; a resident physician who had been criticized by his chief of staff became angry with his patient.*

Displacement occurs more easily when the secondary object is in some way actually or symbolically related to the original one. A patient who has unresolved angry feelings toward his mother may be prone to feel angry with the nurses because the nurturant, caretaking (mothering) aspects of the nurse's role evoke conflictual memories and feelings about the mother.

Displacement is operative in heterothetic patient behavior. The emotional suffering and anxiety arising from problems of living may be shifted to a physical symptom in instances where contacting the physician for a physical

---

*Behavior akin to displacement appears in animals also (Tinbergen, 1953; Lorenz, 1966). For example, a cat whose aggressiveness has been increased by the sound of a barking dog may attack an inanimate object instead.

symptom is more acceptable to the patient than doing so for emotional reasons.

Projection. This is a mechanism by which unacceptable feelings and thoughts within oneself are attributed to and perceived as belonging to some- one else. A patient may insist that he is consulting the physician only because his wife is upset about his symptoms, though he "knows" that "the symptoms are of no consequence."

Projection is the major defense involved in the development of paranoid feelings and ideas. A patient who develops erotic feelings toward the physician may accuse him of being seductive and/or of making sexual advances. Confusing environmental cues (such as those encountered in intensive care units and recovery rooms) or lowered capacity to put together such cues and percepts (as in organic brain syndromes) facilitate projection formation of paranoid persecutory delusions (see vignette 6). A physician uncomfortable about discussing the prognosis of a serious or terminal illness may feel that the patient does not wish to "know" (see vignette 3).

Introjection. This process, whereby the qualities of an emotionally impor- tant person are perceived as being within or belonging to the self, may lead a patient to regard a part of his body (such as a diseased organ) as if it were someone else. For example, a patient with cancer felt as if the cancer within her were her mother persecuting her from within her own body (see Chapter 19). This may occur at a conscious or unconscious level. If conscious, it constitutes a frank delusion. If unconscious, it may give rise to neurotic attitudes about the illness or its treatment.

Constriction of Awareness (Constriction of the "Ego"). This is a proc- ess whereby the person reduces his sphere of awareness to exclude unpleas- ant situations from becoming conscious. This is usually achieved by focusing all of one's awareness on some limited aspects of one's life at the expense of other aspects. For example, a patient with extensive and severe burns may focus his attention exclusively on his pain in order to avoid becoming aware of the possibility of being seriously disfigured.

Terminally ill patients often use constriction of awareness—being con- cerned and preoccupied with minor symptoms allows them to be unconcerned with (the implications of) the illness itself. Students are often surprised at the excessive concern over minor discomforts and seeming lack of concern about prognosis in seriously ill patients.

Defense Mechanisms That Manifest Their Main Effects in the Internal Processing Subsystem

Repression. This is the mechanism which underlies forgetting of unpleas- ant things—it bars unwanted impulses, memories, desires, thoughts, etc., from consciousness. Mental content so "forgotten" subjectively no longer seems to exist, but that it does remain in existence in the "unconscious" is evidenced by the fact that there are circumstances under which it may again become conscious, such as

1. when critical functions of the mind are weakened, as in toxic states of the brain (drugs, severe fatigue, fever, etc.). For example, a patient with organic brain syndrome may use obscene language and may alarm the nurses with "improper suggestions." (Normally unacceptable impulses being expressed due to reduced repression.)
2. when the critical functions of the mind are suspended, as in sleep (dreaming) or under hypnosis.
3. when the balance of forces between strength of repression and strength of the impulses is upset by an upsurge in pressure of the impulses such as occurs in puberty, after long periods of abstinence, or when life circumstances are particularly stimulating or seductive.

Repression operates unconsciously. There is a (probably related) conscious mechanism called *suppression* which refers to a conscious (intentional) effort to forget something or put it out of one's mind. The accessibility or recovery into consciousness of forgotten material may vary from being *relatively* recoverable (e.g., momentary forgetting; see below) to being deeply and firmly barred from recall, as is the case with highly charged traumatic events. The latter may exert considerable influence on behavior, including that involved with health and illness. One striking example is the phenomenon known as the *"anniversary reaction,"* in which it has been observed that patients may become ill (e.g., suffer a heart attack) on the forgotten anniversary date of a highly charged painful event such as the death of a loved one (Weiss and English, 1957).

The simplest example of repression at work is *momentary forgetting*—the forgotten thought is often shown to be related to unpleasant feelings, either directly or indirectly. Other somewhat more long-lasting examples would be the patient in vignette 1 who conveniently forgot an important doctor's appointment and the case of a patient who, on Monday, was told by his physician that he had cancer and, by Tuesday, had forgotten that he had seen his physician the previous day. Further discussion of this defense and its ramifications would take us beyond the scope of this work; appropriate references should be consulted by those who are interested.

You can imagine for yourself the myriad ways in which emotionally determined forgetting could affect illness and sick role behavior (forgetting to take medication, etc., etc.).

Rationalization. This is a process whereby a person "explains away" anxiety-provoking situations or meanings. He may advance rational-sounding explanations for behaviors which were motivated by unacceptable or undesirable feelings or thoughts. The "rational explanations" usually have some degree of validity.

A woman who felt a lump in her breast did not consult a physician, having rationalized that it was due to the menstrual period she was having at the time of discovery. A patient with organic brain syndrome and memory difficulty may attribute his faulty memory to the medications he is taking (which may or may not be partially true). A hospital may require unrealistic working hours and case loads of its house staff "for their training experience," when actually this may be motivated by the need for service.

Intellectualization. This defense is closely related to rationalization and refers to the use of intellectual processes to master anxiety-provoking information and situations. After developing a serious illness, a patient may spend much of his time reading about the illness in medical journals and textbooks. Under similar circumstances, another patient may read philosophy books in an attempt to develop a stoic attitude toward the illness.

Physicians invariably and naturally use intellectualization in their professional activities. Without it, constant exposure to illness and death might well be unbearable. Furthermore, it is knowledge and understanding that render the physician capable of practicing medicine. The wisdom, the skill, and the professionalism of the physician, as well as the objective and impartial attitude toward patients, all presuppose and, to an extent, require the use of intellectual defenses.

As intellectualization is often an effective defense, physicians may wish to encourage some patients to use it and to provide them with detailed information about the disease, references to appropriate books, etc.

Isolation. Isolation as a psychological defense mechanism refers to the process whereby unpleasant feelings are dissociated from the cognitive process. Thus, a person recognizes a situation or memory without experiencing painful or anxious feelings associated with it. Through this mechanism, a patient may be able to give the physician a detailed narrative of a painful experience, such as protracted pain, without becoming overly emotional. Survivors of catastrophes such as accidents and fires often use isolation when remembering the experience—calm, newspaper-report-like accounts of frightening experiences.

This defense is obviously utilized a great deal by physicians. On occasion, excessive use of isolation on the physician's part gives the impression to the patient that he is uncaring and hostile. Excessive isolation on the patient's part sometimes gives the impression to the physician that the patient is really not suffering or that he is displaying "bizarre" affect.

Fantasy and Daydreaming. These are mechanisms through which (partial) gratification is achieved through imagination. They may also serve to distract attention away from unpleasant reality. Fantasy may concern or be stimulated by real situations; for example, a physical examination may stimulate the fantasy that the physician will meet the (unfulfilled) sexual needs of the patient. Although the content of daydreams is conscious, not all fantasies are. Patients are often unaware of the fantasy gratification they derive from medical experiences and procedures; for example, painful procedures may satisfy unconscious guilt and/or masochistic wishes. In extreme cases, this may even lead to the patient's repeatedly seeking operative procedures as if addicted to them. In such cases, the fantasy is acted out through a substitute activity which disguises the true nature of the underlying wishes and needs.

Reaction Formation. Through reaction formation, an unacceptable thought, feeling, or impulse generates its intensely felt opposite in consciousness. Thus, strong affection may be felt instead of hate, great respect instead of contempt, strong affinity instead of repulsion. A patient with unrecognized hostile feelings toward his doctor may become especially cooperative and even ingratiating. A physician may show extra concern toward a patient about whom he might feel hostile. On the other hand, it is also possible for hostility to replace or defend against love or erotic attraction which must be repressed. It should be emphasized again that these mechanisms operate without awareness—what the individual actually feels is the (often exaggerated) opposite of the feeling against which he is defending himself.

Defense Mechanisms That Manifest Their Main Effects in the Output (Action) Subsystem

Counterphobic Maneuvers. These refer to the process by which a person exposes himself to or becomes involved in the very activity or situation he fears. The anxiety may be replaced or made up for by a sense of mastery. The lion tamer in the circus and the reformed alcoholic who has become an abstemious bartender are extreme examples. The patient who reads voluminous books about his illness is behaving counterphobically and using intellectualization as a defense.

An advanced cancer patient, upon being informed of her diagnosis, established a local chapter of the American Cancer Society within a short time and contributed greatly to a cancer early-detection program in the community. A patient with angina pectoris regularly jogged every day, against his doctor's advice—he felt reassured when his chest pain after jogging did not reach unbearable intensity.

Undoing. This refers to an act that symbolically nullifies a previously committed act or thought. Rituals and ceremonial acts may be considered to be examples of undoing.

A physician may become oversolicitous and/or may overmedicate a patient in whose treatment he has made an error.

For some patients, the suffering accompanying illness may serve the role of "undoing" actions or feelings about which they feel guilty.

Sublimation. Through this mechanism, wishes and impulses which were originally unacceptable can find gratification through acceptable channels. Thus, aggressive drives may be channeled into such socially acceptable activities as surgery; sexual curiosity may find expression in the practice of psychiatry. Sublimation is also important in many creative activities, including intellectual and artistic endeavors.

In the course of development, sublimations may become independent of their defensive (and substitute gratification) role and continue to be pursued and perfected in their own right—for pleasure, for accomplishment, and for productivity. Each time the surgeon operates, each time the sculptor "attacks" a block of marble, he or she is not necessarily deriving covert gratification of aggressive impulses, even though such may once have been the case and can on occasion again be so.

Activity and Acting Out. Engaging in any sort of activity may help relieve or reduce anxiety or tension in a nonspecific way, and this may be very useful and adaptive. The term "action-out" refers to a specific form of covert gratification, or discharge of unconscious wishes, or reenactment of forgotten experiences through acting which is unaccompanied by explicit recognition of its inner meaning. As in pantomime, the inner meaning may be obvious to the observer, but in acting out, it is not recognized by the "actor." A patient who convinces (seduces) doctors repeatedly to perform unnecessary exploratory operations for esoteric and vague symptoms may be acting out a forgotten conflictual memory of having been painfully and sadistically attacked or molested.

Withdrawal and Avoidance. These are psychological mechanisms by which a person avoids the occurrence of painful emotions by declining to engage in new interpersonal relationships and disengaging from old ones. Behavioral withdrawal and social isolation often follow. Some patients stop interpersonal contact after being informed of a serious illness because they anticipate and fear social rejection; others actively withdraw by choice in order to avoid ending up later in a position where the disability will leave them no choice and *force* them to limit interpersonal relationships. Withdrawal and avoidance may enable a patient to achieve a state of "comfortable" emotional detachment. When this is not effective, however, painful affective states such as depression may ensue; in fact, withdrawal and depression are often observed to occur together when the defense is only partially effective.

Defense Mechanisms Whose Main Effects Are More Evenly Distributed in All the Subsystems by Affecting the Decider or Executive Subsystem Itself

Regression. In this mechanism, cognitive and behavioral aspects of earlier stages of development are reexperienced or reenacted, usually in the mode of an epoch during which the individual enjoyed rather full gratification and relative freedom from anxiety. When regressed, one may in many ways feel and act as if he were a child, or even an infant. Regressive behavior is a prominent feature of the psychopathology of some major psychopathological disorders, for example, in certain stages of schizophrenia. It can also be observed in medical patients, virtually invariably when the illness is severe and/or of long duration. Since the patient is expected to entrust his life and welfare to the health care personnel (doctor, nurse, etc.), he must assume a childlike dependent role. The medical care setting is especially conducive to the appearance of this phenomenon; in fact, hospitalized patients find themselves literally infantilized—deprived of privacy, being bathed and fed, having to carry out excretory functions in bed, etc. Given all of this, added to the basic anxiety of being ill and in a hospital, in fact, a certain amount of regression is probably necessary to function in the patient role in the hospital.

Along with regression, forgotten memories, conflicts, and feelings of childhood often reappear and lead patients into inappropriate acting out of childhood or infantile conflicts. A patient who without provocation accuses a particular nurse of being hostile to him may be reexperiencing old conflicts over dependency on his mother, whom he had as child perceived as uncaring and hostile. In such a case, the particular nurse might even have some characteristics of appearance or temperament that are reminiscent of the patient's mother; this would facilitate the process but is not a necessary condition for its occurrence. The experiencing of feelings that were associated with an important person in childhood as belonging to someone in the present is the *"transference phenomenon."* Transference phenomena are regressive in nature and may utilize additional mechanisms such as displacement and projection.

Identification. Through this mechanism, a person takes on (with only partial or no realization that he is doing so) the characteristics of another person; that is, he *becomes like* the other person—perceiving, processing information, and behaving like the other. This is considered to be a major defense against the anxiety connected with separation from the loved person; that is, if you are (like) the person you love, you do not lose him. *Imitation* is seen as a precursor to identification. Through identification, a person learns a wide variety of values, attitudes, mannerisms, and behavioral characteristics, including illness behavior, sick role behavior, and help-seeking behavior.

Identification may also be with a feared person (*"identification with the aggressor"),* in which case the motivating force may be to reduce the fear of the person by becoming like him. Another motivating force for identification may be guilt; taking on a hated person's suffering or symptoms may serve as "just" or "deserving" punishment and so relieve feelings of guilt. An example of this is a patient who developed unexplained shortness of breath and chest pain shortly after his mother's death from chronic lung disease.

As noted earlier, identification plays an important role in healthy growth, development, and learning. The educational development of the physician includes a large element of progressive identification with faculty who act as preceptors and role models. Patients also tend to form partial identification with their physicians, for example, in adopting the physician's attitude and outlook concerning the illness. (In vignette 3, many patients of the surgeon identified with him, taking on his cheerfulness.)

Defense Mechanisms, Anxiety, Character, and Coping Styles

Although the psychological mechanisms intrinsic to the defenses are extensively used in reducing anxiety, most of them—some more than others (e.g., fantasy)—seem to be inherent in human beings and may manifest themselves even in the absence of anxiety or anxiety-provoking situations. Some defense mechanisms are more closely related to particular personalities and psychiatric disorders than others. However, everybody uses some of the defense mechanisms in a habitual way, and, as noted earlier, this habitual pattern of defensive maneuvers forms the basis of "character." The term "personality" involves all the behavioral characteristics of a person, including the "character." These terms, however, are often used synonymously (see Chapter 15 for further discussion).

The defense mechanisms are also closely related to the concept of "coping styles." The latter refers to a person's habitual ways of dealing with clearly defined, conscious anxiety-provoking situations, such as hospitalization or impending surgery. Many defense mechanisms, alone or in combination, enter into the development of the coping styles (see Chapter 12, p. 229).

Summary

Help-seeking behavior often occurs in the presence of anxiety. Human beings have a tendency to prevent feeling anxiety by the automatic (unconscious) use of certain psychological processes called "defense mechanisms." The function of the defense mechanisms is to reduce or prevent the generation of anxiety, a common pathway to distress, by keeping stimuli that signal or could lead to danger situations out of conscious awareness or by inducing a sense of mastery.

The processes can be classified, on the basis of the functional subsystems primarily affected, into (1) those affecting input (perception); (2) those affecting internal processing (cognitive and affective processes); (3) those affecting output (action); and (4) those affecting all subsystems evenly by affecting the "decider" or "executive" function of the personality system.

Defense mechanisms commonly used in medical settings include denial, displacement, projection, introjection, constriction of awareness, repression, rationalization, intellectualization, acting out, counterphobic maneuvers, undoing, sublimation, nonspecific activity, regression, and identification.

Implications

For the Patient

The defense mechanisms that a patient uses exert a major influence on when and whether he seeks help for a particular symptom; how he will respond emotionally to the medical treatment and to information provided by the health care team; and how he will cope with illness, procedures, and recovery process. For example, excessive use of denial and repression is likely to result in delayed help-seeking behavior, noncompliance with the doctor's instructions, and frequent conflict with the health care personnel. On the other hand, the ability to deny anxiety to a limited degree and under certain circumstances, for example, in the acute phase of myocardial infarction, may exert a salutary effect.

For the Physician

In Terms of Understanding the Patient. An assessment of the habitual defense mechanisms used by the patient is essential for understanding the patient and for planning treatment approaches. The recognition that defense mechanisms are geared to ward off anxiety (and thus distress) should help the physician in learning how to cope with them. Defenses should not be attacked frontally—this would only cause excessive mobilization of anxiety and distress. The physician in vignette 2 would have understood his patient better if he had been acquainted with the concept of denial, and he might even have wondered whether the excessive denial on the patient's part could have been related to a "priming experience," such as exposure to someone else who had a lump or ulceration on the breast. Regression is a common phenomenon in the hospital, where a certain amount of actual infantilization takes place. Recognition of this phenomenon will help the physician in understanding why some patients may manifest infantile or childlike behavior in the hospital and also why some patients develop irrational feelings concerning members of the health care team, including the doctors and nurses. This understanding is important if the unrealistic or irrational feelings expressed by patients are not to be "taken personally" but rather to be understood as part of the process of being ill and as belonging not to the current health care personnel but to important figures in the patient's past. Habitual defense mechanisms may serve as guides to *strategies in clinical management.* For example, patients showing a tendency to intellectualize may respond well to the provision of reading material concerning the illness or proposed procedure; patients who tend to show denial may respond better to blanket reassurances than to detailed information when anxiety reduction is indicated; patients who use repression excessively may not remember the doctor's instructions or explanations; patients accustomed to using activity as a major defense mechanism may find it unbearable to be confined in the hospital without activity, and for such patients, physical therapy may be indicated as well as early ambulation whenever possible.

In Terms of Understanding Self. In the doctor–patient relationship, the defense mechanisms used by the physician, too, play a major role. In dealing with patients, it is helpful for physicians to be aware of their own habitual defense mechanisms and to understand how they may interact with the patient's defensive style. One clue that may alert us to the fact that defense mechanisms may be "overworking" (i.e., that we are really quite anxious) is to feel a strong overwhelming conviction without being able to explicate the reasons for it. For example, a physician who feels strongly (and stubbornly) that radical surgery should be performed on a patient when, in fact, the objective indications for the operation are equivocal may be using the mechanisms of denial and activity as a way of reducing feelings of helplessness, impotence, and anxiety (vignette 5). Self-awareness could help him to refrain from insisting on an unnecessary, and perhaps dangerous, surgical procedure. Learning to *wait, to observe,* and to *listen*—rather than feeling compelled to *do* something (anything as long as it is active)—is one of the hardest "skills" physicians have to acquire. The social expectation that physicians will not exploit patients for their own needs includes an implicit dictum against treatments that serve mainly as ways of reducing anxiety in the physician.

For the Community and Health Care System

Why do millions of people still smoke cigarettes despite the quite visible and rational warnings by the surgeon general and the medical profession?

Surely, denial, counterphobic maneuvers, rationalization, etc., must play a role in the otherwise inscrutable smoking behavior of many individuals.

Refinement and extrapolation of principles based on understanding of psychological defenses in individual behavior in order to design programs of group and public health education, health care delivery, and preventive medicine constitute a major challenge in our society.

Recommended Reading

Freud A: *The Ego and the Mechanisms of Defense*. New York, International Universities Press, 1966. A classical monograph describing the phenomenology and development of defense mechanisms as an "ego function." Easy to read, succinct, and full of actual illustrations of defense mechanisms in action.

Hackett TP, Cassem NH, Wishnie HA: The coronary care unit: An appraisal of its psychologic hazards. *N Engl J Med* **279**:1365–1370, 1968. The psychologic environment of the coronary care unit. Patients who used major denial had a better hospital course than those who were not using much denial.

Meissner WW, Mack JE, Semrad EV: Structure of the psychic apparatus, in Freedman AM, Kaplan HI, Sadock BJ (eds): *Comprehensive Textbook of Psychiatry,* ed 2. Baltimore, Williams & Wilkins, 1975, vol 1, chap 8.1 (Classical psychoanalysis), pp 528–540. An up-to-date account of the psychoanalytic concept of the psychic apparatus: the id, ego, and superego. Defense mechanisms are discussed in terms of the development of the ego and functions of the ego. The ego is a hypothetical construct of the mind representing a "coherent organization of functions," whose task it is to avoid displeasure through the regulation of the "instinctual drives" and the demands of external reality. This chapter contains a classification of defense mechanisms into narcissistic, immature, neurotic, and mature defenses.

Sachar EJ, Kanter SS, Buie D, *et al.*: Psychoendocrinology of ego disintegration. *Am J Psychiatry* **126**:1067–1078, 1970. In a psychoendocrinologic study of four acute schizophrenic males, the authors found great activation of the adrenocortical hormones when the defense mechanisms were failing. When defense mechanisms were functioning, even if they were pathological defenses such as projection and delusion formation, the hormonal activity was not increased.

References

Freud A: *The Ego and the Mechanisms of Defense*. New York, International Universities, 1966.

Hackett TP, Cassem NH, Wishnie HA: The coronary care unit: An appraisal of its psychologic hazards. *N Engl J Med* **279**:1365–1370, 1968.

Lorenz K: *On Aggression*. New York, Bantam Books, 1966.

Meissner WW, Mack JE, Semrad EV: Classical psychoanalysis, in Freedman AM, Kaplan HI, Sadock BJ (eds): *Comprehensive Textbook of Psychiatry, II,* ed 2. Baltimore, Williams & Wilkins, 1975, vol 1, pp 482–566.

Sachar EJ, Kanter SS, Buie D, *et al.*: Psychoendocrinology of ego disintegration. *Am J Psychiatry* **126**:1067–1078, 1970.

Tinbergen N: *Social Behavior in Animals*. New York, John Wiley & Co, 1953.

Weiss E, English OS: *Psychosomatic Medicine: A Clinical Study of Psychophysiologic Reactions*. Philadelphia, WB Saunders, 1957, p 214.

CHAPTER 6

Depression

1. A 43-year-old married woman, the mother of two children, ages 21 and 18, consulted her physician at the urging of her husband. She complained of fatigue, headaches, and vague aches and pains in many parts of her body. She had developed progressive difficulty in sleeping over the last month or so, with the onset of the vague symptoms. She would often wake up at 3:00 A.M. and think about how empty and meaningless life was. She would feel sad and burst into tears, but lately she felt that her tears had dried up. She neglected her personal appearance and seemed to feel extremely guilty about "not being a good mother, or a wife, or even a housemaid." Her sexual activity decreased to zero. In the last month, she lost 15 pounds. When urged to eat, she would say that food had no flavor, like cardboard. She was also convinced that she had a fatal disease, "Cancer of an internal organ, maybe the stomach." She would not, however, see a doctor because she "might as well be dead, being such a no-good person . . . anyway, the cancer has spread all over me, there is nothing they can do."

2. While making rounds in the morning, a 28-year-old medical resident was noticed to be loud, inappropriate, and irritable. For example, he would crack intimate jokes with the patients in full view of other patients and staff, ask questions of the attending physician in a condescending manner, and propose radical, potentially dangerous, and unnecessary procedures for the patients. When the proposals were not accepted, he became irritable and accused the others of being incompetent, again in front of patients and staff. When he further stated that he now possessed a secret method of healing that would cure any disease without the need for any diagnostic tests, his colleagues decided that he had to receive psychiatric help on an emergency basis.

On admission, the patient was talking incessantly in a loud voice. He stated to the psychiatrist that he came to the psychiatric unit so that he

91

could teach the staff how to cure schizophrenia using his secret method. He would also give electroshock treatments to all the patients on the unit with his bare hands, which were "charged with electricity." He also asked for a dictaphone in his room because he was in the middle of writing five articles at once, including his proposal to the hospital on how to make more money, a "Nobel-prize-winning article on new, secret medical therapeutics for all diseases," and an autobiography. During the first day of hospitalization, he attempted to date all the nurses he saw on the unit.

3. A 64-year-old successful executive of a major company became depressed and despondent after his wife's death about three years ago. His work efficiency decreased, and he began drinking excessively. He often talked about life being meaningless and about how empty success was. The only things in life that really gave pleasure, according to him, were things of beauty, like the collection of original paintings he had in his study, which was his lifetime hobby. Since about two years ago, however, he did not purchase any more paintings, which was unusual for him. He seemed to be especially brooding and generally irritable since about three months ago and was absent from work for several days, which was again, unusual. Since about a week ago, his spirits seemed to have lifted considerably. He tidied up his office, and he seemed to socialize more, calling up his friends and giving them as gifts his prized painting collection. He even gave his secretary an expensive original painting that was hanging in his office. Last night, he shot himself in the head.

4. A 50-year-old married woman was admitted to the psychiatric unit because of tearfulness, suicidal thoughts, and fatigue. Since approximately four or five weeks prior to admission, she became progressively depressed, with less interest in such activities as watching television, bridge, and reading—all of which she had enjoyed doing in the past. She developed a feeling of impending doom—as if everything would crumble about her. She lost all interest in sex, and food had no taste or flavor. She lost ten pounds during this period. She had difficulty in falling asleep and also in staying asleep through the night. She felt guilty about minor things and felt that she was not a worthwhile person to be allowed to live. She withdrew from her family and friends.

Upon admission to the psychiatric unit, she was treated with antidepressant medications with equivocal results. She continued to lose weight. A thorough medical workup in the hospital revealed that the patient had a carcinoma of the pancreas. Her depression abated following surgical removal of the diseased pancreas.

5. A few days ago, a 25-year-old medical student began to feel sad, blue, and dejected. He felt like crying from time to time and seemed to feel less pleasure in usual activities. During conversation with a friend, it suddenly occurred to him that the anniversary of his mother's death had just passed. He had been so busy with schoolwork that this had completely escaped his mind. With this recognition, he understood the reason for his sadness.

Affect, Mood, and Depression

Like anxiety, depression in its milder form is a ubiquitous experience. We feel sad in the face of loss and sometimes helpless and inadequate when we realize that we are not up to meeting the tasks required of us. On the other hand, when we have accomplished a task well, we feel joyous, and even elated. In the company of a good friend, and perhaps with a glass of good wine, we feel content and euphoric.

The emotional feeling tone of an individual, such as sadness, joy, depression, and elation, is called an *affect* (see Chapter 4 for further discussion of affect or emotion). When the affect is prolonged and colors the whole emotional life of the person, it is called a *mood*. Thus, a person may be in a blue mood, an elated mood, or a depressed mood.

Very simply, one can consider good and bad moods. On the bad side, such descriptions as feeling down, blue, sad, miserable, depressed, down in the dumps, are used, while, on the other hand, one can think of being happy, high, joyous, euphoric, elated, exulted, ecstatic, and manic. While all of us experience varying gradations of these moods, the extremes of moods, the depressive syndrome and mania, are not experienced except in pathological conditions.

Phenomenology of Depression and the Depressive and Manic Syndromes

The subjective feeling of sadness is the most common experience of depression in everyday life. This feeling is usually experienced after suffering a loss or failure—the loss of a loved one, possession, or prestige. The loss may be purely imaginary, and even the anticipation of a loss may cause sadness. Depression, in this sense, is closely related to grief, the specific emotional suffering related to loss, and separation, a common antecedent to grief. Separation and grieving processes will be discussed in a later section of this chapter.

The term *"depression"* is a confusing one, because it is used to denote the whole gamut of unpleasant moods, and exactly what degree of severity is referred to is not clear by the term itself. When psychiatrists use the term "depression," it almost invariably means the *depressive syndrome,* which is very different, indeed, from feelings of sadness associated with, say, the moving away of a good friend. This is somewhat similar to the difference in the use of the term *"hypertension"* between the lay public and the medical profession. When a patient talks about having hypertension, he may mean that he (1) has high blood pressure, (2) tends to become tense and nervous, or (3) both. Of course, there are precise blood pressure levels and procedures for the diagnosis of hypertension in medicine. What, then, is meant by depression when the term is used in a medical context?

The *depressive syndrome* [major affective disorder according to the *Diagnostic and Statistical Manual of Mental Disorders* (DSM III), draft, of the American Psychiatric Association, 1978] is characterized by a period of either *depressive mood* or *a pervasive loss of interest or pleasure*. The patient, as in vignette 1, often feels *sad, hopeless, helpless,* and *empty. Guilt* feelings are prominent, and there is a loss of *self-esteem*. Feeling discouraged and "down in the dumps" is common. The patient typically *withdraws* from family and friends, and activities and hobbies that used to give him pleasure no longer interest him. There is usually some *sleep disturbance,* usually early-morning awakening (EMA), but middle-of-the-night awakening (MNA) and difficulty in falling asleep (DFA) are not uncommon, especially if anxiety is also prominent. *Loss of appetite* is quite common, with concomitant weight loss, although in some patients, there may be an increase in eating with weight gain. The patients often show *psychomotor agitation* or *retardation*. In agitation, pulling out hair, pacing, wringing hands, inability to sit still, incessant talking, and shaking of hands and feet often occur. Psychomotor retardation is characterized by slowing of speech, slowed body movements, or even muteness.

In the depressive syndrome, patients often manifest *cognitive disturbances* (disturbances in thinking). This includes inability to concentrate, indecisiveness, and generally slowed thinking processes. Often, patients feel that they do not have enough energy to think out a simple problem. They feel tired, fatigued, and exhausted in the absence of physical exhaustion. They may experience vague pains, aches, and discomfort, without any physical basis; headaches, toothaches, backaches, and muscle aches are especially common.

Patients often suffer from feelings of *inadequacy, worthlessness,* and sometimes completely unrealistic *low self-esteem*. The smallest task may appear impossible or monumental. There may be excessive guilt feelings concerning current or past failings, most of them minor, or even delusional conviction of sinfulness or responsibility for some untoward tragic event.

Suicidal ideations are frequent and may take the form of fears of dying, the belief that the individual or others would be better off if they were dead, or suicidal desires or plans. Often, there is a *diurnal variation*—the symptoms are worse upon waking up in the morning and improve slightly as the day progresses.

When the symptoms are mild, temporary improvement often occurs in the presence of positive environmental stimuli. In severe cases, the syndrome is not affected by environmental change to any extent. (Specific diagnostic criteria for the depressive syndrome are found in the section on Evaluation of Depression.)

At the opposite pole of the depressive syndrome in mood is the *manic syndrome*. As sadness and grief are experienced by most people from time to time, the pleasurable moods of euphoria and elation, short of mania or hypomania, fall within the normal range of mood. In euphoria, there is a positive feeling of emotional and physical well-being. In elation, there is a definite feeling of joy with increase in self-confidence, motor activity, and energy level. These states can be induced by drugs such as alcohol, narcotics, and amphetamines.

Mania and hypomania (which is a somewhat less severe form of mania), on the other hand, form a syndrome, like the depressive syndrome, with definite features and signs.

The essential feature of the *manic syndrome* is a distinct period when the predominant mood is elevated, expansive, or irritable and is associated with other symptoms of the manic syndrome. They include hyperactivity, excessive involvement in often indiscreet and foolish activities without recognizing the high potential for painful consequences, pressure of speech, flight of ideas, inflated self-esteem, decreased need for sleep, and distractability (DSM III, 1978).

The patient may describe the *elevated mood* as being euphoric, unusually good, or high. The good mood may have an infectious quality, so that the physician or others in contact with the patient may find themselves feeling expansive and often humorous. The patient may show *indiscriminate enthusiasm* in relating to people or planning things, so that he may start a dozen projects at once, call up distant relatives and bare acquaintances all over the globe, and go on a buying spree. On the other hand, the mood may be characterized by *irritability* rather than joyfulness, especially when the patient's expansiveness is thwarted. The patient then becomes touchy and domineering. The *hyperactivity* is often generalized, including participation in multiple activities which may be sexual, occupational, political, or religious. The patients often have *poor judgment,* and the activities are disorganized, flamboyant, and bizarre (see vignette 2).

Manic speech is usually *loud, rapid,* and *difficult to understand.* It is often full of jokes and puns and is theatrical, with singing and rhetorical mannerisms. In the irritable mood, there may be hostile comments and angry outbursts. Abrupt changes from topic to topic based on understandable associations and distracting stimuli often occur (flight of ideas). When severe, the speech may be incoherent. Distractibility is usually present.

Self-esteem is usually inflated, with unrealistic and uncritical self-confidence and grandiosity. For example, the patient may give advice on matters about which he has no expert knowledge whatever—such as how to perform an operation or how to run the federal government. Grandiose delusions may occur, such as, "I have a special hot line with God."

When an individual has episodes of *both* depression and mania, this is called manic—depressive or *bipolar illness.*

Separation, Bereavement, and Grief

Phenomenology

The phenomenology of acute grief following separation and bereavement has much in common with that of depression. Lindemann described the symptomatology of acute grief in his classical paper based on bereaved persons, including those who lost their relatives in the Coconut Grove fire (Lindemann, 1944). The symptoms of normal grief include sensations of *somatic distress* occurring in waves lasting from 20 minutes to an hour at a time, a feeling of tightness in the throat, shortness of breath, frequent sighing, an empty feeling in the stomach, lack of muscular power, and an intense subjective distress described as tension or mental pain. These waves of distress can be precipitated by mere mention of the deceased. There is often a loss of appetite.

In addition to the somatic distress, grieving persons have an *intense preoccupation with the image of the deceased* — to the point where they may look for the deceased person in a crowd or almost feel the presence of the deceased in the room. *Guilt feelings* are also common. The bereaved searches the time before the death for evidence of failure to do the right things. Self-accusation of negligence and exaggeration of minor omissions are common. The bereaved tends to become *irritable and hostile* to friends and relatives who are making a special effort to show sympathy.

There is often a change in the *patterns of conduct*. The bereaved finds it difficult to initiate and maintain organized patterns of activity, simply going through the motions of carrying out normal activity. The bereaved is surprised to discover how large a part of his customary activity was done in some meaningful relationship to the deceased and has now lost its significance. The bereaved feels restless and unable to sit still. He tends to move about in an aimless fashion, as if in search of something to do.

In addition to the five symptoms described by Lindemann to be pathognomonic for acute grief, some bereaved persons develop an *identification* with the deceased, manifested by the taking on of the manner or speech or gait of the deceased or even the development of symptoms of the deceased's last illness in the absence of evidence of the disease.

Course

The *course* of bereavement was studied extensively by Parkes (1972). He described *three phases* of bereavement: the phase of numbness, followed by the phase of pining, which, in turn, is followed by the phase of depression.

The first phase described by Parkes is a period of *numbness* that may last for a few hours up to a few days. This phase may be punctuated by moments of panic and distress, including the somatic distress described above. The second phase of *pining* is characterized by *anxious searching,* with preoccupation with the thoughts and images of the deceased. This phase includes the somatic distress described by Lindemann, as well as feelings of anger and guilt. Guilt alternates with and eventually gives way to feelings of depression. The anxious searching phase peaks in two to four weeks and leads to the phase of *depression and despair.* This period is also characterized by apathy and aimlessness, with loss of patterns of control.

The course of normal acute grief is approximately four to eight weeks (Huston, 1975), but a substantial proportion of the bereaved continue to report distress up to one or two years after the death of a spouse.

Pathological Grief Reactions

Lindemann described two types of pathological grief reactions, the *delayed* grief reaction and the *distorted* grief reaction.

The delayed grief reaction is characterized by a postponement of the grieving process. When an individual is in the middle of performing important tasks, or when it is necessary to maintain the morale of others, there may be no overt sign of grief after loss for weeks, months, or even years. The full-blown picture of acute grief may be precipitated, however, by the serendipitous mention of the deceased or by a situation that reminds the bereaved of the loss. Such precipitating events may be the anniversary of the loss or the individual's attaining the same age as the deceased's at the time of death.

Distorted reactions may occur during any phase of grief or as a delayed reaction. They include overactivity, no sense of loss, the acquisition of symptoms belonging to the last illness of the deceased, severe alteration in relationship to friends and relatives, excessive hostility against specific persons, lasting loss of initiative, self-destructive activities, and the development of the full-blown depressive syndrome.

Separation in Children

Spitz described the phenomenon of *"anaclitic depression"* in infants in the latter half of the first year upon separation from their mothers (Spitz, 1942). This syndrome consisted of crying, apprehension, withdrawal, psychomotor slowing, dejection, stupor, insomnia, anorexia, weight loss, and gross retardation in growth and development. "Anaclitic" means dependence, and the depressive syndrome was presumed to be due to the absence of the mother, a figure to depend on.

Bowlby studied the effects of separation from mothers of somewhat older children (Robertson and Bowlby, 1952; Bowlby, 1960) and described three phases. The first is a *"protest"* phase, characterized by a frantic searching for the mother with restlessness and tearfulness, followed by a *"despair"* phase in which the child withdraws from others and appears apathetic. Parkes' later staging of the grief reaction in adults, discussed above, has much similarity to these stages described by Bowlby. When the child is reunited with the mother, some children ignore the mother or actively reject the mother for a period. This was called the "detachment" stage by Bowlby.

Although separation in infants results in a syndrome similar to grief in adults, a causal relationship between early separation and later vulnerability to depression is as yet unproven (Akiskal and McKinney, 1975). Further, there is evidence that substitute mothering can, to a large extent, alleviate whatever damage may occur following separation from the mother.

Separation in Infant Monkeys

The separation reaction described by Bowlby occurs in nonhuman primates as well. Separation of seven-month-old infant monkeys from the mother resulted in initial *"violent protest"* with crying and searching behavior, followed by a *"despair"* phase with decreased activity, withdrawn behavior, and occasional crying (Figure 9) (Seay and Harlow, 1965; Kaufman and Rosenblum, 1967).

Harlow and Harlow demonstrated the effects of isolation from mothers and peers from birth in rhesus monkeys (Harlow and Harlow, 1962, 1966a,b). The Harlows' experiments showed that tactile sensation was an important element of attachment behavior. Some monkeys were given inanimate "surrogate mothers" made of terry cloth or wire. The infant monkeys would choose "terry-cloth mothers," which were mechanical devices with soft terry cloth, over "wire mothers," which were equipped with a feeding apparatus but without any soft terry cloth. Monkeys who were socially isolated in this way early in life developed difficulties in later life, especially in socialization and sexual activity. These difficulties were, to a large measure, alleviated, however, if peers were present during infancy and childhood.

Significance of Bereavement and Depression

Many recent epidemiologic studies indicate that the experience of bereavement or grief is associated with an increased risk of becoming ill or, in fact,

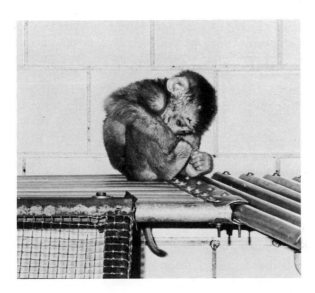

Figure 9. Depressed captive pigtail infant monkey showing characteristic posture of despair including head between legs. (From Kaufman and Rosenblum, 1967. Courtesy of the authors. Reproduced with permission.)

dying. Grief was accepted as a cause of death in prescientific medicine, as evidenced by Table 2. The pathophysiologic mechanism by which the experience of bereavement, grief, or, for that matter, depression leads to morbidity and mortality by such diseases as coronary disease and cancer still remains unclear (see Chapter 4).

The *increased mortality rate* in the bereaved seems to be two to seven times that of the expected rate in age- and sex-matched nonbereaved persons during the first year of bereavement. The risk of mortality is greater for men than for women for all ages. The major effect of bereavement in terms of mortality seems to occur in the first two years after the death of a spouse and, in men, almost exclusively in the first six months (Jacobs and Ostfeld, 1978). The

Table 2. Dr. Heberden's Classification of the Causes of Death in London during the year 1657 [a]

Flox and smallpox	839
Found dead in the streets, etc.	9
French pox	25
Gout	8
Griefe	10
Griping and plague in the guts	446
Hang'd and made away 'emselves	24

[a] As quoted by Parkes (1972), Chapter 2. Copyright 1972 by Tavistock Publications, Ltd. Reproduced with permission from the author and Associated Book Publishers, Ltd., London.

cause of death of men is accounted for by tuberculosis, influenza and pneumonia, cirrhosis of the liver and alcoholism, suicides and accidents, and heart disease. For women, elevated mortality occurs from tuberculosis, cirrhosis of the liver and alcoholism, heart disease, and cancer.

In addition to increasing the risk of morbidity and mortality from *medical diseases* such as tuberculosis, heart disease, and cancer, *bereavement precipitates a depressive syndrome* in a significant number of persons. Clayton and her associates studied 109 randomly selected bereaved subjects (Clayton *et al.,* 1972; Bornstein *et al.,* 1973). At one month after bereavement, 35% of the sample were definitely or probably depressed; at 13 months, 17%. Thirty-nine percent had a depressive syndrome at some time during the period.

Depression unassociated with bereavement has also been shown to be associated with increased morbidity and mortality. For example, in one study, subjects who had acute myocardial infarction and died had higher depression scores on the Minnesota Multiphasic Personality Inventory (MMPI) than those who had acute myocardial infarction and survived (Lebovitz *et al.,* 1967).

Preoperative depression is known to be a predictor of increased postoperative behavioral problems and mortality in cardiac surgery patients (Kennedy and Bakst, 1966; Reiser and Bakst, 1975). Based on studies of illness-onset situations, Schmale and Engel postulate that a feeling of helplessness and hopelessness (the *"giving up—given up complex")* may provide a "permissive" setting for the development of a medical disease (Schmale, 1972). This permissive setting, which has many features of depression, was found to occur in patients who had leukemia, lymphoma, diabetic ketosis, cervical carcinoma, bronchial asthma, etc.

Function of Depression

The phenomenology of mild forms of depression is indistinguishable from that of grief reactions to losses of varying degrees. Thus, depression as an affect can be conceptualized as a response to loss or separation, actual or symbolic, which may have an adaptive function. The depressive syndrome, in this light, may be seen as a disregulation syndrome of the depressive affect.

The feeling of depression signals that a loss or separation has occurred or is in the making. In cases of threatened loss, anxiety will occur together with depressive affect and prepare the individual to deal with the loss (including, in certain instances, avoidance of the loss).

The protest phase of the separation reaction in infants and young monkeys serves the function of drawing the attention of the mother or other members of the social group to the separated infant. The crying of the baby may suddenly remind the mother that it has crawled into another room while she was not watching. *Social support* is often mobilized for an infant who is lost or separated from its mother.

When the separation is prolonged, the infant proceeds into the stage of despair, with reduction in activity and behavioral withdrawal. This state may serve the *conservation* function previously described—in the face of adversity, the organism might withdraw and tend to conserve energy and strength by reduction of activity, so that there might be strength at a later date. Thus, the behavioral patterns of depression may have biologically and socially adaptive functions.

The affect of depression related to helplessness in childhood and threat of loss may play an important role in the *socialization* and *learning* of infants and children. Somewhat like anxiety, which has an optimal level for performance, certain amounts of depressive experience may help the learning process.

Brain Mechanisms of Depression

Certain diencephalic areas in the brain are known to be associated with the experience of pleasure and displeasure. Among others, electrical stimulation of the *medial forebrain bundle* is considered to be pleasurable and reinforcing to the animal, while electrical stimulation of the *periventricular system* is considered to be unpleasant (see Figures 10–12). It is reasonable to suppose, then, that these structures are somehow involved in the experience of depression (Akiskal and McKinney, 1975). The biogenic amines norepinephrine and serotonin are both involved in the modulation of the function of the medial forebrain bundle and the periventricular system.

Biogenic Amines

Much information on the brain mechanisms of depression is based on the study of patients with the fully developed depressive syndrome and their pharmacologic treatment. The two classes of antidepressants effective in the treatment of the depressive syndrome, the *tricyclics* and the *monoamine oxidase inhibitors*, both essentially increase the functional levels of biogenic amines in the brain. The biogenic amines thought to be involved in the brain are the catecholamines (mainly norepinephrine and dopamine) and the indoleamine, serotonin. Reserpine, used in the treatment of hypertension, depletes biogenic amines (both catecholamines and indoleamines) in the neurons and can cause the depressive syndrome in 10–15% of patients receiving it. The

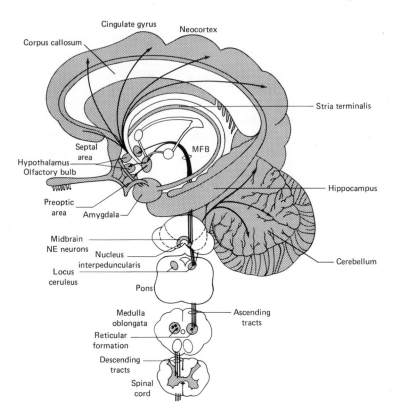

Figure 10. Noradrenergic (NE) systems. Sagittal projection of NE pathways arising from cell groups in medulla oblongata and pons. The NE tracts are both descending and ascending. Descending fibers arise from cell bodies in the medulla oblongata and innervate the gray matter of the spinal cord. Ascending neurons are derived primarily from cell bodies in the medulla oblongata (reticular formation) and pons (locus ceruleus) and enter the medial forebrain bundle (MFB). These fibers innervate the hypothalamus, stria terminalis, preoptic area, septal area, amygdaloid cortex, cingulate gyrus, and neocortex. The cerebellum is also innervated by NE neurons from the medulla and pons. A smaller number of NE neurons arise from an area surrounding the nucleus inter-peduncularis. (From *Neuropsychopharmacology, 1: The Monamine Systems*, 1976. Reproduced with permission from Roche Laboratories, Nutley, N.J.)

catecholamine hypothesis of depressive disorders (Schildkraut and Kety, 1967) postulates that in mania, there is an increased functional level of norepinephrine in the noradrenergic synapses in the brain, whereas in depression, there is a decreased functional level of norepinephrine in the brain. The cell bodies of the norepinephrine-containing neurons are in the brain stem, especially in the *locus ceruleus* in the pons (see Figures 6 and 10). The axons ascend in the medial forebrain bundle to supply the hypothalamus and areas of the limbic system as well as the entire cerebral cortex (Sweeney and Maas, 1978).

The pharmacologic evidence may be equally strong for a *serotonin* theory, which is especially widely accepted in Great Britain. The cell bodies of the serotonergic neurons are in the medial raphe nuclei in the mesencephalon and upper pons (Figure 12). Their axons ascend in the medial forebrain bundle, giving off terminals to various parts of the brain, including the hypothalamic areas and the cerebral cortex. There is evidence that depressed patients have low levels of 5-hydroxyindoleacetic acid, a serotonin metabolite, in the cerebrospinal fluid (Bowers *et al.*, 1970; Åsberg *et al.*, 1973). Low levels of serotonin and 5-hydroxyindoleacetic acid were found in the autopsied brains of suicidal patients (Davis, 1977). L-Tryptophan is the precursor of serotonin in the brain, and the brain level of serotonin seems to be determined by the blood level of L-tryptophan. There is evidence that L-tryptophan may

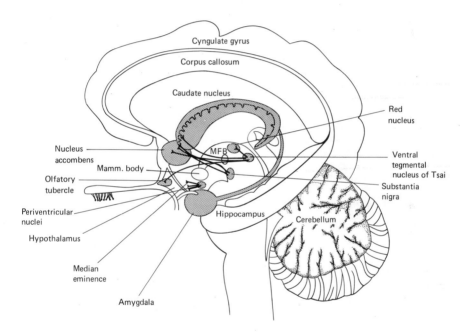

Figure 11. Dopaminergic (DA) systems. Sagittal projection of the DA pathways arising from cell groups in the midbrain. The DA neurons form at least three definable systems. One pathway consists of the nigrostriatal tract, which arises from cell bodies in the substantia nigra and terminates on small interneurons of the neostriatum (caudate nucleus and putamen). (Note: Putamen cannot be seen from sagittal view.) A second major pathway arises from the ventral tegmental nucleus of Tsai (located about the cranial portion of the nucleus interpeduncularis), enters the medial forebrain bundle (MFB), and terminates anterior to the caudate nucleus in the nucleus accombens (nuclei nervi vestibulocochlearis), olfactory tubercle, and red nucleus of the stria terminalis (the limbic striatum). A third pathway involves DA cell bodies from the arcuate and anterior periventricular nuclei which terminate in the median eminence of the hypothalamus and appear to have a role in regulating gonadotropin secretion. (From *Neuropsychopharmacology, 1: The Monamine Systems,* 1976. Reproduced with permission from Roche Laboratories, Nutley, N.J.)

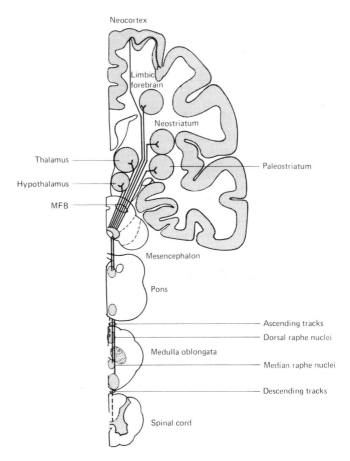

Figure 12. Serotonergic (5-HT) systems. Diagrammatic representation of 5-HT pathways arising in the mesencephalon, entering the medial forebrain bundle (MFB), and innervating rostral nuclei along with NE neurons. The 5-HT neurons tend to have a distribution similar to the NE system. Descending pathways innervate the gray matter of the spinal cord; cell bodies are located primarily in the lower raphe nuclei of the pons. Ascending neurons arise from cell bodies in the medulla, primarily the medial and dorsal raphe nuclei, and accompany the NE neurons to the hypothalamus, limbic forebrain, neostriatum, paleostriatum, and neocortex. (From *Neuropsychopharmacology, 1: The Monamine Systems,* 1976. Reproduced with permission from Roche Laboratories, Nutley, N.J.)

improve the symptoms of both mania and depression in some patients (Davis, 1977). Prange and others (1974) postulate a *"permissive theory"* of affective disorders which states that in all affective disorders, there is an abnormally *low level of functional serotonin* in the brain; in addition, in the case of *depression,* there is a *decrease* in the functional level of norepinephrine in the brain and in *mania,* an *increase* (see Chapter 8 for serotonin's role in sleep).

Other investigators believe that there may be *two different kinds of depressive syndromes,* one associated with *decreased functional levels of norepinephrine* in the brain and the other, with *decreased functional levels of serotonin.* The urinary excretion of *3-hydroxy-4-methoxyphenylethylene glycol* (MHPG), a metabolite of norepinephrine largely produced in the brain, is found to be low in some depressed patients but not in others. Those who have low levels of MHPG tend to respond better to imipramine, a tricyclic antidepressant that increases the brain levels of norepinephrine and, to a lesser extent, serotonin, whereas those who do not have low levels of MHPG tend to respond better to amitriptyline, a tricyclic that increases brain serotonin levels more than imipramine (Maas, 1978).

Acetylcholine

In addition to the biogenic amines norepinephrine and serotonin, acetylcholine is also probably involved in depression. There is evidence to indicate that the brain cholinergic function may be high in depression and low in mania (Janowsky *et al.,* 1972, 1973). Physostigmine, a substance that inhibits cholinesterase, the enzyme that breaks down acetylcholine, was shown to convert mania to depression and to make depression worse.

Three major neurotransmitters in the brain, acetylcholine, norepinephrine, and serotonin, then, seem to be involved in at least some forms of depression. Another way of conceptualizing the relationship between the neurotransmitters and depression is that the central nervous system must function as a system in which there is an equilibrium of neurons using different transmitters. Such a system may become disregulated if any of the components malfunctions, and the overall equilibrium of the neurotransmitters may shift, producing abnormalities in more than one subsystem. At the same time, in one disregulated system, one may find particularly low levels of one component (say, norepinephrine), while in another disregulated system with the same behavioral characteristic, one finds low levels of another component (such as serotonin).

Brain norepinephrine levels may be reduced in cats in states of heightened emotionality, regardless of whether the state is pleasurable or aversive (Bliss and Zwanziger, 1966; Bliss *et al.,* 1966).

Other Putative Neurotransmitters and Neuromodulators

Numerous other substances, among them the endorphins and enkephalins (see Chapters 4 and 7) and, possibly, histamine, have been suspected of being involved in mood states, but the findings are still too preliminary to warrant full discussion.

Intracellular Sodium

In both depression and mania, there seems to be an increase in residual sodium (intracellular sodium plus the sodium in bone). In depression, the magnitude of increase is 50% and in mania, 100%. This increased intracellular sodium (hypothesized for the brain) may lower resting membrane potential and increase neuronal irritability and thus "arousal." There may be central hyperarousal in both depression and mania, as evidenced by insomnia, especially reduction in the delta (deep) sleep, and lowered threshold for arousal (Whybrow and Mendels, 1969).

Parenthetically, alcohol also increases intracellular sodium and potentially aggravates depression.

Psychological Aspects

Early psychoanalytic formulations concerning depression focused mainly upon object loss and *turning inward of hostility* which had originally been directed toward an ambivalently loved person who had been lost through death or separation (actual, threatened, or symbolic). Later, "ego psychologists" such as Bibring added the formulation that depression is a state in which the individual recognizes his inadequacy and *helplessness*—loss of self-esteem (Bibring, 1965). Beck (1967) postulates an altered *cognitive style* characterized by negative expectations to be the basis of depressive states. His theory, then, gives primacy to the cognitive or thinking aspects of depression—negative conception of the self, negative interpretations of one's experiences, and a negative view of the future. From these cognitive changes arise helplessness and hopelessness and the mood of depression. The "learned helplessness" model of Seligman (Seligman and Maier, 1967) provides an interesting model for depression. Many animals that had been exposed to multiple sessions of inescapable shock showed impaired ability to avoid shock even when it was avoidable—as if they had "learned" that the shocks were not avoidable.

According to Wolpe (1971), chronic anxiety resulting from chronic frustration in one's personal or professional life causes *hopelessness* concerning the reduction of anxiety. Related to these theories are the observations that, antecedent to a depressive episode, there is often a lack of environmental rewards (positive reinforcement) to formerly successful behaviors.

A Hypothetical Integrated Model (Figure 13)

Depression may be conceptualized as expressing a state of the central nervous system with accompanying neuroendocrine and physiologic changes. This state of depression may have a *final common pathway*, which might be the state of diencephalic neuronal systems concerned with reinforcement and pleasure. Environmental, symbolic, and genetic–chemical factors would contribute to and influence this final common pathway to varying degrees. For example, the basic vulnerability of the neurotransmitter (and perhaps reinforcement) systems in the brain may be determined by genetic (and early experiential) factors.

Psychosocial stresses such as separation and loss might be translated in the brain into neuronal impulses and neuroendocrine responses, which, in

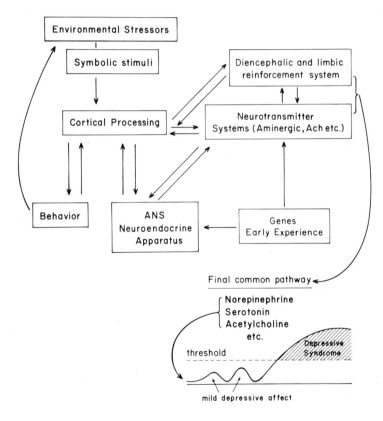

Figure 13. An integrated model of depression.

turn, may change the activity of neurons in the neurotransmitter and re-inforcement–pleasure systems. Vulnerability to depression may be concep-tualized as related to a hypothesized threshold in the central nervous system. Given a large *genetic loading* (low threshold) for depression, only a minimal amount of symbolic stimuli may be sufficient to trigger off a severe depressive state. On the other hand, in some individuals with no genetic loading (high threshold), even catastrophic losses conceivably might not result in a detecta-ble depressive state. Once a depressive state occurs, it may further aggravate depression through behavioral changes (e.g., social withdrawal) and cognitive changes (e.g., pessimistic outlook).

On the basis of clinical studies, it seems that once a severe *depressive syndrome* has developed, no matter what the precipitating event, it reaches a phase that has an autonomous course which can be modified only by time or somatic intervention, such as antidepressants or electroshock therapy. Thus, one might postulate a threshold for the final common pathway for depression—once the threshold has been reached for the depressive syn-drome, a process similar to a stress-induced disease in other organs (such as stress-induced peptic ulcers) may ensue. This threshold might speculatively be related to the functional level and balance of norepinephrine and acetylcholine available to specific receptor sites in diencephalic and limbic areas related to reinforcement and pleasure. Seen in this light, depression would be a stress-related disease with the brain as the target organ (Figure 13).

Physiology and Endocrinology of Depression

Depression is associated with a specific pattern of facial muscular pattern-ing (Izard, 1977) that is identifiable in monkeys and humans and across cultures. This characteristic facial expression, together with the specific be-havior patterns (such as protest and despair), is probably associated with the adaptive significance of depression discussed above.

In states of *sadness,* there seems to be agreement that the parasympa-thetic nervous system is activated, with concomitant physiologic alterations. The latter include lacrimation and decrease in blood pressure and heart rate (Izard, 1972). In the *depressive syndrome,* however, the physiologic changes are quite complex. In patients with established depressive syndrome, the heart rate may be increased, and increased blood pressure has been associated with depression (Heine *et al.,* 1969; Altschule, 1953). The increased sympathetic activity found in the depressive syndrome may be associated with the central arousal and anxiety often accompanying the syndrome.

Neuroendocrinology

Endocrine changes have been studied primarily in patients with the full-blown depressive syndrome. A number of typical endocrine changes accompanying depression have now been identified, and it is also known that primary endocrinopathies may cause secondary depressive syndromes or depressive symptomatology (see section on Evaluation of Depression). In general, the endocrine changes found in the depressive disorder (depressive syndrome) are the kinds of changes that might be anticipated on the basis of the effect of functionally decreased levels of brain norepinephrine on the hypothalamic releasing and inhibitory hormones.

Adrenocorticotropic Hormone and Cortisol. Adrenocorticotropic hormone (ACTH) seems to be synthesized and released in response to the hypothalamic corticotropin-releasing factor (CRF). Under normal conditions, CRF secretion appears to be tonically inhibited by the higher brain centers through a noradrenergic (norepinephrine) influence.

In the depressive syndrome, there may be a severe *disinhibition of the hypothalamic–pituitary–adrenal* function. Thus, in depression, there is a marked elevation in the plasma cortisol levels throughout the day and night, obliterating the normal circadian rhythm of cortisol secretion (Ettigi and Brown, 1977; Sachar, 1975a). Depressive patients with elevated cortisol secretion often do not show normal suppression of cortisol production after the administration of *dexamethasone,* a potent synthetic corticosteroid. Dexamethasone normally suppresses pituitary ACTH secretion and thus lowers plasma cortisol. The depressive patient's dexamethasone suppression test usually returns to normal when depression improves (Carroll, 1972).

Although nonspecific emotional arousal can also result in increased cortisol levels, the increase accompanying the depressive syndrome seems to be fundamental and not secondary to arousal, as evidenced by elevated cortisol levels in sleeping patients and apathetic patients.

Growth Hormone. Growth hormone secretion is probably controlled by a hypothalamic releasing factor (GHRH) and an inhibiting factor (somatostatin). Growth hormone release normally occurs in response to hypoglycemia, exercise, stress, arginine infusion, and slow-wave sleep.

There is evidence to suggest that catecholamines (norepinephrine and dopamine) mediate growth hormone secretion. In depression, there appears to be a *decreased growth hormone response* to hypoglycemia.

Other Hormones. In addition to corticosteroids and growth hormone, whose levels are probably altered in depression, other hormone systems, such as luteinizing hormone, thyroid hormone, and prolactin, might also be altered in depression, although this is not yet well established.

The endocrine changes in mania are not well established and are, at best, controversial.

Physiologic Signs of Depression (Depressive Syndrome)

In severe depression (depressive syndrome), there is often a loss of appetite, decreased sexual interest and drive, profound loss of interest in and experience of pleasure, constipation, and weight loss. In some individuals, there may be an increase in appetite and weight gain, especially when depression is not severe. Sleep disturbances are common, especially early-morning awakening. There may be profound psychomotor retardation or agitation. Vague physical symptoms such as aches and pains may be present.

Evaluation of Depression

When the physician suspects that a patient is depressed, specific types of further evaluation should be made. The kinds of things the physician must decide in the course of this evaluation are the *severity* and *nature* of depression, *suicidal risk, advisability* of *hospitalization,* and *management plans.*

We mentioned earlier that depressive affect is usually generated in response to a loss and that it may have adaptive significance. In cases of mild depressions (or rather, sadness), recognizing the loss suffices in the evaluation, as the loss can be dealt with by the patient alone or with the support of his family, friends, or the physician. The same is true in grief reactions, in which the nature of the loss is clear. Grief reactions often occur in medical setting in anticipation of the *loss of function* or of an organ, such as in amputations. Grief over the patient's own impending death also occurs. Duration of depression is an important factor to be considered. A patient who has become seriously depressed in the last month, for example, needs a different management plan from another patient who has been depressed for the last five years.

The following specific questions, then, should be answered in the comprehensive evaluation of a patient with suspected depression:

1. Questions concerning the *phenomenology* of depression
   Sad affect, loss of interest
   Difficulty with concentration
   Crying
   Guilt feelings
   Hopelessness and helplessness
   Low self-esteem
   Decreased libido

      Anorexia
      Constipation
      Dry skin
      Dry mouth
      Vague aches and pains
      Sleep pattern
      Suicidal thoughts or plans

2. Observation of *behavior and appearance*
      Sad or apathetic appearance
      Evidence of self-neglect
      Agitation or psychomotor retardation
      Cognitive disturbances

3. Questions concerning *history of depression*
      Duration of the depression
      Past history of depression or mania
      Family history of depression, mania,
         suicide or alcoholism

4. Questions concerning *medical history*
      Possible concurrent disease
      Drugs

5. Questions concerning *environmental factors*
      Losses
      Separations
      Anniversary of above

Once mild sadness and grief reactions have been ruled out, the physician should determine whether the depression is *chronic* or *acute*.

Chronic depressive disorder (depressive personality) is defined as moderate to severe depression with a duration of *longer than two years without remission*. With these patients, sad feelings and some of the other psychologic and physiologic signs of depression seem to be a *character style*. Depression in this case, then, is a trait that cannot be expected to be easily removed by treatment.

If the patient's depression does not fall under the chronic depressive disorder, then the presence or absence of the depressive syndrome (depressive episode) has to be determined. An acute *depressive syndrome* can be diagnosed by the criteria shown in Table 3.

Once the diagnosis of the *depressive syndrome* is made, completely or partially (although not all criteria are met, sufficient criteria are fulfilled to cause reluctance in ruling out this possibility), then it is helpful to make a further decision as to whether or not the depressive syndrome is associated with a known antecedent or cause such as a medical disease, exogenous toxins (e.g.,

Table 3. Diagnostic Criteria for
Depressive Syndrome (Depressive Episode)[a]

1. Dysphoric mood or loss of interest or pleasure in all or almost all usual activities and pastimes. The dysphoric mood is characterized by symptoms such as the following: depressed, sad, blue, hopeless, low, down in the dumps, irritable, worried. The disturbance must be prominent and relatively persistent but not necessarily the most dominant symptom. It does not include momentary shifts from one dysphoric mood to another dysphoric mood, for example, anxiety to depression to anger, such as seen in states of acute psychotic turmoil.

2. At least four of the following symptoms:
   a. Poor appetite or weight loss or increased appetite or weight gain (change of one pound a week or ten pounds a year when not dieting)
   b. Sleep difficulty or sleeping too much
   c. Loss of energy, fatigability, or tiredness
   d. Psychomotor agitation or retardation (but not mere subjective feelings of restlessness or being slowed down)
   e. Loss of interest or pleasure in usual activities or decrease in sexual drive
   f. Feelings of self-reproach or excessive or inappropriate guilt (either may be delusional)
   g. Complaints or evidence of diminished ability to think or concentrate, such as slow thinking or indecisiveness (do not include if associated with obvious signs of schizophrenia)
   h. Recurrent thoughts of death or suicide, or any suicidal behavior, including thoughts of wishing to be dead.

3. Duration of period of illness of at least two weeks from the time of the first noticeable change in the individual's usual condition

4. None of the following which suggest schizophrenia is present:
   a. Delusions of being controlled or thought broadcasting, insertion, or withdrawal
   b. Hallucinations of any type throughout the day for several days or intermittently throughout a one-week period unless all of the content is clearly related to depression or elation
   c. Auditory hallucinations in which either a voice keeps up a running commentary on the individual's behaviors or thoughts as they occur, or two or more voices converse with each other
   d. Delusions or hallucinations for more than one month at some time during the period of illness in the absence of prominent affective (manic or depressive) symptoms (although typical depressive delusions, such as delusions of guilt, sin, poverty, nihilism, or self-deprecation, or hallucinations of similar content are permitted)
   e. Preoccupation with a delusion or hallucination to the relative exclusion of other symptoms or concerns (other than delusions of guilt, sin, poverty, nihilism, or self-deprecation, or hallucinations with similar content)
   f. Marked formal thought disorder if accompanied by either blunted or inappropriate affect, delusions or hallucinations of any type, or grossly disorganized behavior

5. Not due to any organic mental disorder (organic brain syndrome)

6. Not superimposed on schizophrenia, residual subtype (history of schizophrenia)

7. Excludes simple bereavement following loss of a loved one if all of the features are commonly seen in members of the individual's subcultural group in similar circumstances

[a]Quoted, with minor modifications, from the Diagnostic and Statistical Manual of Mental Disorders (DSM III), draft (1978). Reproduced with permission from the American Psychiatric Association.

drugs), or psychological stress such as bereavement. Table 4 presents a partial list of medical conditions that must be ruled out in a depressed patient.

It is because of this frequent association of the depressive syndrome with serious medical diseases that a thorough *medical workup* with physical examination and laboratory tests is a *must* in the evaluation of a depressed patient. Once depression secondary to a medical condition is established and the underlying disease diagnosed, the depressive syndrome usually abates when the underlying disease has been satisfactorily treated (vignette 4). If a thorough medical evaluation rules out possible underlying disease, then the possibility of primary depression should be entertained.

Depressive syndrome is an integral part of a psychiatric disorder called *major affective disorder* (primary depressive illness, endogenous depression, manic–depressive illness). In this disorder, the symptomatology of the patient is usually severe enough to fully meet the criteria for diagnosis of the depressive syndrome. In addition, there is often a positive *family history* of depression, mania, suicide, or alcoholism. About 15–20% of the first-degree relatives of patients with major affective disorders have histories of similar illnesses. History of a previous depressive episode is common, since in 95% of patients, one or more episodes of depression can be expected to occur within ten years after the

Table 4. Partial List of Medical Conditions Often Associated with Depression

Endocrinopathies
    Hyperparathyroidism (hypercalcemia)
    Cushing's syndrome
    Hypothyroidism
    Premenstrual tension syndrome
Viral disease (often during incubation and convalescence)
    Influenza
    Infectious mononucleosis
    Infectious hepatitis
    Any other viral infection
Malignancies
    Occult abdominal malignancies, especially cancer of the tail of the pancreas
    Any other malignancy
Drugs that may cause or aggravate depression
    Corticosteroids and ACTH
    Oral contraceptives
    Reserpine
    Alpha-methyldopa (Aldomet)
    Propranolol (Inderal)
    Alcohol
    Benzodiazepines (e.g., diazepam or chlordiazepoxide)

initial episode. The first episode may occur at any age but is most common in middle age. In some patients, depressive episodes may alternate with, or be associated with, manic episodes (bipolar affective disorder). It appears that the *unipolar* and *bipolar disorders* have different genetic vulnerability, so that a depressed patient who has a relative who had manic episodes may eventually have a manic episode as well.

A depressive episode due to major affective disorder is usually self-limiting, the average duration without treatment being about six to nine months (in bipolar disorder, somewhat shorter; in unipolar, somewhat longer).

Physical Symptoms in Depressive Syndrome Associated with Major Affective Disorders

Certain physical and physiologic symptoms and signs are often present in the depressive syndrome. In fact, some of the physiologic signs, such as loss of appetite and weight loss, sleep disturbance, and loss of sexual interest, are part of the diagnostic criteria. In addition, many patients have *vague pains* and *discomfort* in various parts of the body, perhaps associated with a turning inward of attention with depression. To complicate matters even more, some patients who have the depressive syndrome have *primarily* physical symptoms, with relatively mild to moderate depressive affect, and may seek help for physical symptoms such as vague toothaches, headaches, and back-aches (related concepts are "depressive equivalents" and "masked depression"). In some, this may be a heterothetic help-seeking behavior (see Chapter 1). In patients complaining of vague physical pains and discomfort whose medical workup is negative, the physician should consider the possibility that the symptoms may be associated with the depressive syndrome. Careful questioning about affect and other associated symptoms and signs and history will usually disclose more features of the depressive syndrome.

Evaluation of Suicidal Potential

An important consideration in evaluating a depressive patient is the suicidal potential. Approximately 15% of depressive patients ultimately commit suicide (Pokorny, 1977). In a study of 134 consecutive suicides, Robins and associates found, on the basis of interviews with relatives and medical records, that about 45% of the suicides probably had a depressive disorder (Robins *et al.,* 1959a,b).

Risk Factors

In a classic book called *Le Suicide* (1897/1966), the French sociologist Emile Durkheim studied the sociological factors influencing suicide rates in different cultural conditions. He found that suicide rates were higher in the Protestant areas of Europe as opposed to the Catholic areas, which he attributed to the spirit of free inquiry and individualism among the Protestants. Durkheim postulated that loosening of the individual's ties with the society, as in the case of Protestants and unmarried persons, tends to lead the individual to question the purpose of life itself and, thus, to a heightened risk of suicide. This type of suicide was called the "egoistic suicide." Durkheim also described the "altruistic suicide," occurring in an opposite cultural setting. Altruistic suicide occurs in settings of excessive lack of individualism, such as the suicide of women on the death of their husbands in some cultures. In this type of suicide, there is a sense of duty, a social prescription for the suicide. Durkheim also included religious suicides, such as self-immolation occurring in certain Buddhist sects, in the category of altruistic suicide.

Anomie and *anomic suicide* are important concepts proposed by Durkheim. He noted that the suicide rate increased at times of relative peace and financial prosperity. He also noted that the suicide rate was high in the European countries where the divorce rates were high. He postulated that at times of peace, relative financial prosperity, and following divorce and separation, there is a loss of regulation in one's life—that is, the individual feels lost without a sense of purpose and demands. He called this state of lack of regulation "anomie," and the resultant suicide occurring in some individuals, "anomic suicide" (Durkheim, 1897/1966).

Current statistics show that suicide is the second leading cause of death for white men between the ages of 10 and 55 in the United States. It is one of the ten leading causes of death for both men and women up to the age of 75. The rate of actually committed suicide is higher for men than women (3 to 1), and more women than men attempt suicide (2 to 1).

Suicide is common among certain professions, especially physicians. Under the age of 40, suicide is the leading cause of death among physicians, psychiatry leading other medical fields (Schneidman *et al.*, 1975).

In the United States, the rate of suicide in the *general population* is approximately 1 in 10,000. The risk for successful suicide is higher in *single, separated,* or *divorced persons;* in *men;* and in *older persons.* Suicide risk is higher in patients who have pain, who are *depressed,* or who have a history of a depressive syndrome. Patients who live *alone,* who *drink heavily,* and who have experienced a *recent stressful event* are also at a higher risk for suicide.

About 80% of persons who commit suicide give *definite warnings about their intent* (Motto, 1975). Suicides often occur during a phase *when the person's depression seems to be lifting.* When a depressed patient has decided to commit suicide, there may be a sudden lifting of depressive affect, with a sense of resolution (vignette 3). With antidepressant therapy, the suicide risk rises initially as the patient becomes more energetic and able to contemplate the execution of a suicidal plan. Many persons intending to commit suicide indicate this decision by such actions as making out a will, getting insurance, and giving away personally valued possessions (as in vignette 3).

Many people who ultimately commit suicide have recently *engaged in help-seeking behavior.* (Seventy percent of depressed persons committing suicide were in touch with a physician within 30 days of their death, and nearly half during the preceding week.)

To recap, then, suicidal potential should be evaluated by asking specific questions about the risk factors listed in Table 5.

Suicidal Attempt

The physician usually encounters the suicidal patient in two contexts: the patient who is depressed and therefore a suicidal risk and the patient who comes to the physician's attention because of a suicidal attempt. The latter is an especially important problem encountered in the emergency rooms and intensive care units.

It used to be said that suicidal attempters seldom actually commit suicide—this is *not* true. Approximately 1% of suicidal attempters who were admitted to the hospital complete suicide *each year* (Weissman, 1974). Although not all suicidal attempters ultimately wind up committing suicide, the suicidal attempt is usually an indication of serious suffering, which may be alleviated if proper help is offered by the physician.

Table 5. Suicide Risk Factors

1. Presence of a depressive syndrome, including suicidal thoughts; especially, has the patient planned how he would do it?
2. Demographic risk factors: religion (high in non-Catholics), marital status (higher in single, divorced, and separated persons), older age, male sex
3. Presence of a painful condition or other medical disorder
4. Living conditions—living alone increases risk
5. Alcohol use—heavy use increases risk
6. Behavioral warnings of suicide—seeking help (including medical), talking about suicide, giving away possessions, putting personal affairs in order, hoarding drugs, buying weapons, etc.
7. Apparent lifting of depression—suicide occurs more often following this
8. Ready availability of the means of suicide, for example, large quantities of prescribed medication or a rifle hanging in the den
9. Previous suicide attempt, history of depression, family history

In contrast to completed suicides, suicidal attempters tend to be *young* in age (peak age, 20–24 years), 50% of the attempters being under 30 years of age (Weissman, 1974). Again, unlike completed suicides, women outnumber men by 2 to 1 among the suicide attempters.

Suicide attempt often occurs in the context of *interpersonal difficulties.* Although it is more common among separated and divorced persons, suicidal attempt is also common among married persons and single persons (especially in the younger age group, where this is the norm). Although, as Durkheim pointed out, suicidal mortality is lower in countries that have a large number of Roman Catholics, suicidal attempt does not seem to be infrequent among Catholics (Weissman, 1974).

The most common form of suicidal attempt is drug overdosage (70–90% of all attempts). Barbiturates, tranquilizers, and antidepressant medications are among the drugs commonly used in suicidal attempts.

Evaluation of Suicidal Attempt

In evaluating a patient who has attempted suicide, we have to consider (1) the current context, including the immediate reason for the attempt; (2) the recent context or recent events or changes that culminated in the patient's attempt; and (3) the background factors, such as the patient's personality, cultural forces, and the meaning of suicide. (For a detailed discussion of these contexts, see Part III.)

Current Context Factors. *Method of Suicidal Attempt.* The *lethality* of the method is an important consideration. A patient who attempts suicide by using a gun is obviously more serious in his attempt than someone who ingests ten tablets of aspirin. However, one has to consider the patient's own ideas about the lethality of the method used. For example, a patient who attempts suicide with aspirin believing it to be very lethal is more serious than someone who takes an overdose of antidepressants believing that antidepressants could not seriously endanger life. (In fact, antidepressants are highly lethal.)

Although ingestion of drugs may not be immediately as lethal as shooting, this is still the most common method of suicidal attempt and completed suicide. Whether the patient has any *further supply* of the drug (which might be used in a repeat attempt) and *where the patient* obtained the drug should be ascertained. In one study, over half of the patients who committed suicide by overdosage had received a prescription for a fully lethal amount of hypnotic medication which the patient ingested, or an unlimited prescription for it, from their physicians (Murphy, 1975a). The *physician should be alerted to* the patient's suicidal attempt as soon as possible if the patient is brought directly to the hospital.

Emotional State of the Patient. This includes the seriousness of *suicidal intent,* presence or absence of *intoxication* or *overwhelming emotion* at the time of the attempt, and degree of impulsivity. The seriousness of the suicidal intent is best evaluated by direct questions of the patient, such as, "What did you have in mind when you took the pills? Did you seriously want to die?" "What ideas did you have about what would happen after you died?" Alcohol or other drug intoxication, presence of rage, or an impulsive suicidal attempt militate against the patient's suicidality being prolonged beyond the current attempt. However, the presence of depressive affect or apathy on a continuing basis indicates continuing suicidal risk.

Patient's Behavior and Psychological State around and after the Attempt. If the patient went to a secluded place before ingesting an overdose, the seriousness of the suicidal risk should be considered grave, even if the method of attempt was less serious (e.g., aspirin). Making a phone call to a friend after ingestion of an overdose probably indicates the presence of ambivalence and a wish for rescue.

Recent Context Factors: Recent Events, Changes, Stresses. *Depression.* Eighty percent of suicidal attempts are *clinically depressed* (i.e., have the depressive syndrome) at the time of the attempt (Silver *et al.,* 1971). The patients should be *asked specific questions* concerning mood, loss of interest, libido, sleep patterns, appetite, weight loss, fatigue, etc., to determine whether the suicidal attempt is a part of the depressive syndrome.

Interpersonal Conflict. This includes recent marital problems, arguments with lovers, and separations. In certain situations, the interpersonal conflict may be resolved after a suicidal attempt, for example, marital reconciliation. In other situations, no interpersonal change occurs, and the *risk may continue.*

Help-Seeking Behavior and Pain. Suicidal attempt occurs often in patients with *chronic or severe pain.* Pain can also be a symptom of a depressive syndrome. Help-seeking behavior of any kind occurs often before a suicidal attempt. Understanding the help-seeking behavior pattern of the patient will help the physician to recognize future suicidal potential. For example, increased frequency of visits to the doctor with complaints of vague pains may be the most prominent symptom of increasing depression for a patient, culminating in a suicidal attempt.

Termination Behavior. Persons who have decided on suicide engage in activities indicating this, such as giving away prized possessions and making out a new will (vignette 3).

Previous Suicidal Attempts. Over two-thirds of those who eventually commit suicide have histories of suicidal attempts or threats (Murphy, 1975b). Positive findings in any of the recent context factors indicate that the attempt was a serious one requiring thoughtful management.

Background Context Factors: Personality, Constitution, Culture. *De-*

mographic Data Related to the Risk Factors. The risk for completed suicide increases (if the patient attempts suicide again) with increasing age; in men; in persons whose marital status is single, divorced, or separated; in non-Catholics; in certain professions (e.g., physicians); etc.

Cultural Views on Suicide. Culture often influences the desirability of suicide as an option (e.g., in Japanese culture) and the method of suicide. The latter is obviously related to the lethality of the attempt. Culture and early history also often influence the psychological meaning of suicide. For example, death by suicide may mean reunion with a loved one, liberation from pain and suffering, or eternal fire and brimstone.

Personality of the Patient. Impulsive personality style tends to increase the risk for impulsive suicide. On the other hand, patients who tend to be orderly and controlling (see Chapter 15) are more likely to be successful in a suicidal attempt because of their tendency for careful planning. In the past, "hysterical personality" was considered to have a low risk for actual suicide—this is *not* true. Suicidal attempts are very common in hysterical personality, and completed suicide is not uncommon.

Constitutional or Genetic Factors. These are important in that the depressive syndrome has a genetic predisposition. Family history of suicide increases the risk for the patient's having a major affective disorder and for suicide.

The background context factors provide information on the broad background factors for assessing a patient's suicidal risk.

Management of Depression

A comprehensive evaluation of the depressed patient is the first step toward management. This includes the nature and severity of the depressive affect as well as the life situation of the patient.

Mild depressive affect occurring in response to loss or separation usually does not require specific treatment. In severe *grief reactions,* a generally supportive environment and empathic attitude by the family, friends, and physician usually allow the "grief work" to proceed to resolution in time. On occasion, the grieving person may be *frightened* about the very vivid images of the deceased that he or she may experience or, occasionally, by *hallucinations* concerning the deceased. Reassurance by the physician that these are normal phenomena occurring in the course of bereavement or grief is effective and enlightening. Antidepressant medications are generally *not* indicated and ineffective in uncomplicated grief reactions. If the sleep disturbance is severe or anxiety symptoms are prominent, mild sedatives or tranquilizers may be of transient benefit, for example, 15 mg flurazepam at bedtime for sleep when necessary.

For *chronic depressive disorder,* the recognition of the chronic nature of the depression as a personality style is the key to management. Depressive ways of looking at things, relating with people, and feeling are unlikely to change easily or promptly. The health care personnel should consider this as a limiting factor in management. Long-term psychotherapy or restructuring of the patient's life may be effective in some instances, but this requires extensive investment of time, money, and effort. When the physiologic symptoms and signs of depression are prominent in a chronic depressive disorder, antidepressants may be transiently effective, but the chronic characterological aspects are unlikely to respond.

Once the presence of an *acute depressive syndrome* has been recognized, the physician should determine whether it is due to or associated with a medical disease such as an occult carcinoma or an endocrinopathy. If this is the case, the *underlying medical disease* should be treated. In the meanwhile, if the depressive symptomatology is very severe, including serious suicidal ideations, a *protective psychiatric hospitalization* may be necessary. (The medical disease should be treated in the psychiatric unit, or, if surgery is needed, the patient could be transferred for the operation after initial admission to psychiatry.) Antidepressants are not usually effective in depressive syndromes due to medical diseases.

If the diagnosis of a *major affective disorder* is made in a patient with the depressive syndrome, then specific treatments for this disorder are to be considered.

Before embarking on a specific treatment regimen for the depressed patient, a decision should be made as to whether the patient should be *hospitalized.* If the patient is at high risk for suicide, has active suicidal thoughts or plans, is unable to function at work or home, or cannot care for himself, then hospitalization is definitely indicated.

Psychotherapy as a general measure is valuable and often by itself sufficient in milder cases. Psychotherapy in this context should begin as a supportive relationship with a physician who understands the patient's experience of the illness, who has a hopeful and confident attitude, and who encourages the patient to share and discuss his problems. More ambitious or active psychotherapy with such patients should be undertaken only by a specialist. The frequency of such psychotherapy can be flexible, but initially, it should be at least once a week. If the patient is to be treated as an outpatient, the physician should determine whether the patient needs hospitalization at the time of each therapy visit, as the need may arise in the course of treatment.

In addition to the type of psychotherapy described above, specific treatment for the depressive syndrome that is a part of the major affective disorder may include *antidepressants, lithium carbonate,* or *electroconvulsive therapy*

(ECT). In patients with bipolar disorder, lithium is helpful in treating the acute manic episode and especially in the prevention of recurring manic episodes. Lithium also has the beneficial effect in unipolar depressions of reducing the frequency and severity of recurrent depressive episodes.

Antidepressants include the *tricyclic antidepressants* and the *monoamine oxidase inhibitors*. Because the monoamine oxidase inhibitors have many interactions with other medications and certain foods (any food containing tyramine, such as aged cheese, wine, and pickles), tricyclic antidepressants are more commonly used, especially in patients with concurrent medical problems. The use of antidepressants and lithium is described in more detail in Chapter 18.

Electroconvulsive therapy (ECT) is an effective treatment for depression. It is usually performed on hospitalized patients who are very agitated and suicidal. Contrary to popular belief, ECT therapy is quite painless. (The patient is anesthetized with sodium pentothal, and muscles are relaxed with a relaxant like succinylcholine during ECT.) ECT is a safe procedure. The only absolute contraindication to ECT is increased intracranial pressure or recent cerebrovascular accident.

Generally, *antidepressant medications* should be tried first in conjunction with psychotherapy to treat the depressive syndrome. Antidepressant drugs should be used in adequate doses for an adequate amount of time (at least two to three weeks) before the effectiveness is determined. Since antidepressants are potentially lethal medications, however, the prescription for an outpatient should not exceed more than one week's supply (another reason why the doctor should see the patient at least every week—to give new prescriptions). If the antidepressant is not effective, or if the patient is acutely suicidal and agitated, the patient may need hospitalization and, possibly, ECT.

With antidepressant therapy and/or ECT, 80–90% of patients with the depressive syndrome will respond dramatically within four to six weeks of treatment. Antidepressant drugs should, however, be continued for at least about six months (for the duration of the natural history of the depressive syndrome, which is about nine months without treatment). For some patients, more intensive long-term psychotherapy for underlying chronic unresolved conflicts that may contribute to depressive episodes may be indicated.

The management of *suicidal states* should also be based on comprehensive evaluation. Depression, intoxication, and other acute psychological and medical states should be managed with specific treatment, protection, and general supportive measures. Acutely suicidal patients should be hospitalized, by commitment if necessary. Long-term management and prevention should be based on each of the factors described in the section on Evaluation of Suicidal Potential.

Summary

Sadness is an affect usually associated with loss, failure, or separation. Although sadness and grief are normal experiences, the extreme form, depressive syndrome, is a pathological condition. At the opposite pole of the depressive syndrome in mood is the manic syndrome, also a pathological condition. There are specific features and criteria for the diagnosis of the depressive syndrome.

Grief reaction is a response to acute loss. The symptomatology includes somatic distress, intense preoccupation with the image of the deceased, guilt feelings, irritability, and change in patterns of behavior. The course of bereavement or the grief reaction has been described as consisting of three phases: numbness, pining (anxious searching), and depression and despair. The course of the normal acute grief reaction is approximately four to eight weeks, but a substantial portion of the bereaved continue to feel some distress up to one or two years after the death of a spouse. Pathological grief reactions consist of delayed and distorted grief reactions. Depressive syndrome may also ensue.

Studies of young children separated from their mothers show three phases: protest, despair, and detachment. Phenomena similar to those occurring in the protest and despair phases have also been described in infant monkeys that are separated from their mothers. Monkeys that are socially isolated from early life also develop difficulties in later life, especially in social and sexual activity.

There is an increased morbidity and mortality due to many causes in depressed patients and in the bereaved population.

Depressive affect may be adaptive. It serves as a signal of a loss or separation. The typical expression and behavior pattern (such as protest or despair) may mobilize social support and nurturance. Reduction of activity and withdrawal may facilitate conservation of energy and resources in the face of adversity. In childhood, the threat of sadness resulting from loss of love and approval by the parents and others may help the socialization and learning process.

The *brain mechanisms* of depression are not completely understood. Presumably, there is a dysfunction of the brain areas involved with pleasurable and unpleasurable affects, including the medial forebrain bundle and the periventricular system, respectively, and, perhaps, the whole limbic brain. The major neurotransmitters implicated in depression include norepinephrine, serotonin, and acetylcholine. The catecholamine theory of affective disorders postulates that there is an increase in the functional level of norepinephrine in the brain in mania and a decrease in its level in depression. Psychological aspects include possible turning inward of aggression, altered cognitive style due to repeated failures, and the response to the recognition of the inadequacy of the individual to perform a task. An integrated model postulates multiple factors (environmental, psychological, genetic, and neurophysiological) that may lead to a final common pathway of dysfunction in the reinforcement system of the brain.

In depression, there is often a marked increase in the corticosteroids and an abnormal dexamethasone suppression test. Growth hormone response to hypoglycemia is often decreased in depression.

The *evaluation* of depression should consider the severity and nature of depression, suicidal risk, advisability of hospitalization, and management plans. *Medical conditions* that may cause depression, such as endocrinopathies and occult malignancies, should be carefully ruled out.

An important consideration in the evaluation of depression is the patient's suicidal potential. The risk factors for suicide include male sex, single, separated, or divorced marital status, older age, certain professions, lack of social support, heavy drinking, recent stressful event, anomie, certain religious groups, and, most importantly, presence of depression and past history of suicidal attempt. Among the signs of increasing suicidal risk are help-seeking behavior, including contacting a physician for medical problems, seeming lifting of depression, giving away possessions, and reference to suicide.

Suicidal attempt is much more common than completed suicides. The uncompleted suicidal attempters tend to be younger and female as compared to completed suicides. A suicidal attempt often results in the context of interpersonal conflict. It is a serious cry for help and should be evaluated systematically.

The *management* of *grief reactions* includes supportive interpersonal environment and reassurances concerning the symptomatology when indicated. Antianxiety agents might be indicated transiently in some cases. *Chronic depressive disorder* should be considered a characterological style which is not amenable to rapid change but should be a consideration in managing the patient for concurrent medical problems.

Acute depressive syndrome due to major affective disorder should be treated with psychotherapy (doctor–patient relationship) and a specific treatment such as antidepressant medications or electroconvulsive therapy. In bipolar disorders, lithium carbonate is indicated.

The *underlying medical disease* should be treated in depressive syndrome associated with a medical condition.

An important clinical decision in managing a depressed patient is whether or not to hospitalize. Suicidality and inability to function are indications for hospitalization.

Implications

For the Patient

Depression is often a natural response to a medical illness or hospitalization with attendant loss of autonomy and function. Severe depression (depressive syndrome), however, colors every aspect of the patient's life, including his thinking process (slowed and lacking concentration), outlook (hopeless), and behavior (self-defeating or unable to act). Thus, depressed patients often do *not* consult a physician in the presence of serious symptoms or signs of disease and may have an unrealistically pessimistic outlook on existing disease. On the other hand, a relatively mild depression may increase the tendency for help-seeking behavior, especially when accompanied by vague pains and preoccupation with bodily parts. Depression and bereavement are often contributing factors to disease. Depression increases morbidity and mortality in the presence of medical disease and following surgical procedures.

For the Physician

As depression is common among medical patients, but often not recognized by the physician (Murphy, 1975b), doctors should deliberately evaluate a patient for possible depression. Since depression can be caused by an underlying, undiagnosed medical disease such as occult carcinoma and endocrinopathies, a thorough medical workup should be performed on the patients who are depressed. When patients appear mentally slowed or especially apathetic or pessimistic about the medical condition, the possibility of concurrent depressive syndrome should be entertained.

Physicians should also be aware that fatigue, vague pains and aches, insomnia, and somatic preoccupation may be symptoms of the depressive syndrome. In these cases, specific questions should be asked to establish or rule out the presence of the syndrome.

For the Community and Health Care System

Since mild depression responds to environmental stimuli, hospitals should provide a cheerful physical and environmental situation for the patients. This may also have a preventive effect. More research by the medical profession is needed to increase our understanding of the mechanisms by which depression and bereavement increase morbidity and mortality.

Recommended Reading

Akiskal HS, McKinney WT: Overview of recent research in depression. *Arch Gen Psychiatry* **32**:285–305, 1975. A thorough review of recent research findings on depresssion. The authors propose a unified model of depression. Extensive references.

Flach FF, Draghi SC (eds): *The Nature and Treatment of Depression.* New York, John Wiley & Sons, 1975. A comprehensive volume with chapters on various aspects of depression, including the interpersonal, psychodynamic, and environmental, as well as consideration of different age groups; the biological aspects of depression and various treatment modalities also presented.

Freud S: Mourning and melancholia, in Strachey J (ed): *Standard Edition of the Complete Psychological Works of Sigmund Freud.* London, Hogarth Press, 1957, vol 14, pp 237–260. Also in *Collected Papers of Sigmund Freud.* London, Hogarth Press, 1925, vol 4, pp 152–170. (Originally published, 1917.) A classic work on the early psychoanalytic understanding of depression, in which Freud postulates the turning inward of aggression.

Jacobsen E: *Depression.* New York, International Universities Press, 1971. A detailed, up-to-date, psychoanalytic treatise on depression.

Parkes, CM: *Bereavement: Studies of Grief in Adult Life.* New York, International Universities Press, 1972. A comprehensive discussion and description of the bereavement process. Recommended because so many patients and their families are at risk for bereavement.

References

Akiskal HS, McKinney WT: Overview of recent research in depression. *Arch Gen Psychiatry* **32**:285–305, 1975.

Altschule MD: *Bodily Physiology in Mental and Emotional Disorders.* New York, Grune & Stratton, 1953.

Asberg M, Bertilsson L, Tuck D, *et al.:* Indolamine metabolites in the cerebrospinal fluid of depressed patients before and during treatment with nortriptyline. *Clin Pharmacol Ther* **14**:277–286, 1973.

Beck A: *Depression: Clinical, Experimental, and Theoretical Aspects.* New York, Harper & Row, 1967.

Bibring E: The mechanism of depression, in Greenacre P (ed): *Affective Disorders.* New York, International Universities Press, 1965, 13–48.

Bliss E, Zwanziger J: Brain amines and emotional stress. *J Psychiatr Res* **4**:189–198, 1966.

Bliss E, Wilson V, Zwanziger J: Changes in brain norepinephrine in self-stimulating and "aversive" animals. *J Psychiatr Res* **4**:59–63, 1966.

Bornstein PE, Clayton PJ, Halikas JA, *et al.:* The depression of widowhood after thirteen months. *Br J Psychiatry* **122**:561–566, 1973.

Bowers MF, Heninger GR, Gerbode F: Cerebrospinal fluid 5-hydroxyindolacetic acid and homovanillic acid in psychiatric patients. *Int J Neuropharmacol* **8**:255–262, 1970.

Bowlby J: Grief and mourning in infancy and early childhood. *Psychoanal Study Child* **15**:9–52, 1960.

Carroll BJ: The hypothalamic–pituitary axis: Functions, control mechanisms, and method of study, in Davies B, Carroll BJ, Mowbrary RM (ed): *Depressive Illness: Some Research Studies.* Springfield, Ill., Charles C Thomas, 1972.

Clayton PJ, Halikas JA, Maurine WL: The depression of widowhood. Br J Psychiatry 120:71–78, 1972.

Davis JM: Central biogenic amines and theories of depression and mania, in Fann WE, Karacan I, Pokorny AD, et al. (eds): Phenomenology and Treatment of Depression. Jamaica, NY, Spectrum Publications, 1977, pp 17–32.

Diagnostic and Statistical Manual of Mental Disorders (DSM III), draft. Washington, DC, American Psychiatric Association, 1978.

Durkheim E: Suicide, New York, The Free Press, 1966. (Originally published in French, 1897.)

Ettigi PG, Brown GM: Psychoneuroendocrinology of affective disorders: An overview. Am J Psychiatry 134:493–501, 1977.

Freud S: Mourning and melancholia, in Strachey J (ed): Standard Edition of the Complete Psychological Works of Sigmund Freud. London, Hogarth Press, 1957, vol 14, pp 237–260. (Originally published, 1917.)

Harlow H, Harlow M: Social deprivation in monkeys. Sci Am 207:137–146, 1962.

Harlow H, Harlow M: Learning to love. Am Sci 54:244–272, 1966a.

Harlow H, Harlow M: Affection in primates. Discovery 27:11–17, 1966b.

Heine BE, Sainsbury P, Chynoweth RC: Hypertension and emotional disturbance. J Psychiatr Res 7:119–130, 1969.

Huston PE: Psychotic depressive reaction, in Freedman AM, Kaplan HI, Sadock BJ (eds): Comprehensive Textbook of Psychiatry, II, ed 2. Baltimore, Williams & Wilkins, 1975, vol 1, pp 1043–1055.

Izard CE: Patterns of Emotions. New York, Academic Press, 1972.

Izard CE: Human Emotions. New York, Plenum Press, 1977.

Jacobs S, Ostfeld AM: An epidemiological review of the mortality of bereavement. Psychosom Med 39:344–357, 1978.

Janowsky DS, El-Yousef MK, Davis JM, et al.: A cholinergic–adrenergic hypothesis of mania and depression. Lancet 1:632–635, 1972.

Janowsky DS, El-Yousef MK, Davis JM: Parasympathetic suppression of manic symptoms of physostigmine. Arch Gen Psychiatry 28:542–547, 1973.

Kaufman IC, Rosenblum LA: The reaction to separation in infant monkeys: Anaclitic depression and conservation–withdrawal. Psychosom Med 29:648–675, 1967.

Kennedy JA, Bakst H: The influence of emotions on the outcome of cardiac surgery: A predictive study. Bull NY Acad Med 42:811–845, 1966.

Lebovitz BZ, Shekelle RB, Ostfeld AM, et al.: Prospective and retrospective psychological studies of coronary heart disease. Psychosom Med 29:265–272, 1967.

Lindemann E: Symptomatology and management of acute grief. Am J Psychiatry 101:141–148, 1944.

Maas J: Clinical and biochemical heterogeneity of depressive disorders. Ann Intern Med 88:556–563, 1978.

Motto JA: The recognition and management of the suicidal patient, in Flach FF, Draghi SC (eds): The Nature and Treatment of Depression. New York, John Wiley & Sons, 1975, pp 229–254.

Murphy GE: The physician's responsibility for suicide: I. An error of commission. Ann Intern Med 82:301–304, 1975a.

Murphy GE: The physician's responsibility for suicide: II. Errors of omission. Ann Intern Med 82:305–309, 1975b.

Neuropsychopharmacology, 1: The Monoamine Systems. Nutley, N.J., Roche Laboratories, 1976.

Parkes CM: Bereavement: Studies of Grief in Adult Life. New York, International Universities Press, 1972.

Pokorny AD: Suicide in depression, in Fann WE, Karacan I, Pokorny AD, et al. (eds):

Phenomenology and Treatment of Depression. Jamaica, NY, Spectrum Publications, 1977, pp 197–216.

Prange A, Wilson I, Lynn CW, *et al.:* L-Tryptophan in mania: Contribution to a permissive hypothesis of affective disorders. *Arch Gen Psychiatry* **30:**56–62, 1974.

Reiser MF, Bakst H: Psychophysiological and psychodynamic problems of the patient with structural heart disease, in Reiser MF (ed): *American Handbook of Psychiatry,* ed 2. New York, Basic Books, 1975, vol 4, pp. 618–652.

Robertson J, Bowlby J: Responses of young children to separation from their mothers. *Courr Cent Int Enfence* **2:**131–142, 1952.

Robins E, Gassner S, Kayes J, *et al.:* The communication of suicidal intent: A study of 134 consecutive cases of successful (completed) suicide. *Am J Psychiatry* **115:**724–733, 1959a.

Robins E, Murphy G, Wilkinson R, *et al.:* Some clinical considerations in the prevention of suicide based on a study of 134 successful suicides. *Am J Public Health* **49:**888–889, 1959b.

Sachar EJ: Endocrine factors in depressive illness, in Flach FF, Draghi SC (eds): *The Nature and Treatment of Depression.* New York, John Wiley & Sons, 1975a, pp 397–411.

Schildkraut JJ, Kety SS: Biogenic amines and emotion. *Science* **156:**21–30, 1967.

Schmale AH: Giving up as a final common pathway to changes in health. *Ad Psychosom Med* **8:**20–40, 1972.

Schneidman ES: Suicide, in Freedman AM, Kaplan HI, Sadock BJ (eds): *Comprehensive Textbook of Psychiatry, II,* ed 2. Baltimore, Williams & Wilkins, 1975, vol 2.

Seay B, Harlow HF: Maternal separation in the rhesus monkey. *J Nerv Ment Dis* **140:**434–441, 1965.

Seligman M, Maier S: Failure to escape traumatic shock. *J Exp Psychol* **74:**1–9, 1967.

Silver MA, Bohnert M, Beck A, *et al.:* Relation of depression at attempted suicide and seriousness of intent. *Arch Gen Psychiatry* **25:**573–576, 1971.

Spitz R: Anaclitic depression: An inquiry into the genesis of psychiatric conditions in early childhood. *Psychoanal Study Child* **2:**313–342, 1942.

Sweeney DR, Maas JW: Specificity of depressive diseases. *Annu Rev Med* **29:**219–229, 1978.

Weissman MM: The epidemiology of suicide attempts, 1960–1971. *Arch Gen Psychiatry* **30:**737–746, 1974.

Whybrow, P, Mendels J: Toward a biology of depression: Some suggestions from neurophysiology. *Am J Psychiatry* **125:**45–54, 1969.

Wolpe J: Neurotic depression: Experimental analog, clinical syndromes, and treatment. *Am J Psychother* **25:**362–368, 1971.

CHAPTER 7

Pain

1. A 59-year-old man came to the emergency room complaining of crushing pains in the chest. He was immediately admitted to the coronary care unit with a diagnosis of myocardial infarction (heart attack). Morphine was given by injection to relieve the pain.

2. A 23-year-old married woman was admitted to the obstetrics ward today as she developed labor pains. As he was waiting for her to deliver the baby, the husband also experienced severe crampy pains in his abdomen, which disappeared after his wife's delivery.

3. A 20-year-old single woman is still in severe pain after two weeks in the hospital. This is her seventh admission to the hospital in three years because of severe pains in the abdomen. During the first admission, an operation was done to rule out acute appendicitis. Her appendix was normal. She had two additional operations on the abdomen, as adhesions from the first operation were suspected of causing the pain. All tests so far during this hospitalization have been normal, but she continues to have severe crampy pains and is asking for frequent pain medications. When she asks for pain medications, she has been receiving saline injections (placebos) at the orders of the physician, who believes that she is addicted to narcotic pain medications. The injections seem to help her for a couple of hours, but then she cries for more injections. According to the nurses, she seems to be always bitter and cynical.

4. A 27-year-old man who is a surgical patient in the hospital is complaining of severe shooting and stabbing pains in his right leg and foot. The patient had an amputation of the right leg and foot four weeks ago, after an industrial accident which crushed his right foot. This is an example of "phantom limb" pain—pain felt as coming from a limb which is no longer there.

These are only some of the examples of patients with pain frequently seen in the hospital. Many patients with pain obviously do not present themselves to the physician, and almost all of us have had some pain from time to time in some part of the body which we were able to ignore or which could be relieved with aspirin. It should be obvious from the foregoing cases that pain is not a simple phenomenon; it is determined and influenced by many factors. What, then, are the mechanisms and functions of pain, and what are the factors that affect this familiar but sometimes puzzling entity?

Definitions and Functions of Pain

Pain is an abstract concept which refers to a personal, private sensation of hurt, often as a result of a harmful stimulus which signals current or impending tissue damage, and an accompanying pattern of responses which operate to protect the organism from harm (Sternbach, 1968).

At a concrete level, pain is a perceptual experience like hearing or vision, but, unlike vision or hearing, pain experience is determined or modified to a greater extent by a multiplicity of factors such as the psychological set of the individual, including expectations, suggestions, previous experiences, and sociocultural environment.

The function of pain is protective; it is usually a signal that tissue damage is occurring, and it alerts the organism to take appropriate action or get away from it if possible. In this sense, pain as a signal of impending threat is analogous to anxiety. Anxiety occurs in anticipation of the threat, while pain occurs when the threatening situation is actually causing damage to the organism. Unlike anxiety, pain is usually perceived as emanating from a part of the body—it is *localizable*.

Like anxiety, pain may signify the presence of a *psychological state* without actual tissue damage. Pain *metaphors* describing emotional states are common, such as the "pain of loneliness" and "heartaches." In fact, descriptions of pain occurring from tissue damage are often also quite metaphorical, such as "splitting headaches," "stabbing pain" and "heartburn." These linguistic uses clearly indicate close association between the experience of pain and the *symbolic* meanings in the mental life of human beings. Thus, it is not surprising that some individuals perceive certain psychological states as physical pain, attributable to a body organ.

Pain often generates anxiety; in many situations, anxiety is generated as a signal that a potentially painful process is in the making. *Anxiety may also generate pain;* pain is the most common heterothetic symptom resulting in doctor–patient contact.

Anxiety and pain are probably associated through a learning process (see

Chapter 4). In childhood, physical punishment (pain) often occurs in a situation where the child has anxieties about the possible loss of parental love; fear of the loss of bodily parts in injury is also accompanied by the sensation of pain. For many individuals, therefore, pain is often associated with anxiety and anxiety with pain.

Qualities of Pain

Many different adjectives have been used to describe the qualitative aspects of pain. These include, among others, throbbing, pounding, shooting, stabbing, tender, aching, splitting, stinging, and grueling. Melzack and Torgerson (1971) classified 102 such descriptors into three major classes:

1. Words describing the *sensory* qualities of the experience, such as temporal, spatial, pressure, and thermal properties—pricking, scalding, etc.
2. Words describing the *affective* qualities, such as tension and fear, and autonomic properties—sickening, exhausting, frightening, wretched, etc.
3. Words *evaluating* the subjective overall intensity of pain—miserable, unbearable, etc.

Quality of pain reported by patients is most important in helping the physician in diagnosis. For example, the crushing pain reported in vignette 1 is typical of a coronary disease, while a dull, aching pain in the same location (chest) is more likely to be from the chest wall, not the heart. Elaborate metaphorical quality in the description of pain, such as "feeling as if someone is sitting on my stomach, cutting bowels out with a knife," often indicates that the pain is associated with elaborate fantasies of the patient.

Neurophysiological experiments show that pain sensation emanating from tissue damage can be classified into three major types:

1. Pricking pain: the type of pain caused by a needle pricking the skin or by incision of the skin. Strong irritation of a large area of the skin can also cause this sensation.
2. Burning pain: the type of pain felt when the skin is burned. This is often excruciating.
3. Aching pain: a low-intensity pain usually felt deep inside the body, not on the surface.

Pricking pain is conducted through small myelinated type A delta nerve fibers, while burning and aching pains are conducted by even smaller unmyelinated type C nerve fibers.

Nature of Pain

Phenomenologically, pain is a *subjective experience* and falls into the realm of "private" data; that is, the experience of pain *cannot be shared* by others but can only be reported. This is an important point, since physicians may tend spuriously to objectify pain, as if it were identical in degree with the degree of pathology causing it.

Although certain events, such as injury, are usually associated with pain, under some circumstances, whether pain is experienced or not, and if so, how much, is dependent on factors other than tissue damage; for example, Beecher (1959b) reported that two-thirds of the badly wounded men in a World War II battle did not complain of pain or ask for medications for it.

Beecher proposed that there are two *components* to a pain experience, a primary *sensory* component and a reactive *psychological* component. The primary component is the pain sensation itself, which includes the perception, discrimination, and recognition of the noxious stimulus. The secondary component is the suffering aspect of pain, which is an emotional aspect including anxiety. The reactive component is not always commensurate with the primary sensation. Physiologic changes associated with pain, such as change in heart rate, blood pressure, and skin conductance, are thought to be related to the reactive component of pain.

Neurophysiology of Pain

The "pain receptors" are considered to be free nerve endings which are stimulated by tissue damage and stimuli that can cause tissue damage. The exact mechanism by which tissue damage stimulates the pain receptors is not known. There seem to be in the free nerve endings receptors that respond only to very strong mechanical stimuli and strong thermal stimuli evoking pain sensation. Also, various chemicals, such as lactic acid formed in the muscle due to lack of oxygen; polypeptides, such as bradykinin formed as a tissue breakdown product; amines (serotonin and histamine); and prostaglandins are known to cause intense pain.

The nerve impulses arising from the pain receptors (nocioceptors) travel through two types of nerve fibers in the sensory nerve: the type A delta fibers and the type C fibers. The A delta fibers have a conduction velocity of 3–20 m/sec, while the C fibers transmit impulses at 0.5–2 m/sec. As mentioned earlier, the pricking type of pain is transmitted by the A delta fibers and the burning, aching pain, by the type C fibers. Thus, a sudden painful stimulus can result in two perceptions, an initial pricking sensation followed by an aching or burning sensation a second or so later. The cell bodies of the pain fibers are in the dorsal root ganglia, and most pain fibers enter the spinal cord through the dorsal roots, then ascend or descend one or two segments in Lissauer's tract, terminating in the neurons in the gray matter of the dorsal horns (see Figures 14 and 15). Recent evidence has shown that significant numbers of unmyelinated C fibers enter the spinal cord via the ventral roots and then project to the dorsal horn.

In the dorsal horns, the signals pass through one or more short-fibered neurons, the last of which give rise to long fibers which cross to the contralateral side and ascend in the spinal cord as the *spinothalamic* and *spinoreticular tracts.*

In the brain, the ascending pain pathway separates into two separate pathways, the "pricking pain pathway" and the "burning pain pathway" (Guyton, 1976). The pricking pain pathway terminates in the caudalmost part of the ventrobasal complex of the thalamus. There are neural connections between this complex and the somatosensory cortex and other areas of the thalamus.

The burning pain pathway terminates in the reticular formation of the brain stem and the intralaminar nucleus of the thalamus. The reticular formation and the intralaminar nuclei are parts of the reticular activating system (RAS) (see Figure 7), whose function it is to regulate the level of arousal of the entire central nervous system. The pain signals activate this system, sending activating signals to the entire cortex, entire brain stem, thalamus, and hypothalamus, which controls the autonomic and neuroendocrine systems. Thus, through the RAS, pain causes a central nervous system state of arousal, promoting defensive reactions to get rid of the noxious stimulus (see Chapter 5).

Pain sensations from various parts of the body are represented in the thalamic nuclei in a somatotopical fashion somewhat like that in the sensory cortex. Although sensory modalities other than pain require intact sensory cortex to be perceived, the perception of pain seems to require the functional integrity of the nervous system *only up to the thalamic level.* The states of other parts of the nervous system, however, have a major impact on the degree of perception and on the interpretation of the perception and the organism's response to it. The cerebral cortex may affect the state of the neurons in the spinal column through efferent nerves, which might, in turn, affect the sensation itself.

The localization of pain seems to depend to a large extent on the simultaneous stimulation of tactile receptors. The signals transmitted by type C fibers are localizable only very grossly, as this pathway terminates very diffusely in the brain. As mentioned earlier, pain is a subjective experience which cannot be measured objectively. It is possible, however, to measure the least amount of stimulus on the skin necessary to elicit the report of pain from an individual *(pain threshold).* This threshold can be measured by applying a beam of

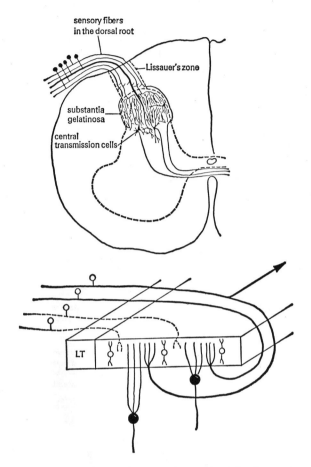

Figure 14. Top: Schematic drawing of the substantia gelatinosa in relation to somatosensory fibers and dorsal horn cells that project their axons across the cord to the anterolateral pathway. (After figure originally published in A.A. Pearson, *Arch. Neurol. Psychiatry* **68**:515, 1952. Copyright 1952 by American Medical Association.) Bottom: Main components of the cutaneous afferent system in the upper dorsal horn. The large-diameter cutaneous peripheral fibers are represented by thick lines running from the dorsal root and terminating in the region of the substantia gelatinosa; one of these, as shown, sends a branch toward the brain in the dorsal column. The finer peripheral fibers are represented by dashed lines running directly into the substantia gelatinosa. The large cells, on which cutaneous afferent nerves terminate, are shown as large black spheres with their axons projecting deeper into the dorsal horn. The open circles represent the cells of the substantia gelatinosa. The axons (not shown) of these cells connect them to one another and also run in Lissauer's tract (LT) to distant parts of the substantia gelatinosa. (Adapted from figure originally published in P.D. Wall, *Prog. Brain Res.* **12**:92, 1964. Courtesy of Oxford University Press.) (From Melzack, 1973. Copyright 1973 by Ronald Melzack and reproduced with his permission.)

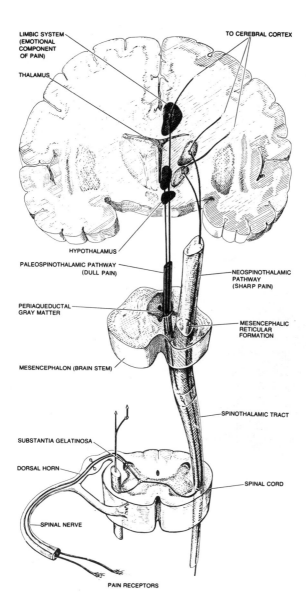

Figure 15. Pain pathways carrying information from the periphery of the nervous system to the brain are separated into two types: the laterally located neospinothalamic pathway, which transmits sharp, localized pain, and the medially located paleospinothalamic pathway (shaded), which transmits less localized burning pain. Burning pain is best relieved by opiates, and opiate receptors have been found to be concentrated in the substantia gelatinosa and in the central thalamus. (From Snyder, 1977. Copyright 1977 by Scientific American, Inc. Reproduced with permission.)

radiant heat on the skin. The skin temperature at which pain is first perceived is remarkably uniform in different people, regardless of their ethnic or cultural background, sex, age, etc. Most people begin to feel the sensation of pain when the skin temperature reaches almost exactly 45°C.

This uniformity of the threshold for pain, however, is valid only in precisely controlled laboratory situations, where the environmental factors are kept constant. The perception of pain is markedly modified in natural conditions by the psychologic state of the individual, such as anticipation, attention, or suggestion. Pain threshold is lowered in injured skin reddened by vasodilatation. Sensitization of pain receptors occurs also when a very strong stimulus is initially applied (Perl, 1976). "Adaptation" to stimuli also occurs, so that there is a decrease in pain sensation after repeated stimuli.

Historical Neurophysiologic Theories of Pain Perception

Historically, there are three theories concerning the neurophysiologic basis of pain perception. They are the (1) specificity theory, (2) pattern theory, and (3) gate control theory.

The *specificity theory* is the oldest theory postulating a specific pain receptor with specific pathways leading to a particular nucleus in the thalamus. In other words, according to this theory, the free nerve endings responsible for pain sensation have no function other than to detect pain, and there is no mechanism for detection of pain other than stimulation of these free nerve endings (receptors). The thalamus is considered to be the primary organ for the integration of pain sensation, according to this theory. In its classic form, this theory cannot account for pain phenomena in which there is no stimulation of the specific pain receptors, as in phantom pain (vignette 4) (see Figure 16).

The *pattern theory* postulates that particular types of input, whether or not they came from specific receptors, would set in motion a particular firing pattern in *reverberatory circuits* in the spinal cord internuncial neurons. This self-propagating nerve impulse in the dorsal horns would then send volleys of impulses to the brain, which are perceived as pain. This theory can explain phantom limb pain, as the initial damage to the limb, or the amputation procedure itself, could initiate abnormal firing patterns in the reverberatory circuits in the dorsal horns. There is not good evidence, however, that reverberatory circuits initiating and perpetuating pain exist in the spinal cord.

The *gate control theory* was proposed by Melzack and Wall (1965). This is an attempted integration of the theories concerning pain and postulates the following: A neural mechanism in the dorsal horns of the spinal cord acts like a gate which can increase or decrease the flow of nerve impulses from peripheral

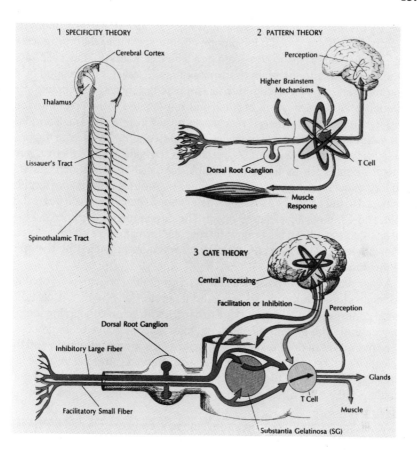

Figure 16. Schematic representation of three theories of pain transmission and perception. The earliest was the specificity theory (1), which held that pain stimuli enter the spinal cord through spinal nerves and synapse ipsilaterally, then rise several levels in Lissauer's tract. They then cross the cord and ascend to the thalamus where they synapse again and rise to the cerebral cortex where pain is perceived. The pattern theory (2) postulates stimuli entering from nerves through dorsal root ganglia into the spinal cord. The so-called T cell is in the lateral horn of the spinal cord. It sets up a response, part of which results in an impulse to higher brain stem mechanisms. These, in turn, modulate the response by action on the T cell, which fires and sends impulses to the brain, causing perception, and to striated muscle, facilitating response. The gate theory (3) depends on the concept of two "parallel" fibers, both with cell bodies in the dorsal root ganglia. The large fiber has basically an inhibitory effect on pain perception, the small fiber basically a facilitatory effect. The large fiber acts upon the substantia gelatinosa (SG) and stimulates it. Such stimulation will prevent firing of the T cell, which is necessary for pain perception. The small fiber can overcome or modify the large fiber's influence on the SG, and/or it can directly stimulate the T cell to fire. The large fiber may also act directly on the brain's central processing mechanisms, although the pathways of this action have not been defined. Impulses may be either inhibitory or facilitatory. If the latter, the result will be firing of the T cell, producing pain perception and endocrine and muscle responses. (From Pearson, 1976. Reproduced with permission from HP Publishing Co., Inc. Original publication was made possible by an educational grant from Pfizer, Inc., New York.)

fibers to the central nervous system (Melzack, 1973). Once signals from receptors (which are specific for pain, as in the specificity theory) reach the spinal cord, their transmission from the afferent fibers to the cells giving ascending output into the brain (transmission, or T, cells) is modulated by the gating mechanism. The gating mechanism was thought to be located in the *substantia gelatinosa*, a group of small neurons located at the tip of the dorsal horn. The substantia gelatinosa receives impulses from many small and large fibers entering the spinal cord as well as from descending fibers from the brain, such as the reticulospinal tract. According to the gate control theory, large-diameter fibers, such as those responsible for position and touch, have an inhibitory effect on the gate control mechanism, reducing the flow of impulses transmitted to the brain. The small-diameter fibers, such as the pain fibers (both A delta and C), have a facilitatory effect. The descending fibers from the brain have an inhibitory effect; the brain stem reticular formation is also considered to exert a powerful inhibitory control over information projected by the spinal cord transmission cells.

A specialized system of large-diameter, fast-conducting fibers (probably in the dorsal column of the spinal cord and its projections), which is called the "central control trigger," is postulated to carry information concerning the pain (e.g., location). This system is considered to activate selective brain processes, such as memories of prior experiences, before the perception of pain and then to selectively exert control over the sensory input by modulating the gate control system through descending pathways and/or by modulating the receptivity of the cortical neurons to the stimuli coming up more slowly through the pain pathways.

According to this theory, phantom limb pain can be explained on the basis of release from inhibition; the loss of large-diameter fibers from the amputated organ "opens the gate control mechanisms," so that the T cell fires at a very low threshold level or even spontaneously. This theory can also explain the pain-relieving effect of counterirritation (such as liniment and acupuncture), which stimulates the inhibitory large-diameter fibers.

There is controversy concerning the existence of such a gating mechanism and the exact nature of the T cells. More recent findings indicate that there is a specific system of nocioception in which specific receptors that are activated only in case of tissue damage (e.g., high-intensity pressure) give rise to impulses in corresponding specific afferent nerves (high-threshold neurons as opposed to low-threshold neurons such as those subserving touch sensation), leading to activation of specific nociceptive areas of the central nervous system (Kerr and Wilson, 1978). It is, however, also clear that this specific nociceptive system is influenced and modified by many factors other than tissue damage, especially through descending fibers from the brain (see below).

Descending Influences from the Brain

A number of descending systems from the brain influence the state of the spinal cord. Brain stem stimulation can cause a change in the excitability of spinal cord cells (Wall, 1976). Stimulation of the sensorimotor cortex inhibits low-threshold neurons, but the high-threshold units are unaffected (Coulter *et al.*, 1974). A cold block of the spinal cord rostral to the recording site has a tonic inhibitory effect on nociceptive neurons (Handwerker *et al.*, 1975).

Electrical stimulation of certain areas of the brain produces potent analgesia, called stimulus-produced analgesia (SPA). SPA can also be produced by stimulation of peripheral nerves, although not as consistently as by brain stimulation. The areas of the brain that produce analgesia upon stimulation include the periaqueductal gray, the dorsal raphe nucleus, the nucleus raphe magnus of the medulla, the gray matter surrounding the third ventricle, and the septal area (Kerr and Wilson, 1978) (see Figure 15). The analgesia produced by brain stimulation specifically inhibits the activation of the nociceptive neurons in the dorsal horn without affecting the low-threshold neurons (Beall *et al.*, 1976; Oliveras *et al.*, 1974). SPA produced by brain stimulation is effective against visceral as well as somatic pain.

Injection of very small amounts of morphine into some of the brain areas that can cause SPA also produces a marked elevation in pain threshold, and the analgesia produced by electrical stimulation of the brain areas is reversed by the administration of or pretreatment with naloxone, an opiate antagonist (Kerr and Wilson, 1978).

Role of Endorphins in Pain Mechanism

When specific receptors binding morphine were discovered in the human brain in the early 1970s, people wondered why human beings might have developed receptors to an alkaloid made by, of all things, the poppy plant. Obviously, a more likely explanation was that these receptors were for some morphine-like substance made by our own brains. Recently, a number of substances that possess morphine-like properties have been identified in the brains and pituitary glands of many animals and humans. These properties include, among others, analgesia, respiratory depression, euphoria, and addictiveness. The chemical structures of these substances have been studied, and all were found to be peptides. The generic name for the peptides with opiate-like properties is "endorphins." "Enkephalins" refers to certain specific pentapeptides belonging to the class of endorphins. Some large-molecule endorphins, such as beta-endorphin, a potent opioid peptide containing 31 amino acids, contain in their structures the shorter 5-amino-acid sequences of the enkephalins.

All of the endorphins, including enkephalins, are antagonized by narcotic antagonists such as naloxone. Thus, their actions seem to be mediated by binding to the opiate receptors discovered earlier. In addition to properties similar to those of morphine, some endorphins have other important behavioral and physiologic effects when injected into the brain or the cerebrospinal fluid. For example, beta-endorphin and metenkephalin (which forms a fragment of the structure of beta-endorphin) cause catatonic behavior in rats, with a decrease in body temperature. These effects are reversible with naloxone (Bloom *et al.,* 1976).

The opiate receptors, the presumed site of action of both the endorphins and narcotic analgesics, are especially heavily distributed in the limbic brain, in the central thalamus, and in the substantia gelatinosa of the spinal cord. As previously discussed, these areas of the central nervous system are especially concerned with the perception of pain. The importance of the limbic brain in the perception of the emotional component of pain should be obvious from our discussion in Chapter 4. It is possible that the euphoriant effect of narcotics is closely related to the concentration of opiate receptors in the limbic system. The opiate receptors are also abundant in all areas the stimulation of which causes analgesia.

The endorphins and the smaller enkephalins (which have a weaker and shorter duration of action) may be neurotransmitters or neuromodulators modifying the perception of pain. The mechanism of action seems to be through inhibition of neurons related to pain perception by means of a rather unusual mechanism of blocking the sodium influx elicited by excitatory neurotransmitters (Snyder, 1977).

Many forms of analgesia may occur through the release of endogenous endorphins, as demonstrable by their reversal by naloxone. These endorphin-dependent analgesias include: brain-stimulation analgesia, acupuncture and some forms of placebo anesthesia, and nitrous oxide anesthesia. Although endorphins may play a role in the inhibition of pain perception during stress, hypnoanesthesia has not been reversed by naloxone (Goldstein, 1976; Marx, 1977).

It seems, then, that endorphins play an important role in the *self-regulation* of the perception and tolerance of pain by the brain through their action on pain at the *spinal cord* all the *way up* to the emotional *reactions* to the pain sensation mediated by the limbic system. In chronic pain, the endogenous endorphin levels may be elevated; on the other hand, insufficient endorphin release due to genetic or other reasons might predispose an individual to feel excessive pain. *Some individuals may require* greater amounts of narcotic analgesics for control of minor pain because of insufficient or depleted endorphin release mechanisms in the central nervous system.

Central Neuropharmacology of Pain

Biogenic amines play an important role in pain perception. Tetrabenazine, a substance that depletes brain monoamines, reduces markedly the analgesia produced by stimulation of the periaqueductal gray in rats (Akil and Liebeskind, 1975). This effect can be reversed by the administration of serotonin or L-dopa.

Dopamine and *serotonin* seem to decrease pain mechanisms in the brain. Stimulation of dopamine receptors in the brain by apomorphine produces a marked increase in brain-stimulation-induced analgesia, while the blockade of dopamine receptors with pimozide impairs the analgesia. The administration of *para*-chlorophenylalanine, an inhibitor of serotonin synthesis, results in decreased brain-stimulation analgesia. This effect is reversed by the administration of the serotonin precursor 5-hydroxytryptophan.

Brain *norepinephrine* seems to have the opposite effect on pain mechanisms as compared to dopamine and serotonin. Disulfiram, a substance that blocks norepinephrine synthesis from dopamine, causes a significant increase in brain-stimulation-induced analgesia.

The effect of morphine and endorphins may be modulated by the brain monoamine levels. For example, reserpine antagonizes experimental morphine anesthesia (Kerr and Wilson, 1978).

Substance P is a peptide that has striking depolarizing effects on neurons. It is present in large concentrations in the dorsal roots and substantia gelatinosa, as well as in the hypothalamus and substantia nigra. Many nocioceptive neurons in the spinal cord respond to substance P.

Glutamate, another substance found in high concentrations in the dorsal roots and ganglia, may be a neurotransmitter concerned with nocioception.

Somatostatin (growth-hormone-release-inhibiting hormone) is also a peptide recently found to be in some small-sized neurons in the dorsal root ganglia. There appears to be a dense plexus of somatostatin-containing fibers in the substantia gelatinosa also. It has potent depressant activity on neuronal firing and may be an inhibitory transmitter for the perception of pain.

Psychosocial Factors Influencing Pain Experience

Although the pain sensation threshold seems to be more or less the same for most people in laboratory situations, as described earlier, the *response* to pain, perceptual intensity, and meaning of pain in natural situations are influenced by a number of psychosocial factors. Even in laboratory situations, persons of differing backgrounds show marked differences in pain *tolerance,* the level of pain at which the subject refuses to tolerate any more pain.

Cultural expectations are known to exert a powerful influence on the experience of pain. In some cultures, for example, childbirth is perceived to be quite painful, while in others, especially in the South American cultures that practice *couvade* (Kroeber, 1923), it is accompanied by no visible distress to the woman. In the latter cultures, the woman often works in the field until the time she is about to deliver, and after the delivery of the baby with no signs of pain, she returns to the field to complete her work. Her husband, however, takes to bed while his wife is delivering and moans and groans as if he were in severe pain. Even in our culture, symptomatic variants of "couvade syndrome" are occasionally seen (vignette 2). In some parts of India, a religious ritual is still practiced in which a chosen man hangs on two steel hooks inserted into the back, which are suspended by a rope, and blesses the children and crops. During the ritual, the man reportedly does not feel pain but rather a "state of exaltation" (Kosambi, 1967) (see Figure 17).

One study in the United States showed that whites tolerated more pain than Orientals, with blacks occupying an intermediate position (Woodrow *et al.,* 1972). In a study of pain involving Old American, Irish, Italian, and Jewish housewives (Sternbach and Tursky, 1964), those of Italian origin were found to have a lower pain tolerance to electric shocks, and the Old Americans showed a more rapid physiological adaptation to repeated shock. Other studies, however, failed to demonstrate such ethnic differences in pain tolerance (Merskey and Spear, 1964; Winsberg and Greenlick, 1967). Ethnic differences in the attitude toward pain have already been discussed (Chapter 1).

What is the mechanism by which cultural and psychosocial factors influence pain experience? Although the exact mechanisms are not known, the descending influences and the recent discovery of the role of endorphins in pain inhibition mechanisms provide a conceptual framework in which the state of the central nervous system, such as attention, anxiety, depression, and past experiences, and values ingrained in the mind and brain can influence the perception of pain.

Age may also affect pain experience. Tolerance to cutaneous pain is reported to increase with age, while tolerance to deep pain decreases with age (Woodrow *et al.,* 1972).

The *personality* of the individual has an important effect on his reaction to pain; conversely, the experience of prolonged or severe pain may also have an effect on the personality. For example, extroversion is associated with greater pain tolerance and, at the same time, with a tendency to exaggerate the pain experience, as compared to introversion (Lynn and Eysenck, 1961; Eysenck, 1961).

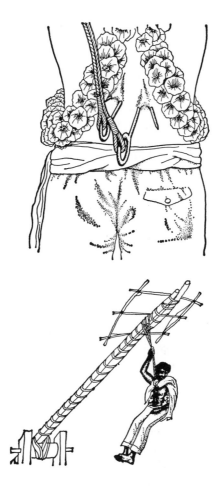

Figure 17. The annual hook-swinging ceremony practiced in remote Indian villages. Top: Two steel hooks are thrust into the small of the back of the "celebrant," who is decked with garlands. The celebrant is later taken to a special cart which has upright timbers and a crossbeam. Bottom: The celebrant is shown hanging on to the ropes as the cart is moved to each village. After he blesses each child and farm field in a village, he swings free, suspended only by the hooks. The crowds cheer at each swing. The celebrant, during the ceremony, is in a state of exaltation and shows no sign of pain. (Originally published in Kosambi, 1967.) (From Melzack, 1973. Copyright 1973 by Ronald Melzack and reproduced with his permission.)

Persistent pain is common in psychiatric disorders, especially those characterized by anxiety, such as neuroses (Merskey, 1965a,b). Chronic pain is also thought to *increase anxiety* and "neuroticism" of patients (Bond, 1971), whether the pain is "organic" or "psychiatric" (Woodforde and Merskey, 1972). Patients with chronic pain also tend to develop a feeling of being out of control of their life and a sense of suspicion and anger toward others, whom they attempt to "manipulate and control" (Timmermans and Sternbach, 1974). *Depression* is also a common consequence of chronic pain (Robinson *et al.,* 1972). These findings indicate that evidence of depression, anxiety, or "neurotic tendencies" in a patient with pain does not justify an automatic diagnosis of "psychogenic" pain.

Among the psychological states affecting the experience of pain are *depression* and *expectancy.* Physical sensations can be accentuated in a state of depressive withdrawal, when the individual's attention is directed toward himself and his bodily sensations. In this instance, any minor discomfort can become magnified and be experienced as serious pain. Depression also tends to result in a vicious cycle of pain escalation—pain causes depression, and then, because of the depressed state, the intensity of pain is accentuated. In cases of pain with signs of depression, antidepressant therapy might be useful to halt this vicious cycle as well as, in some cases, to alleviate the precipitating cause of the pain (see Chapter 6).

Pain has been shown to be associated with *aggression.* In patients with persistent pain, there are often heightened feelings of hostility which are not overtly expressed (Sternbach, 1968). Pain is also implicated in triggering off aggressive behavior in animals. It may be an *unconditioned stimulus for aggressive behavior* (Ulrich *et al.,* 1965). Aggression induced by pain can be conditioned, for example, at the presentation of a tone (Vernon and Ulrich, 1966) (see Chapter 4 for a discussion of conditioning). These studies imply that pain may be exacerbated or exaggerated when patients are angry and that pain may, in turn, provoke angry feelings and aggressive behavior. A non-anxiety-non-aggression-provoking environment, then, would seem to contribute to *prevention* of these undesirable problems of exacerbation of pain or aggressive behavior.

Expectations concerning pain play a major role in the person's experience of pain. In experimental pain situations, subjects who were told to expect severe pain had better pain tolerance than those who were not so prepared (Kanfer and Goldfoot, 1966), and when subjects had an opportunity to obtain information concerning forthcoming electric shocks and, in fact, requested such information, they tended to have decreased anxiety concerning the anticipated shock (Jones *et al.,* 1966).

Another dimension related to expectations concerning pain is the placebo effect, which we will discuss next.

Placebo Effect

Although a placebo is a substance that is considered to be pharmacologically inert, it is by no means "nothing." According to Beecher, it is a powerful therapeutic tool, on the average about one-half to two-thirds as powerful as morphine in the usual dose (10 mg/70 kg body weight) in relieving severe pain (Beecher, 1955). Although the placebo effect is most often described in pain relief, it occurs in many other situations, such as depression and anxiety. It can produce relief from any or all symptoms for which it is given (Sternbach, 1968).

A placebo, like any other pharmacologic agent, can have *"side effects,"* and the side effects may be "toxic" in appearance at times.

The placebo effect is not always consistent. In one study, about 50% of patients receiving both morphine and placebos for postoperative pain were relieved of the pain when the dispensing of the medication was not prolonged (Lasagna *et al.*, 1954). Of the patients who had *more than one dose of placebo, only 14%* consistently obtained relief from the placebos, 55% had inconsistent responses, and 31% consistently never received relief.

It is now recognized that approximately *one-third of the general population are placebo responders* in clinical situations, whether the pain is from surgery, angina pectoris, cancer, or headache (Beecher, 1959a, 1960). There are no generally accepted tests to differentiate placebo responders from non-responders. Although placebo reactors were reported to be more anxious, dependent, self-centered, emotionally labile, and preoccupied with internal bodily processes than nonreactors by the Rorschach test (Lasagna *et al.*, 1954), there were no superficial behavioral characteristics—that is, the reactors were not "whiners" but rather had less "self-critical inhibition" of expressing dependency needs. The placebo reactors might be able to receive considerable pain relief through the comfort from nursing care as well as from the confidence in the efficacy of the medications. In fact, the study found that the reactors had a less painful postoperative course and received fewer medications than the nonreactors.

Placebo responses are not simply alterations in the mental state of affective response to pain. Placebo administration can also produce physiologic responses (Sternbach, 1968).

The *mechanism* for the placebo effect is probably quite complex, including psychological and psychodynamic factors. The basic neurophysiologic mechanism probably includes the *endorphin* pain inhibition system as well as other systems. In one recent study, placebo analgesia was reversed by the administration of naloxone (Levine *et al.*, 1978). Psychologically, gratification of dependency needs in the form of a medication may play a role. On the other hand, Herrnstein (1962) formulated a simple classical conditioning model of the placebo response. In rats, scopolamine depressed lever-pressing behavior, while saline alone did not. When saline was followed by scopolamine in a conditioning paradigm, saline resulted in depression of the lever-pressing behavior. He postulated that a similar type of *conditioned placebo response* might also occur in humans, although increased in complexity.

This model suggests that relief of pain was associated in childhood with certain persons and behaviors as well as affects. Love, comfort, and caring, as well as reduction of anxiety, are related to relief from pain, as are such behaviors as "mother kissing the hurt and making it better." Taking a pill is also often associated with the relief of pain. When exposed to a situation similar to those in which relief was obtained in the past, such as taking a pill or being cared for by a mother-like person (nurse), the pain may disappear (as in conditioned response).

Sternbach (1968) hypothesizes that the production of an "approach–avoidance conflict" concerning reaction to pain might contribute to the inconsistencies in the response to placebos.

In early childhood, complaining of pain usually brings about comfort and relief. In the course of growing up, however, a child learns that complaining about pain is seen negatively by others, such as, "Don't whine like a crybaby." This may result in a classical approach–avoidance conflict. In clinical situations, there is both pain and the sick role expectation of being in a passive and dependent position. This is conducive to *regression* (discussed in Chapter 5)—and evocation of the approach–avoidance conflict.

Thus, patients may experience a conflict between the wish to complain of pain, to experience pain relief and comfort, and the fear that this would be seen as immature and "being like a sissy," etc. Some of these patients may become angry and particularly resistant to pain relief even with active drugs.

Although the placebo effect has been considered to be similar to hypnosis, it appears that there is in susceptible individuals a specific hypnotic analgesic effect over and above the placebo effect (McGlashan *et al.,* 1969).

Use of Placebos in Medical Practice

It should be clear from the discussions above that favorable nonspecific effects brought about by the patient's coming into contact with the health care system might very well be considered to be related to the placebo effect. This general type of response is an inherent part of medical practice and may be related to what Parsons called "unconscious psychotherapy" (see Chapter 3).

Placebos in a narrower sense, such as saline injections with specific symptoms as targets, may also be administered in a medical treatment setting, but they are more often than not misused.

The most common *misuse* of placebos is as *a diagnostic tool.* A surgeon had asked the psychiatrist to see a patient who was suspected of having pain as a hysterical conversion symptom. When the surgeon was told by the nurses that a saline injection had brought on relief of the patient's pain, he turned to the psychiatrist and exclaimed, "Q.E.D.! Now you don't even have to see her; you can just transfer her to the psychiatry ward." This was an incorrect conclusion. Even patients with severe pain caused by demonstrable tissue damage (e.g., such as that associated with metastatic cancer to bone) frequently respond to placebos. *Placebos should never be used to make a differential diagnosis between an "organic" and a "functional" pain, since it is impossible to make such differentiation with placebos* (Shapiro, 1969).

As previously mentioned, placebos may also have *side effects.* In addition to expected "pharmacologic" side effects such as nausea, blushing, and tachycardia, there is an important social interpersonal side effect that can occur with the use of placebos in a medical setting. An atmosphere of *"trickery"* and deception often develops when placebos are used to treat a patient with persistent pain. When a saline injection is ordered for a patient, the nurse's attitude and feelings are often affected; that is, a feeling of "tricking" the patient, and perhaps anger at the patient for being put in such a position, may ensue. Such an attitudinal change often is sensed by the patient, who then feels deceived and badly treated (vignette 3). Patients with guarded, suspicious personality styles may become quite angry and upset in this situation and may even leave the hospital prematurely ("against medical advice").

Psychological Meanings of Pain

We have already mentioned that pain is often associated with anxiety and anxiety-provoking situations in childhood. Such associations are, of course, unique to individual patients, and the specific meanings of a particular pain will be also unique to the individual. Punishment, threat, loss, and even reward are "meanings" that pain may acquire. Pavlov (1927, 1928) found that dogs can be conditioned to *associate pain with pleasure* (food). Dogs normally have violent negative reactions to electric shock applied to a paw. Shock regularly presented to a hungry dog before feeding changed the reaction—the animal would salivate and start to wag his tail and turn toward the food dish immediately after the shock. In these experiments, the electric shock experience acquired the meaning of a signal of rewards to follow (food). Such learning might account for the behavior of some individuals who seem to be deliberately seeking painful experiences and suffering, for example, patients who are "addicted to surgery" (vignette 3). The "secondary gain" of being sick might be a powerfully motivating "reward experience" for some patients. Sexual excitation may be associated with painful experiences, for example, genital stimulation with pain, an association that may have first been experienced during spanking.

Pain is a *regressive stimulus*. In the presence of severe pain, the individual's thoughts and actions tend to become like those of children. Sternbach (1968) writes:

> It is not only that we cry with the pain; what we say, aloud and to ourselves, is childlike. We ask what we have done to deserve such pain, and think back to make a connection between some action of ours and the onset of the pain. We implore others to help us, to take away the hurt. We promise that once the pain is removed we will be different—we will be kinder to others, do good works. We beg for forgiveness, we say we are sorry. We ask God for help, we ask Him to save us.

Many memories of childhood, associated with pain, with punishment, and with relief of pain, may be reactivated in the presence of pain. Sometimes conflictual feelings about other issues may be activated by the experience of pain. For example, some patients cannot tolerate even small amounts of pain because they are afraid of becoming like a child, the regressive meaning of having pain.

Pain may have *different meanings according to personality type*. For a patient who has a long-suffering, self-sacrificing personality style, pain may be the symbol of expiation of his guilt feelings and justification for receiving care. For a patient with a dramatizing, emotional personality, pain may mean that he is no longer attractive. For a patient with an orderly, controlling personality, pain may mean a loss of control (see Chapter 15).

"Psychogenic" Pain

The terms "functional" or "psychogenic" pain refer to pain experienced without demonstrable peripheral tissue damage; by implication, it may be thought to be "caused" by psychological or psychodynamic factors. Still, pain, no matter what its cause, acquires psychological meaning and may be accompanied by signs of psychological distress. Furthermore, pain may signal early tissue damage or dysfunction that is not yet demonstrable. For these reasons, extreme caution must be exercised in the use of the terms. Nevertheless, there are some individuals who suffer long-standing and severe chronic pain without demonstrable tissue damage, in whom the existence of pain can be explained on the basis of psychological factors (like the hallucinations experienced in dreams) and whose improvement depends largely on successful psychological management. Additionally, there are certain people who experience pain with unusual intensity and frequency, in whom the presence or absence of associated tissue damage is only weakly correlated with the quality and intensity of pain and in whom even removal of the lesion may fail to bring relief from pain. George Engel called such patients "pain prone" and identified a marker of personality characteristically encountered in them (Engel, 1959). He proposed that the physician consider the following questions in evaluating patients with severe pain problems: (1) Are there pathological processes affecting nerve endings and leading to disordered patterns in nerve pathways which would be expected to produce pain? (2) If such processes are present, can the character of the pain experience reported by the patient be fully, partially, or not at all accounted for by the distinctive characteristics of the peripheral pathological process? (3) How are psychological processes operating to determine the ultimate character of the pain experience for the patient and the manner in which it is communicated to the physician? A number of factors and findings may suggest that the pain is psychogenic or psychogenically exacerbated. They include the following:

1. Psychogenic pain tends to be described in a dramatic and metaphorical fashion (such as, "a man sitting on my chest").
2. The location of the pain tends to correspond to the patient's subjective body image rather than to anatomical distribution of peripheral nerves and central nervous system pain pathways.
3. Such pain tends to occur at emotionally charged times (e.g., in anticipation of a loss or at the anniversary of such an event).
4. There is a "complaining" quality to the patient's description of the pain, which is usually exacerbated during an interview when an emotionally charged subject is discussed.
5. Psychogenic pain almost never wakes a patient from sleep.

The past histories of pain-prone patients often include similar episodes of obscure pain in the past in which the pain was used as a means of getting attention and love and/or as a means of atonement for feelings of guilt. The personality style, obviously, is likely to be the long-suffering, self-sacrificing type (see Chapter 15). It is not unusual to find that these patients had been close to someone who suffered from chronic or severe pain and that the patient's pain might even have started shortly after the loss of such a person. In such an instance, identification with the lost person would be an important psychological defense mechanism involved in the development of the symptom (see Chapter 6).

In some cases of psychogenic pain, secondary gain might play an important role. The term "secondary gain" refers to gratification or advantages that accrue to the individual by virture of the illness but did not contribute to its causation. Secondary gains may then reinforce the symptom and make it hard to give up. They include attention- and love-getting, the opportunity to be "unusually" angry and aggressive, and financial gain such as disability compensation payments. In cases where pain occurs as a "depressive equivalent" or in pain associated with the depressive syndrome (see Chapter 6), signs of depression, such as suicidal ideations and guilt feelings, may be found as well as such physiologic signs of depression as sleep disturbance, weight loss, anorexia, constipation, and loss of sexual interest.

We should caution again that while the presence of these indicators should alert the physician to the fact that there may be psychogenic components to the patient's pain experience, these findings in and of themselves *by no means* indicate *absence* of organic pathology. Coexistence of psychogenic and tissue factors in pain is not at all unusual. *One of the most common ways in which psychogenic pain is, in fact, expressed is as an elaboration of pain arising in damaged tissue.*

Management of Pain

The managment of pain obviously requires a comprehensive approach. Relief from pain is important not only as direct relief from suffering itself, but also because of the untoward effects of physiologic concomitants of pain which might be harmful to the patient (such as the increase in cardiac work in myocardial infarction) and the fact that anxiety associated with pain in time may aggravate its intensity as well as the intensity of psychophysiologic reactions to it.

For most acute pain, effective *pharmacologic agents* such as narcotic analgesics are readily available to the physician and should be used in effective doses. There is some evidence, however, that narcotics are *underutilized* in treating acute pain situations for fear of addiction (Marks and Sachar, 1973). Even terminally ill patients with severe pain are often undertreated with narcotic analgesics. It should be pointed out that the actual *risk of causing narcotic addiction in a hospitalized patient with pain is quite negligible* (less than 1%; Marks and Sachar, 1973). Underusage of narcotic analgesics may reinforce the patient's preoccupation with the medication and his drug-seeking behavior, such as calling for the medication before the scheduled time to prevent the development of more severe pain.

Sometimes there may even be an interesting paradoxical pattern in the use of powerful analgesics. The more pain the patient feels, and the more he complains, the less likely he is to receive potent pain medications (Pilowsky et al., 1969). It is no wonder, then, that aggravated aggressive behavior is often found in such patients, especially in view of the fact that pain itself may generate aggressive feelings.

Relief of anxiety is also important in managing pain. This calls not only for a reassuring attitude on the physician's part but also for *informing patients about treatment plans,* especially about procedures that themselves might be painful. Preparing the patient for the pain will help. As pointed out earlier, experimental subjects anticipating severe pain showed a higher tolerance for it and reduced perception of pain when motivated to endure it (Sternbach, 1968).

As mentioned earlier, pain is a powerful regressive stimulus. An unambivalent, caring attitude on the part of the health care personnel, particularly nurses, can prevent or neutralize anxious and defensive reactions in patients who are embarrassed by regressive needs and behavior.

A comprehensive approach is also particularly necessary in managing patients with *psychogenic or psychologically aggravated pain.* In addition to symptomatic and etiologic treatment of underlying disease processes in tissue, the psychological meaning of the pain should be evaluated and a plan for psychological treatment made. This may involve using *antidepressants* (see Chapters 6 and 18) in patients with depression or depressive equivalents, as well as providing interpersonal contact, social support, and psychotherapy when indicated.

Another important reason for recognizing and treating psychogenic pain factors is the prevention of unnecessary surgical and other drastic treatments.

Summary

Pain is one of the most common experiences leading to help-seeking behavior. Pain, like anxiety, subserves a protective function. *Anxiety* often accentuates, and occasionally is perceived as, pain, and pain is, as a rule, accompanied by anxiety.

Quality of pain is important in the diagnosis of the underlying disease. Tissue damage or very strong stimuli result in stimulation of the pain receptors (free nerve endings). The pricking type of pain and burning and aching pain are conducted by separate types of nerve fibers, small type A delta fibers and even smaller type C fibers, respectively. *Pricking pain* is ultimately projected to the brain in the thalamus and the somatosensory cortex, while the aching and burning pain pathways are projected diffusely in the *reticular activating system* of the brain and thus influence not only the state of arousal, but emotional and neuroendocrine responses as well. The nerve impulses conducting pain are modified at the spinal cord level by various influences, including those coming from the brain. Information concerning the nature and location of pain may be transmitted to the brain before the perception of pain, allowing the brain to modify the perception itself (both at brain and spinal cord levels). The discovery of the opiate receptors and *endorphins* in the human central nervous system opens up the possibility of an intrinsic pain control mechanism. The distribution of opiate receptors in the limbic system, thalamus, and spinal cord implies that control of pain perception is closely related to emotional states and memory functions subserved by the limbic system. These mechanisms may provide a basis for known modifying influences on pain perception, such as the psychological state of the individual, his past experiences, and his cultural background.

Although the pain sensation threshold is very similar in most people, tolerance for and reaction to pain may be strongly influenced by psychological and social factors.

The *placebo* effect is found in approximately one-third of the general population. The placebo response is a complex phenomenon which includes suggestion, anticipation, and conditioned responses. Endorphins are probably involved in the placebo response. Placebos are powerful and can *never* differentiate pain arising from tissue damage from "psychogenic" pain. Many nonspecific beneficial effects of the health care system can be attributed to the placebo effect.

Psychogenic pain, pain in the absence of observable tissue damage, is a complex phenomenon. It might be due to increased sensitivity to otherwise mild or negligible pain as a concomitant or equivalent of depression or a conversion mechanism (e.g., symbolization of a psychological meaning). As all pain sensation can be associated with a psychological meaning, the discovery of a psychological meaning or the presence of a "secondary gain" should not exclude the possibility that there might be an underlying "organic" disease in a patient complaining of pain. Pain-seeking behavior may be a conditioned response or may also be a motivated behavior with complex psychological meaning.

The *management* of pain requires a comprehensive approach in the biological, psychological, and social spheres. In addition to the treatment of tissue damage, the cultural and psychological dimensions of the pain should be understood and treated appropriately.

Implications

For the Patient

Pain is a *subjective* experience that cannot be shared objectively. When a patient presents with pain, he is suffering not only from the sensation but also from anxiety that accompanies the pain. His reaction to pain is influenced by a diversity of factors, such as cultural expecations, ethnic background, and personality. Thus, the probability that a certain level of pain will reach the limit of tolerance or anxiety for a given patient to result in help-seeking behavior is determined not only by the actual intensity of the stimulus but also by the social and psychological factors.

For the Physician

The existence of pain or the absence of it can never be proven in a given individual by a physician. Current understanding of the neurophysiology of pain clearly indicates that the *brain* has an important role in the perception of pain and that sensation of pain can occur without peripheral tissue damage. Whenever possible, *alleviation* of suffering from pain, regardless of the underlying pathology, can facilitate the formation of a cooperative doctor–patient relationship.

Attention to the *description* of pain is important in diagnosing the underlying condition.

An understanding of the cultural background and *social expectations,* as well as the personality of the patient, obtained through *questions* and the *demographic data* of the patient, helps the physician understand the differing reactions to pain in different patients and also can help him to anticipate and to take appropriate measure for adverse reactions to pain that some patients might manifest. Adverse reactions may be nonreporting of pain in certain stoic individuals, as well as overreaction to it in others.

Because information about pain increases the tolerance for it, physicians should inform patients about potentially painful procedures and prepare them.

Because relief of pain by *placebos* regularly occurs in patients with severe tissue damage, placebos should *never* be used to differentiate organic from functional pain. The deceptive use of placebos in the hospital often undermines the patient's trust in the health care personnel.

In treating a patient for pain relief, *adequate analgesics* should be given. Since narcotics probably interact with endogenous endorphin systems, some individuals may require more narcotics for the relief of pain from the same stimulus if the endorphin system is inadequate or depleted. Narcotic addiction in the course of treatment with narcotic analgesics for pain is rare indeed, the incidence being less than 1%.

Pain may be experienced in the absence of tissue damage. This perception may be determined by *guilt feelings* (expiation), as a *body language* expression of the need for emotional caring, as a result of *depression* with bodily preoccupation, or as a conditioned response to *anxiety*. Pain-prone patients often come from a background where pain was used as a means of getting attention and love as well as of atoning for guilt feelings. Pain perceived in the absence of peripheral tissue damage is usually attributed to a part of the body according to the body image of the individual and the meaning of the body part, rather than according to the distribution of nerve pathways. Psychogenic pain, however, is often presented as an *added-on* symptomatology to an organic condition, and the presence of secondary gain, or psychological meaning attributable to the pain, should not rule out the possibility that there might be an organic disease yet undetected.

For the Community and Health Care System

Differences in reaction to pain seen in different ethnic and cultural groups often result in a breakdown of communication between the patients and the health care personnel. An understanding of the cultural expectations of the patients by the health care personnel can help overcome this. As anxiety often increases pain perception, hospital *environment* should be such that there is a minimum of anxiety-provoking situations to which the patients are exposed.

The medical community should be aware that the use of narcotics in the treatment of pain is effective and when properly managed is not likely to result in addiction. Medical schools and hospitals should emphasize *adequate relief* of pain through the use of narcotic analgesics rather than overemphasize the possibility of iatrogenic addiction.

Cultural change and assimilation may result in changes in pain experiences, and ethnic differences in reaction to pain may disappear as the cultural stereotypes change.

Recommended Reading

Bonica JJ, Albe-Fessard DB (eds): *Advances in Pain Research and Therapy.* New York, Raven Press, 1976, vol 1. A very comprehensive multiauthored volume on various aspects of pain, from neurophysiology to psychological factors and surgical management. An excellent up-to-date reference.

Engel GL: "Psychogenic" pain and the pain-prone patient. *Am J Med* **26**:899–918, 1959. A classic paper describing the possible nature of "psychogenic" pain and backgrounds of "pain-prone" patients.

Marks RM, Sachar EJ: Undertreatment of medical inpatients with narcotic analgesics. *Ann Intern Med* **78**:173–181, 1973. This is a must for medical students and physicians to understand the degree of undertreatment of pain rampant in our hospitals. The conclusion is based on interviews with patients being treated for pain and on questionnaires completed by house staff physicians in two major hospitals in New York.

Snyder SH: Opiate receptors and internal opiates. *Sci Am* **236**:44–57, 1977. This is a comprehensive and lucid discussion of the endorphins (enkephalins) and their actions by one of the discoverers of the opiate receptors in the human brain. Recommended especially for those who would like to read more about the structures and mechanism of actions of the endorphins and the distribution of opiate receptors.

Sternbach RA: Pain: A Psychophysiological Analysis. New York, Academic Press, 1968. This is a comprehensive and concise monograph presenting clinical and experimental studies concerning pain. A beautifully written, well-integrated book that also deals with the psychology of pain.

References

Akil H, Liebeskind JC: Monoaminergic mechanism of stimulation-produced analgesia. *Brain Res* **94**:279–296, 1975.

Beall JE, Martin RF, Applebaum AE, *et al.*: Inhibition of primate spino-thalamic tract neurons by stimulation in the region of the nucleus raphe magnus. *Brain Res* **114**:328–333, 1976.

Beecher HK: The powerful placebo. *J Am Med Assoc* **159**:1602–1606, 1955.

Beecher HK: Generalization from pain of various types and diverse origins. *Science* **130**:267–268, 1959.

Beecher HK: *Measurement of Subjective Responses*. New York, Oxford Press, 1959b.

Beecher HK: Increased stress and effectiveness of placebos and "active" drugs. *Science* **132**:91–92, 1960.

Bloom F, Segal D, Ling N, *et al.*: Endorphrins: Profound behavioral effects in rats suggest new etiological factors in mental illness. *Science* **194**:630–632, 1976.

Bond MR: The relation of pain to the Eysenck Personality Inventory, Cornell Medical Index, and Whitely Index of Hypochondria. *Br J Psychiatry* **119**:671, 1971.

Coulter JC, Maunz RA, Willis WD: Effects of stimulation of sensory motor cortex on primate spinothalamin neurons. *Brain Res* **65**:351–356, 1974.

Engel GL: "Psychogenic" pain and the pain-prone patient. *Am J Med* **26**:899–918, 1959.

Eysenck SBG: Personality and pain assessment in childbirth of married and unmarried mothers. *J Ment Sci* **107**:417–430, 1961.

Goldstein A: Opioid peptides (endorphins) in pituitary and brain. *Science* **193**:1081–1086, 1976.

Guyton AC: *Textbook of Medical Physiology*. Philadephia, WB Saunders, 1976.

Handwerker HO, Iggo Z, Zimmerman M: Segmental and supraspinal actions on dorsal horn neurons responding to noxious and non-noxious skin stimuli. *Pain* **1**:147–165, 1975.

Hermstein RJ: Placebo effect in the rat. *Science* **138**:677–678, 1962.

Jones A, Bentler PH, Petry G: The reduction of uncertainty concerning future pain. *J Abnorm Psychol* **71**:87–94, 1966.

Kanfer FH, Goldfoot DA: Self-control and tolerance of noxious stimulation. *Psychol Rep* **18**:79–85, 1966.

Kerr FWL, Wilson PR: Pain. *Annu Rev Neurosci* **1**:83–102, 1978.

Kosambi DD: Living prehistory in India. *Sci Am* **216**:105–114, 1967.

Krober AL: *Anthropology*. New York, Harcourt-Brace, 1923.

Lasagna L, Mosteller F, von Felsinger JM, *et al.*: A study of the placebo response. *Am J Med* **16**:770–779, 1954.

Levine JD, Gordon NC, Fields HL: The mechanism of placebo analgesia. *Lancet* **2**:654–657, 1978.

Lynn R, Eysenck HJ: Tolerance for pain, extraversion, and neuroticism. *Percept Mot Skills* **12**:161–162, 1961.

Marks RM, Sachar EJ: Undertreatment of medical inpatients with narcotic analgesics. *Ann Intern Med* **78**:173–181, 1973.

Marx JL: Analgesia: How the body inhibits pain perception. *Science* **195**:471–473, 1977.

McGlashan TH, Evans FJ, Orne MT: The nature of hypnotic analgesia and placebo response to experimental pain. *Psychosom Med* **31**:227–246, 1969.

Melzack R: *The Puzzle of Pain.* New York, Basic Books, 1973.

Melzack R, Torgerson WS: On the language of pain. *Anesthesiology* **34**:50–59, 1971.

Melzack R, Wall PD: Pain mechanisms: A new theory. *Science* **150**:971–979, 1965.

Merskey H: The characteristics of persistent pain in psychological illness. *J Psychosom Res* **9**:291–298, 1965a.

Merskey H: Psychiatric patients with persistent pain. *J Psychosom Res* **9**:299–309, 1965b.

Merskey H, Spear FG: The reliability of the pressure algometer. *Br J Clin Psychol* **3**:130–136, 1964.

Oliveras JL, Besson JM, Builbaud G, *et al.*: Behavioral and electrophysiological evidence of pain inhibition from midbrain stimulation in the cat. *Exp Brain Res* **20**:32–44, 1974.

Pavlov IP: *Conditioned Relfexes: An Investigation of the Physiological Activity of the Cerebral Cortex,* Anrep GV (Tran–ed). London, Oxford University Press, 1927.

Pavlov IP: *Lectures on Conditioned Reflexes,* Gantt WH (tran). New York, International Publishers, 1928.

Pearson DH: Pain pathways: An overview. *Hosp Pract* (special report), Jan 14–18, 1976.

Perl ER: Sensitization of nocioreceptors and its relation to sensation, in Bonica JJ, Albe-Fessard DG (eds): *Advances in Pain Research and Therapy.* New York, Raven Press, 1976, vol 1.

Pilowsky I, Manzop C, Bond MR: Pain and its management in malignant disease. *Psychosom Med* **31**:400–404, 1969.

Robinson H, Kirk RF, Frye RF, *et al.*: A psychological study of patients with rheumatoid arthritis and other painful diseases. *J Psychosom Res* **16**:53–56, 1972.

Shapiro AK: Attitudes toward the use of placebos in treatment. *J Nerv Ment Dis* **130**:200–211, 1960.

Snyder SH: Opiate receptors and internal opiates. *Sci Am* **236**:44–57, 1977.

Sternbach RA: *Pain: A Psychophysiological Analysis.* New York, Academic Press, 1968.

Sternbach RA, Tursky B: Ethnic differences among housewives in psychophysical and skin potential responses to electric shock. *Psychophysiology* **1**:241–246, 1964.

Timmermans G, Sternbach RA: Factors of human chronic pain: An analysis of personality and pain reaction variables. *Science* **184**:806–808, 1974.

Ulrich RE, Hutchinson RR, Azrin NH: Pain-elicited aggression. *Psychol Rec* **15**:111–126, 1965.

Vernon J, Ulrich RE: Classical conditioning of pain-elicited aggression. *Science* **152**:668–669, 1966.

Wall PD: Modulation of pain by non-painful events, in Bonica JJ, Albe-Fessard D (eds): *Advances in Pain Research and Therapy.* New York, Raven Press, 1976, vol 1.

Winsberg B, Greenlick M: Pain response in Negro and white obstetrical patients. *J Health Soc Behav* **8**:222–227, 1967.

Woodforde JM, Merskey H: Personality traits of patients with chronic pain. *J Psychosom Res* **16**:167–172, 1972.

Woodrow KM, Friedman CD, Siegelaub AB, *et al.*: Pain tolerance: Differences according to age, sex, and race. *Psychosom Med* **34**:548–556, 1972.

CHAPTER 8

Sleep and Dreaming

1. A 40-year-old married woman underwent hysterectomy for uterine fibroids. A few weeks after discharge, she began to experience increasing difficulty in falling asleep. She would also awaken frequently in the middle of the night and wake up at 4:00 A.M. unable to fall asleep again. She felt fatigued, irritable, and unable to concentrate. A depressive syndrome ensued.

2. A 60-year-old widower was admitted to the hospital for elective surgery. The intern found out, during history-taking, that the patient had been taking moderately large doses of secobarbital for sleep at night for the past year or so. Also, he would have one or two "shots" of brandy. The intern decided that perhaps the patient should be taken off the sleep medications and, of course, should receive no alcohol in the hospital. The next night, at 3:00 A.M., the patient rushed to the nurses' station, frightened and perspiring, stating that he had had a most vivid and horrible nightmare.

3. A 47-year-old married woman suffering from advanced rheumatoid arthritis became increasingly irritable, complaining of pain and inability to sleep. The irritability subsided when she was prescribed small doses of flurazepam for sleep.

4. Freud's "Dream of the Botanical Monograph": "I had written a monograph on a certain plant. The book lay before me and I was at the moment turning over a folded coloured plate. Bound up in each copy there was a dried specimen of the plant, as though it had been taken from a herbarium" (Freud, 1900/1965).

In vignettes 1 through 3, a sleep disturbance heralded in a psychiatric illness. Changes in drug regimen can cause sleep disturbance involving dreams, as in vignette 2. Vignette 3 illustrates the interaction between a medical disease and sleep difficulties. Vignette 4 is a famous dream of Freud's which was one of the

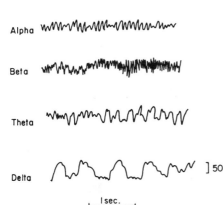

Alpha

Beta

Theta

Delta   ] 50μv

|— 1 sec. —|

Figure 18. Different types of normal electroencephalographic waves. (From Guyton, 1976. Copyright 1976 by W.B.
Saunders Co. Reproduced with permission from the publisher and author.)

first dreams analyzed to show its psychological meanings (see Freud, 1900/
1965).

Sleep was thought to be a relatively simple and uniform state until the
advent of electroencephalographic techniques (see Figures 18–20). During
the waking state, the electroencephalogram (EEG) typically shows low-voltage
fast waves (beta waves, ≥ 14 Hz). When the individual is in a relaxed, awake
state, the EEG may show alpha waves (9–13 Hz), especially when the eyes are
closed. During sleep, the EEG is characterized by slower waves than in the
waking state (see below). Aserinsky and Kleitman (1953) discovered in the
1950s that conjugate, rapid eye movements (REM) appear periodically during
sleep. It soon became clear that dreams, especially visual dreams, occurred
predominantly during the REM periods.

Stages of Sleep

Typically, in a night's sleep, a person goes through a period of non-REM
(NREM) sleep before having his first REM sleep of the night.

NREM Sleep

Electroencephalographically, four stages can be identified during NREM
sleep. They are stages 1 through 4. Stages 3 and 4 are sometimes called *delta*
or slow-wave sleep (see Figures 19 and 20).

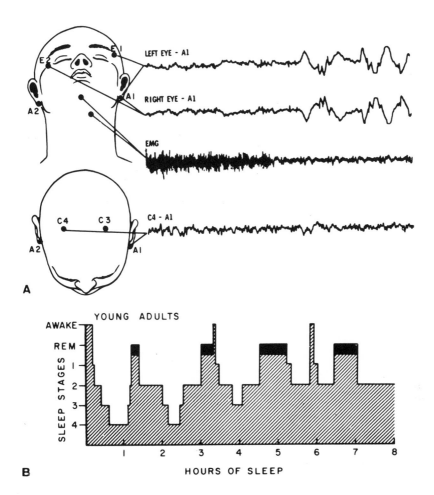

Figure 19. A: Electrode placement in sleep research. The top two tracings show eye movements recorded from electrodes attached laterally to the outer canthus of each eye (electrooculogram) and referred to the ear; this produces out-of-phase deflection in the two tracings for almost all eye movements. The electromyogram (EMG) is recorded from electrodes attached firmly beneath the chin and referred to each other. In the lower tracing, the EEG is derived from a scalp placement referred to the opposite ear. The recordings illustrate the onset of a REM sleep period. First, the EMG decreases sharply; then eye movements appear while the electroencephalographic waves change to low amplitude, mixed frequency. (From Rechtschaffen and Kales, 1968.) B: Nocturnal sleep pattern in young adults. Note the absence of Stage 4 and the decreased length of NREM periods during the latter part of the night and the short first REM period. (From Kales, 1968. Reproduced with permission from American College of Physicians and the author.)

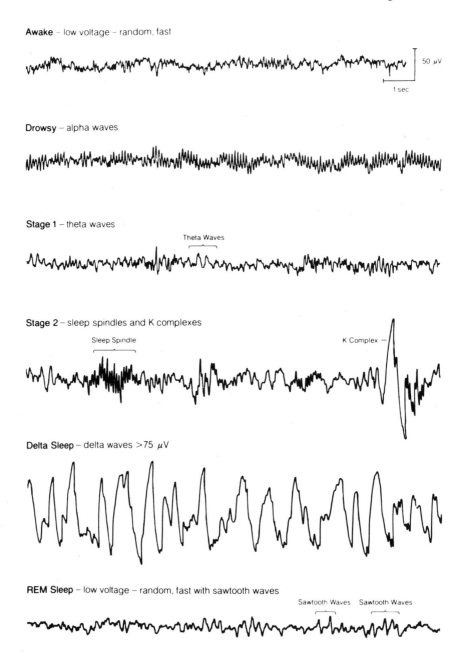

Figure 20. Human sleep stages (From Hauri, 1977. Copyright 1977 by the Upjohn Co. Reproduced with permission from the publisher and author.)

Stage 1. This is a transition phase between wakefulness and sleep. The EEG shows low-voltage, mixed-frequency waves with theta (4–8 Hz) predominating. During this phase, thoughts begin to drift, and thinking is no longer reality-oriented. Short dreams often develop (Foulkes and Vogel, 1965). Many people subjectively feel that they are awake during Stage 1 (Hauri, 1977). Stage 1 is usually quite short, in the range of 0.5–7 min.

Stage 2. As sleep progresses, *"sleep spindles,"* bursts of 12–16 Hz lasting 0.5–2 sec, appear with low-amplitude, fast-frequency activity. K complexes, which are well-delineated, slow, negative EEG deflections followed by a positive component, also appear. Mentation during this stage consists of short, mundane, and fragmented thoughts (Foulkes, 1962).

Delta Sleep (Stages 3 and 4). When the EEG shows at least 20% delta waves (frequency < 4 Hz), delta sleep is reached. Delta sleep may be subdivided into Stages 3 (20–50% delta) and 4 (> 50% delta). The majority of delta-wave sleep occurs early in the night, when sleep is deepest.

REM Sleep

After the person has been asleep for 80–100 min in NREM sleep, REM sleep appears. During this phase, rapid eye movement occurs which can be demonstrated by the electrooculogram (EOG) (see Figure 19). The *EEG shows a desynchronized pattern similar to Stage 1 sleep,* except that "sawtooth" waves are also present (Figure 20). The REM phase is about 5–20 min in duration and alternates with the NREM phase approximately every 90 min. Initially in the night, the REM phase may be skipped or very brief. In addition to *rapid eye movement,* there are several other *characteristic features of REM sleep:* The skeletal muscles are relaxed (Figure 19), although there may be occasional twitches; there is *physiologic activation* manifested by irregular (highly variable) heart rate, respiratory rate, and blood pressure; penile erection also occurs in men. About 80% of subjects awakened during REM are usually able to recall *dreams,* while visual dreams are recalled in less than 20% during NREM awakenings.

The *total time spent in REM* during a typical night is about 20–25% of sleep time; Stage 2, about 50%; Stage delta, about 20%; and Stage 1, 5–10% (see Figure 19B). The amount of *total REM sleep* time *decreases with age,* so that in the neonate, about 50% of total sleep time is spent in REM, in young adults, 20–25%, and in older adults, about 15% (see Figure 21).

Basic Rest–Activity Cycle

Kleitman (1965) proposed that the 90-min REM–NREM cycle represents a *basic rest–activity cycle* (BRAC) which reflects a fundamental periodicity in

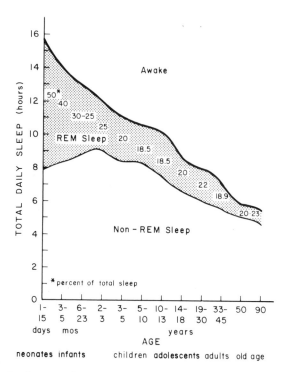

Figure 21. Mean development of human sleep over a lifetime. (From Hauri, 1977. Copyright 1977 by the Upjohn Co. Reproduced with permission from the publisher and author.)

the activity of the central nervous system of homothermal animals. He proposed that this particular cycle was easier to discern during sleep because of the EEG changes. There is some current evidence that certain types of activities, including "oral activity" such as eating, drinking, and smoking, as well as waking gastric contractility, follow 90–120 min ultradian rhythms (Friedman and Fisher, 1967).

Interestingly, the length of the rest–activity cycle seems to be proportional to the size of the animal species, running from 7–13 min in the rat to 2 hr in the elephant (Table 6).

Biological Rhythms

The sleep–wake cycle and REM–NREM cycle represent but two of the many rhythmic activities that characterize life. The period of the rhythm may be a day *(circadian),* such as in the sleep–wake cycle, within the daytime *(diur-*

Table 6. REM State in Various Mammalian Species (Young Adults)[a,b]

Species	Average length of REM period (min)	Average length of cycle (min)	REM time (% of total sleep)
Human	14	80–90	20–24
Monkey	4–10	40–60	11–20
Cat	10	20–40	20–60
Sheep	—	—	2–3
Rabbit	—	24	1–3
Rat	4–7	7–13	15–20
Mouse	—	3–4	—
Opossum	5	17	22–40

[a] Based on data from the work of many authors.
[b] From Hartmann (1970). Copyright 1970 by Little, Brown & Co. Reproduced with permission from the publisher and author.

nal), as in the mood change of depressives between the morning and evening hours, and within the nighttime (nocturnal). The period may be greater than 24 hr (infradian), such as the menstrual cycle, or less than 24 hr (ultradian), as in the REM–NREM cycle.

Many endocrine and metabolic systems follow rhythmic variations, circadian, infradian, or ultradian (Curtis, 1972) (see Figure 22). Circadian rhythms have been observed in cell mitosis of different organs as well as in the susceptibility of the organism to infectious and toxic agents.*

An implication of this observation of rhythmicity in the biological systems is that the time of the day has to be controlled in all biological experiments, measurements, and interventions. For example, animals have been shown to exhibit the fewest toxic effects to pharmacologic agents if they are administered before the sleep period. Changes in the rhythmicity of functional systems may be an early evidence of dysfunction, such as disruption in sleep and REM.

Brain Mechanisms of Sleep

The brain mechanisms of sleep and dreaming are not yet completely understood. Arousal and wakefulness seem to depend on the activity of the ascending reticular activating system, which is predominately cholinergic (see Figure 7). The ascending reticular activating system is distributed diffusely throughout the brain stem and limbic system and determines the general tone

*For a comprehensive review of biological rhythms, the reader is referred to the monograph Biological Rhythms in Psychiatry and Medicine.

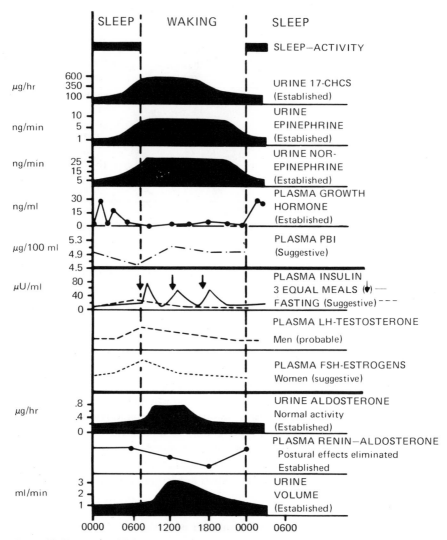

Figure 22. Phase map of daily cycle of endocrine measures and urine volume in humans in relation to habitual sleep and feeding schedule. (From Curtis, 1972. Reproduced with permission from the publisher and author.)

and arousal of the central nervous system. Continuing high activity of the system inhibits sleep.

Sleep does not automatically occur when sensory input is low. *NREM sleep* is an active phenomenon probably brought about by the activation of the serotonergic neurons of the pontine raphe system (see Figure 12). Lesions of the raphe nuclei lead to a state of relatively permanent cortical desynchronization associated with behavioral arousal. Drugs that deplete serotonin levels in the brain, such as *para*-chlorophenylalanine (PCPA), cause a reduction in sleep time in animals, involving both slow-wave and REM sleep (Morgane and Stern, 1974). Jouvet proposed that *serotonergic systems* are involved in *slow-wave sleep* and *noradrenergic* and possibly *cholinergic systems* in *REM and waking* (Jouvet, 1972a,b). Jouvet noted that the types of insomnia caused by lesioning of the serotonergic neurons or by drug-induced inhibition of serotonin synthesis have one common characteristic: The decrease in sleep is not followed by a subsequent rebound of sleep. Insomnia can also be caused by activation of the ascending noradrenergic pontomesencephalic system, either by direct stimulation of the mesencephalon, by nociceptive stimuli, by sleep deprivation, or by drugs such as amphetamines. In these instances, either total insomnia or selective suppression of REM occurs, but never a selective suppression of slow-wave sleep. This type of insomnia is always followed by a rebound of slow-wave and/or REM sleep, the intensity and duration of which is proportional to the duration of the insomnia. This suggests that, in this form of insomnia, there may be an increased activity of the "waking system" that affects the biosynthesis and turnover of the serotonin system. Jouvet noted that both forms of insomnia share one common characteristic: They can be suppressed by the inhibition of the synthesis of catecholamines by α-methyl-*para*-tyrosine (AMPT), which decreases the turnover of central catecholamines. There is also evidence that an increase in the serotonin turnover results in true hypersomnia (increases in both slow-wave and REM sleep).

In cats, intravenous injection of the serotonin precursor 5-hydroxy-tryptophan is followed within minutes by a state resembling slow-wave sleep. Reserpine, which depletes both norepinephrine and serotonin in the brain, can suppress both slow-wave and REM sleep totally in the cat. 5-Hydroxy-tryptophan, when given a few hours after reserpine, will restore slow-wave sleep but not REM sleep. Morgane and Stern (1974) conclude that the *presence of serotonin in the brain* is a *necessary condition* for the *patterns of sleep, both slow-wave and REM, to become fully manifest.*

Jouvet found that lesions in the dorsolateral part of the pontine reticular formation totally suppress REM sleep without interfering significantly with slow-wave sleep (Jouvet, 1972a,b). Since dorsolateral pontine tegmentum contains the noradrenergic nuclei, *locus ceruleus* (see Figure 23 and also Figures 6 and 10) and subceruleus, these structures are considered to be implicated in REM sleep. Bilateral lesions of the caudal part of the locus ceruleus suppress the inhibition of skeletal muscles (relaxation) that occurs during REM sleep. Bilateral total lesions of the locus ceruleus and subceruleus are followed by a decrease in waking and permanent suppression of REM sleep. Following this type of lesion, there is a marked fall in norepinephrine concentration in all parts of the brain.

Hobson (1975, 1977, 1978) postulates *reciprocal interaction* between the

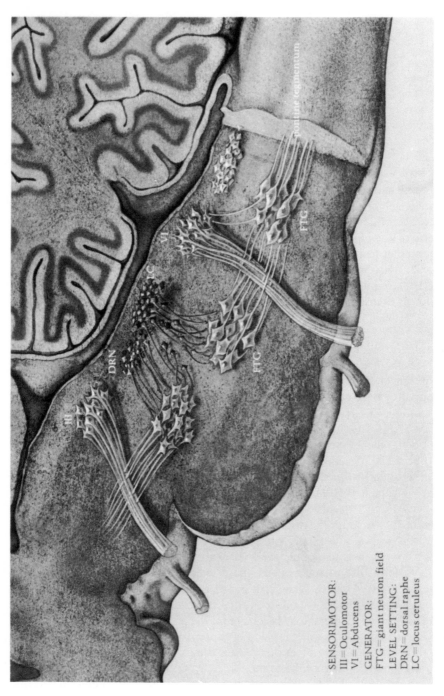

SENSORIMOTOR:
III = Oculomotor
VI = Abducens
GENERATOR:
FTG = giant neuron field
LEVEL SETTING:
DRN = dorsal raphe
LC = locus ceruleus

Figure 23. Schematic view of sagittal section of the midbrain and pons illustrating the "dream-state generator." (From Hobson, 1978. Reproduced with permission from Hoffmann-La Roche, Inc. and the author.)

pontine reticular giant cells (cholinergic) on one hand and the *noradrenergic locus ceruleus* and the *serotonergic raphe neurons* on the other. He proposes that when the pontine reticular giant cells are activated, the REM state occurs. He also postulates that the cholinergic giant cells are excitatory to themselves and also to the group of monoaminergic neurons, locus ceruleus and raphe nuclei. On the other hand, the monoaminergic neurons (locus ceruleus and raphe) are considered to be inhibitory to themselves as well as to the reticular giant cells (see Figure 24). This model results in an oscillation in activation between the cholinergic giant cells and the monoaminergic neurons. Hobson and McCarley (1977) found that microinjection of Carbachol, a cholinomimetic substance, into the pontine giant-cell zone potently enhanced the REM state and simultaneously activated giant cells. Stimulation of locus ceruleus had an inhibitory effect on the giant cells.

Hobson (1977, 1978) discussed the time sequence in the generation of the REM state. In essence, changes in the rate of firing of the pontine reticular giant cells preceded the cortical changes, such as EEG desynchronization, as well as the eye movements. Further, eye movements occurred before EEG desynchronization (cortical activation). The implication of these findings is that the *REM state seems to be primarily generated by the pontine oscillating*

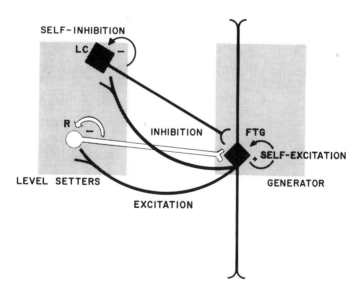

Figure 24. Dream-state generator. Schematic diagram of proposed reciprocal connections between the monoaminergic, "level-setting" neurons in the raphe and locus ceruleus nuclei and the cholinergic, "generator" neurons of the gigantocellular tegmental field. The self-inhibiting and self-exciting collaterals of both groups are also shown. Abbreviations: FTG, giant neuron field; LC, locus ceruleus; R, raphe nucleus. (From Hobson, 1978. Reproduced with permission from Hoffmann-La Roche, Inc. and the author.)

system, and the *eye movements and dreaming* (cortical activation) *seem to be secondary phenomena to the dream (REM) state* (see Figure 25).

Dreams

Freud (1900/1965) proposed that dreams represented *fulfillment of wishes* in the form of hallucinations during sleep, motivated by the sleeper's desire to continue sleep. A thirsty sleeper, for example, would dream of drinking water rather than interrupt his sleep to fetch a glass of water. He further

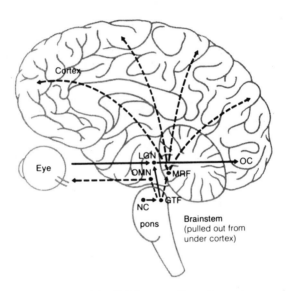

Figure 25. Schematic diagram of the REM system. From the nucleus ceruleus (NC) to the gigantocellular tegmental field (GTF): (1) Discharges from the NC usually inhibit discharges from the GTF during waking and NREM sleep; (2) the neurotransmitter involved in this inhibition appears to be aminergic; (3) this inhibition breaks down just before and during REM, liberating the GTF cells to discharge spikes. From the GTF via the lateral geniculate nucleus (LGN) to the occipital cortex (OC)—the PGO Spike: (1) Discharges from the GTF enter the LGN, a halfway station on the visual pathway from the retina to the OC; (2) via the LGN, these discharges then enter the OC, where they are apparently interpreted as coming from the retina (seen as pictures in our dreams); (3) because the pathway GTF→LGN→OC was the first one discovered, the discharges are called pontine-geniculate-occipital, or PGO, spikes. Other discharges from the GTF: The discharges from the GTF enter a multitude of other neuronal structures, apparently causing many of the typical phenomena related to REM sleep. Only two are outlined here: (1) Discharges enter the oculomotor nuclei (OMN) and cause eye movements; (2) discharges enter the midbrain reticular formation (MRF) and cause general desynchronization of the cortex typical for REM sleep. (From Hauri, 1977. Copyright 1977 by the Upjohn Co. Reproduced with permission from the publisher and author.)

postulated that wishes that were pushed out of one's awareness during waking life because of their unacceptable nature find fulfillment in dreams, occasioned by the weakening of the part of the personality structure concerned with censoring out unacceptable impulses (superego) in the state of sleep. Thus, during sleep, normally forbidden wishes might be fulfilled through hallucinations. According to Freud, the normally unconscious wishes are not directly transformed to dreams, but they undergo distortions and disguises so that they might appear somwhat more acceptable, that is, not to alarm the dreamer's personality system to the extent that he would have to interrupt his sleep.

This process of constructing dreams out of unconscious wishes was called by Freud the "dream work." The dream work involves such processes as compressing several ideas and thoughts into a single image (condensation), displacing feelings from the original object to another object, or reversing feelings or ideas to their opposites. An example of condensation is dreaming of a face that is a composite of features belonging to several different persons. Through reversal, night may be represented in dreams as broad daylight, and very emotional scenes may appear to be quite tranquil.

Recent experiences (especially of the previous day) often appear in dreams, although the particular experience (or image, such as the face of a person) may have been quite incidental. Freud called this the "day's residue." The day's residue was thought to be otherwise neutral images or experiences which could be exploited to represent unconscious wishes, and it was used as a readily available "material" with which to construct the dreams, which are wish fulfillments.

In his classic study of dreams, Freud constructed a purely psychological theory based on psychological data alone. This was because physiologic information concerning sleep and dream states was then largely nonexistent, One of the most important aspects of his discoveries regarding dreams is the demonstration that thoughts rendered in dreams have meaning in relation to the person's ongoing mental life.

Dream research has been revolutionized since the discovery of the association between REM sleep and dreaming. As previously mentioned, in about 80– 90% of REM awakenings, dream reports are elicited. The dreams occurring during the REM periods seem to be especially visual and detailed ones. Some thinking or conscious activity occurs during the NREM periods also, but this type of NREM "mentation" usually lacks the visual and elaborate quality of the REM dreams. NREM "dreams" tend to be more the auditory– thinking type of conscious activity which is usually lacking in detail and vividness.

The contents of dreams collected by REM awakenings in the laboratory are rather mundane and not necessarily as bizarre and fantastic as some of the remembered dreams. Many of the dreams occurring relatively early during sleep have contents that are temporally closer to the present, while dreams occurring later, toward the morning, seem to contain more material related to early life (Van de Castle, 1970).

According to Hobson, the discovery that the brain electrical activity associated with the REM state (pontine discharges) occurs before cortical activation or oculomotor activation seems to prove that *REM is an autonomously generated state* and not a reaction to an internal or external stimulus threatening the continuation of sleep (Hobson, 1977, 1978). According to this scheme, it appears that the *content* of a dream is constructed by the cerebral cortex in the presence of the ascending signals from the REM-state generator in the pons. The dream content, then, is closely linked to the ongoing thought processes of the person, as first noted by Freud.

It is significant that only some dreams are remembered, and it is the remembered dreams that are analyzed in psychotherapy. Perhaps, in psychotherapy, *certain dreams are selectively remembered or not remembered* because their contents are especially related to experiences, wishes, and images that have particularly important meanings in the context of therapy. These psychological meanings, then, can be explored in psychotherapy.

Functions of Sleep and Dreaming

Hartmann (1973) postulates that the function of *slow-wave* sleep is *physiologic restoration.* Studies show that when sleep has been deprived, slow-wave sleep is made up at the first opportunity, followed by restoration of REM sleep. After exercise, slow-wave sleep also increases. Hartmann also hypothesizes that during slow-wave sleep, proteins and/or RNA are synthesized, especially in the central nervous system (Table 7).

According to Hartmann, the functions of *REM sleep* are related to the brain systems having to do with *focused attention,* the ability to maintain an optimistic mood, energy, and processes of *emotional adaptation to the environment.* He also postulates that REM sleep may have a role in *consolidating learning or memory* and in *restoring* the *catecholamine levels in the brain* (Hartmann, 1973).

Sleep Needs

While the need for sleep seems to change with age (see Figure 21), there is a great *individual variation.* Thus, some individuals sleep for 10–12 hr a night, while others habitually sleep for as little as 1–3 hr a night without any ill effects (Hauri, 1977).

Table 7. Functions of Slow-Wave (S) and REM (D) Sleep[a]

Data base	Functions of S	
Hints from physiology– chemistry of sleep	Anabolism: macromolecule (RNA or protein) synthesis	Anabolism and synthesis of macromolecules to be used partially in the functions of D
Sleep deprivation	Prevent lethargy or physical tiredness	
Sleep as a response	Restoration after exercise, pain or injury, or excessive catabolism	
Psychology of tiredness	Restoration after "physical" tiredness	

Data base	Functions of D	
Hints from physiology	Repatterning	Repair, reorganization, formation of new connections in cortex and the catecholamine systems ascending to cortex required for optimal attention mechanisms, secondary process, and self-guidance during waking
Sleep deprivation	Focus attention and keep out extraneous stimuli; maintain ego integrity; restore ability for new learning; repattern or consolidate memories	
Long and short sleepers Variable sleepers	Restoration after new learning and "psychic strain" including anxiety and depression	
Age changes and pathological states	Restoration at times of new learning and at times of irritability and depression	
Sleep as a response	Restoration of catecholamine systems; restoration after reticular stimulation or hypervigilance; restoration after new learning	
Psychology of tiredness	Restore recent, subtle ego mechanisms and secondary process	
The dream	Shunting out for repair (during D) of certain brain systems necessary for flexible attention, subtle feedback regulated emotion, continuing sense of self	

[a] From Hartmann (1973). Reproduced with permission from the publisher and author.

Sleep-Deprivation Studies. Complete sleep deprivation for an entire night usually results in little decrement in performance in young, healthy volunteers (Johnson, 1969). If the total sleep deprivation is continued for two or three nights, small *"microsleeps"* of a few seconds' duration begin to intrude into wakefulness. The microsleeps interfere with attention and, thus, performance. If an individual is totally deprived of sleep for more than three days, microsleeps become longer and more frequent, so that by about ten days, it becomes hard to tell whether a subject is asleep or awake, even if he performs functions normally associated with being awake, such as walking and talking.

When sleep-deprived individuals are allowed to sleep, there is initially an increase in slow-wave sleep. In fact, on the first recovery night, there may be a decrease in REM sleep. Recovery sleep is usually not equal in length to the lost sleep and is usually not taken in one session.

Selective REM Deprivation. When volunteers are deprived of REM sleep by being awakened each time REM starts, *"REM pressure"* builds up; that is, they have a tendency to go into REM sleep before the customary 90-min lag period and spend more time—the REM state ("REM rebound") (see Figure 26). REM deprivation tends to increase agitation and impulsivity. There is some evidence, however, that REM deprivation has an antidepressant effect in severely depressed patients (Vogel *et al.*, 1976).

Selective Slow-Wave-Sleep Deprivation. Delta-sleep deprivation has a different effect from REM deprivation. Volunteers deprived of delta sleep tend to feel physically uncomfortable, with vague physical complaints and changes in bodily feelings. Their muscles become more sensitive to pressure, and they tend to become withdrawn (Hauri, 1977).

Environmental Factors Affecting Sleep

Noise and temperature, among other things, are known to affect sleep. The amount of noise necessary to awaken a sleeper depends on the sleep

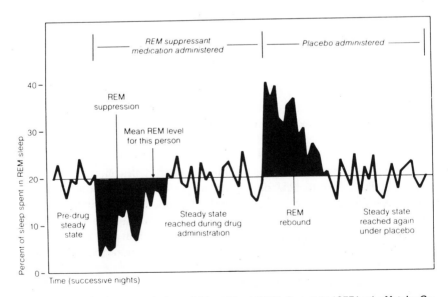

Figure 26. REM deprivation and rebound. (From Hauri, 1977. Copyright 1977 by the Upjohn Co. Reproduced with permission from the publisher and author.)

stage: Stage 1 is the lightest; Stages 2 and REM deeper; and delta sleep the deepest. *During REM sleep, thermoregulation is impaired.* Thus, sleeping in extreme temperatures may have disastrous effects, especially toward the morning when REM periods are longer (Hauri, 1977).

Caloric intake also has an impact on sleep. In experimental animals, weight gain, in general, is associated with longer, uninterrupted sleep, while weight loss is associated with short and fragmented sleep (Jacobs and McGinty, 1971).

Foods containing the serotonin precursor L-tryptophan, such as warm milk, meats, and Ovaltine, increase sleep.

Sleep Disorders

Insomnia

As the need for sleep varies according to individuals, changes in sleep habits are more important than long-term patterns. Insomnia refers to an inability to sleep that interferes with the person's daytime function and sense of well-being, regardless of the amount of hours slept. Of all sleep disorders, insomnia is the symptom most commonly complained about. Insomnia may be subdivided into *difficulty in falling asleep* (DFA), *middle-of-the-night awakening* (MNA), and *early-morning awakening* (EMA) with inability to fall asleep again.

Insomnia is often a *symptom of a medical disease,* including any condition that causes pain and physical discomfort (Kales and Kales, 1974). Thus, the complaint of insomnia should alert the physician to the possibility of an associated medical condition before simply attributing it to psychological stress.

On the other hand, *psychological distress* is the *most common cause* of insomnia. The distress may be related to interpersonal or intrapsychic conflicts or to anxiety associated with a medical disease.

Anxiety and depression are the most common psychiatric syndromes causing insomnia. Anxiety is more often associated with difficulty in falling asleep, while depression is often associated with early-morning awakening. Insomnia associated with other signs of depression, such as loss of appetite, loss of interest, and depressive feelings and guilt, suggests the diagnosis of a depressive syndrome (see Chapter 6). The most common EEG pattern of depressive patients during the night is the waking pattern (insomnia).

A common cause of insomnia is withdrawal from a pharmacologic central nervous system depressant, including the discontinuation of a sleeping medication that the patient had been taking chronically. As many hypnotic agents are also REM suppressants, this may be associated with a REM rebound, including vivid dreams and nightmares (see vignette 2).

Evaluation of Insomnia. Evaluation of insomnia should include a *thorough history and physical examination* to understand the environmental and personal strains as well as to diagnose possible medical conditions causing the insomnia. Attention should be paid to the possibility that the patient may have associated *depression and/or anxiety.* If they are present, psychotherapy may be necessary in conjunction with drug treatment. Drug treatment may be specific for the depression or for the insominia (see Chapter 18).

The possibility of *withdrawal from a central nervous system depressant drug (including alcohol)* should also be considered and a careful history taken. Barbiturates should not be withdrawn abruptly, but rather very gradually.

Hypnotic Agents. Most hypnotic agents are habit-forming and also lose potency with continued use. Thus, the use of hypnotics should be well thought out and not prolonged. Flurazepam (Dalmane), 15– 30 mg, is a relatively safe and effective hypnotic over relatively long periods, but it depresses delta sleep. Barbiturates such as secobarbital, 100 mg, are effective, but they suppress REM sleep. Chloral hydrate does not affect REM sleep, but the therapeutic index is very low (effective dose is 500– 1000 mg and toxicity occurs at as low as 2000 mg). Recently, the serotonin precursor L-tryptophan has been described as a natural hypnotic with minimum toxicity (in 1- to 2-mg doses). L-Tryptophan occurs naturally in meats and milk.

Hypersomnia

Hypersomnia refers to excessive sleep. In contrast to narcolepsy (see below), sleep is not irresistible in hypersomnia, and there are no associated symptoms. Hypersomnic sleep may be from many hours to several days. There is often confusion and extreme difficulty in completely awakening from nocturnal sleep (Rechtschaffen and Dement, 1969). Hypersomnic patients, by and large, have *normal EEG sleep patterns* during sleep, although the heart rate and respiratory rate are often elevated before and during sleep.

Chronic hypersomnia may occur as a *symptom of central nervous system lesions,* such as after head injury, brain tumor, and cerebrovascular accidents (Kales and Kales, 1974). It may also be a symptom of *psychiatric disorders,* such as chronic anxiety and depression, in which sleep represents an escape. Especially in bipolar, manic– depressive disorders, hypersomnia may occur as the patient becomes depressed.

In Kleine–Levin syndrome, hypersomnia occurs in conjunction with bulimia (overeating). In Pickwickian syndrome, hypersomnia occurs with obesity and respiratory disorder.

Narcolepsy

Narcolepsy in an episodic disorder characterized by irresistible *sleep attacks* of a few minutes' duration (usually less than 15 min). The sleep attacks often occur after meals and toward the evening. The patient usually feels refreshed after a sleep attack, and there is usually a refractory period of a few hours before the next attack. In the complete narcoleptic syndrome, in addition to sleep attacks, there are three *associated symptoms*. They are *cataplexy* (sudden loss of muscle tone), sleep paralysis (momentary inability to move while falling asleep or waking up), and *hypnagogic hallucinations* (vivid visual hallucinations while falling asleep).

Cataplexy is the most common associated symptom and is often related to an emotional stimulus, such as *laughter*. Cataplexy may cause serious injuries. Sleep paralysis and hypnagogic hallucinations often occur together. The relative frequency of the narcoleptic tetrad among narcoleptics is as follows (Kales and Kales, 1974):

Sleep attacks	100%
Sleep attacks + cataplexy	70%
Hypnagogic hallucinations as one of the symptoms	25%
Sleep paralysis as one of the symptoms	50%
Sleep paralysis alone	5% or less
Full tetrad	10%

Narcolepsy usually appears during *adolescence* or *young adulthood*. There is evidence that it has a genetic basis, perhaps a single dominant gene. Whether there is a psychological disturbance in narcolepsy is controversial. EEG studies in narcolepsy show that in the majority of patients who had a history of cataplexy, both nocturnal sleep and sleep attacks invariably *begin with REM sleep*. Normals usually have 60–100 min of NREM sleep before going to REM. Only 10% of the narcoleptic patients without history of cataplexy have REM at the onset of their sleep attacks. Rechtschaffen and Dement (1969) proposed that in narcolepsy with associated symptoms, the *sleep episodes are attacks of REM sleep* and that *cataplexy is an attack of motor inhibition* similar to the one seen in REM sleep.

Diagnosis. Establishing the diagnosis of narcolepsy is essential, because narcoleptic patients are often misunderstood to be lazy, irresponsible, or emotionally unstable. Diagnosis is primarily on the basis of characteristic history. Sleep-onset REM on EEG is also helpful. Differential diagnosis includes hypersomnia, Kleine–Levin syndrome, Pickwickian syndrome, sleep-apnea hypersomnia, hypothyroidism, hypoglycemia, coma, and epilepsy (Kales and Kales, 1974).

Management. Central nervous system stimulants such as dextroamphetamine and methylphenidate are effective for sleep attacks. They are also REM suppressants. Imipramine (Tofranil), an antidepressant, is effective for the associated symptoms but not for sleep attacks. Combined therapy with imipramine and dextroamphetamine may be dangerous, as amphetamines release catecholamines while imipramine blocks reuptake and inactivation of catecholamines (see Chapter 18). Thus, in combination, they may cause hypertensive episodes.

Narcoleptic patients whose attacks are not satisfactorily controlled with medications *should not be allowed to perform potentially dangerous activities* such as driving an automobile or operating certain machinery.

Somnambulism (Sleepwalking)

Somnambulism occurs more commonly among *children* and preponderantly among *males.* There is usually a positive *family history* and a higher incidence of *enuresis* among sleepwalkers than in the general population (Kales and Kales, 1974). The sleepwalking episode usually lasts for several minutes, and there is complete amnesia for the incident. EEG studies show that somnambulism occurs exclusively during *NREM sleep,* especially during delta sleep. Thus, somnambulism is *not* associated with dreaming. Most children who sleepwalk tend to cease sleepwalking in a few years. Psychological disturbances are not associated with somnambulism in children, although they are often present in adult sleepwalkers (Sours *et al.,* 1966).

Management. The most important consideration in somnambulism is to *protect the patient from injury.* Contrary to popular belief, a sleepwalker can, indeed, suffer serious injuries. Locking doors and windows, removing potentially dangerous objects, and having the patient sleep on the first floor are among the prophylactic measures to be used. In children, conveying the information that they usually "outgrow" the condition is reassuring and important. In *adults, psychiatric evaluation* and treatment are often indicated. In severe cases, delta-sleep-suppressant medications, such as *benzodiazepines* (e.g., diazepam), may be tried, although their efficacy has not yet been clearly established (Kales and Kales, 1974).

Enuresis (Bed-Wetting)

Bed-wetting is a relatively *common* condition among children. Approximately 10%–15% of all children between four and five years of age continue to wet the bed. Even in adulthood, enuresis occurs in about 1%–3% of the population.

Primary enuresis refers to bed-wetting since infancy, without any period of consistent dryness for at least a few months (Kales and Kales, 1974). There seems to be a *genetic component* to this condition, and *organic disease* is often the cause of primary enuresis. For example, urethral obstruction in males and ectopic ureter in females can cause constant dribbling. Diverticulum of the anterior urethra, epispadias, ectopia vesicae, and cystitis can also cause bed-wetting.

Secondary enuresis is often associated with psychological factors such as regression due to jealousy of a newborn sibling.

EEG studies in enuresis show that bed-wetting occurs predominantly during *NREM slow-wave sleep*. Most of the enuretic episodes occur during delta-wave sleep; then the pattern changes to Stage 2 of NREM sleep. If the subjects are awakened and changed, they do not report any dreams and, on falling asleep, have normal sleep patterns. If the subjects continue to sleep-wet during the ensuing REM periods, however, they tend to incorporate the wetness into their dreams.

Management. First, the physician should determine whether the enuresis is primary or secondary. There may be a "maturational lag" in primary enuresis, especially if there is a family history of enuresis. The child may simply "outgrow" the enuresis in these instances. In secondary enuresis, psychological treatment may be necessary. Parents of enuretic children should be reassured that most affected children eventually outgrow this disorder.

Imipramine (Tofranil) is effective in reducing enuretic frequency if judiciously used. Conditioning devices, such as a bell activated by bed-wetting, may be sometimes helpful.

Night Terrors

The night terror is characterized by a subjective feeling of *intense anxiety* associated with oppressive sensations, severe autonomic discharge, "blood-curdling screams," and practically no recall of specifics. In children, this is also called *pavor nocturnus*, and in adults, *incubus*. The night terrors occur during NREM *delta-wave sleep* (especially Stage 4 sleep). As in somnambulism, *children usually outgrow this disorder*. In adults, psychiatric evaluation may be necessary. Delta-wave-sleep suppressants, such as benzodiazepines (e.g., diazepam), are useful in suppressing night terrors. Reassurance of parents that children usually outgrow this condition is helpful.

Nightmares

In contrast to night terrors, nightmares are dreams occurring *during REM sleep.* Frightening dreams often occur during the *REM rebound,* concomitant to withdrawal of REM-suppressant medications, including barbiturates and alcohol.

Sleep Apnea

Sleep apnea may be a universal occurrence in normal infants between one and three months of age (Kales and Kales, 1974). It also occurs in Pickwickian syndrome, narcolepsy, and insomnia. Sleep apnea may be sub-divided into (1) a central type, (2) a peripheral obstructive type due to upper respiratory tract obstruction, and (3) a mixed type of central apnea followed by upper-airway obstruction.

Sleep apnea in infants occurs mostly *during REM* and is often associated with the *sudden-infant-death syndrome.* Sleep apnea associated with hypersomnia, insomnia, and narcolepsy occurs both during REM and NREM states. Snoring is a common finding associated with sleep apnea due to airway obstruction.

Medical Conditions Affected by REM Sleep

REM sleep often precipitates symptoms in patients with medical illness. For example, nocturnal angina is associated with REM. In patients with duodenal ulcers (but not in normal subjects), there is an increase in gastric secretion rate during REM.

Hyperthyroidism and Hypothyroidism

Delta sleep is markedly *reduced* in *hypothyroidism* and *increased* in *hyperthyroidism.* With treatment of the thyroid disorder, delta sleep gradually returns to normal. Sleepiness is a frequent symptom of hypothyroidism.

Summary

Sleep consists of NREM and REM sleep. NREM sleep is made up of Stages 1 through 4. Stages 3 and 4 are often referred to together as delta or slow-wave sleep. During a typical night, NREM sleep occurs first, followed by REM, whose duration is about 5–20 min. The cycle repeats itself every 90–100 min. Total REM time per night is about 20% of sleep time. REM is associated with *physiologic arousal, skeletal muscular relaxation,* and *visual dreams.*

The sleep-wake and REM–NREM cycles are examples of biological rhythm. Biological rhythms may be circadian, diurnal, nocturnal, infradian, or ultradian. Many metabolic and endocrine systems have rhythmicity.

Brain mechanisms of sleep are not completely understood. Arousal and wakefulness seem to depend on the ascending reticular activating system. Sleep, especially NREM sleep, is probably mediated by the serotonergic neurons arising from the pontine median raphe system. In REM sleep, noradrenergic and cholinergic neurons in the pons (from locus ceruleus and pontine giant cells, respectively) seem to be involved in addition to serotonergic neurons. The electrical activity generated in the pons by the interaction of these systems subsequently result in the eye movements (REM) and the cortical desynchronization, which may give rise to the subjective experience of dreaming.

The *content* of remembered *dreams* may be especially important in the context of ongoing emotional life, especially in psychotherapy. Freud formulated a way of conceptualizing dreams. According to his theory, dreams represent wish fulfillments through hallucinations during sleep. The wishes thus emerging are often unconscious or repressed during waking life because of their unacceptable nature. *"Dream work"* is a term used by Freud to refer to the process of constructing dreams out of the unconscious wishes. It includes condensation, displacement, and reversal.

The *function* of slow-wave sleep seems to be physiologic restoration, including protein synthesis in the central nervous system. REM sleep may be related to processes of emotional adaptation to the environment as well as consolidation of memory and, perhaps, restoration of catecholamines in the brain.

The *need* for sleep appears to depend on the individual, with wide variations. In sleep deprivation, NREM sleep is restored first, followed by REM. After selective REM deprivation, there is a REM rebound.

Environmental factors such as noise, caloric intake, and content of food affect sleep.

Sleep disorders include insomnia, hypersomnia, narcolepsy, and somnambulism. Enuresis, somnambulism, and night terrors characteristically occur during delta sleep (NREM). The autonomic arousal during REM may precipitate medical symptoms. Delta sleep is reduced in hypothyroidism and increased in hyperthyroidism. Many medical conditions, especially painful conditions, interfere with sleep. Sleep disturbance is often an important and early sign of depression and anxiety.

Implications

For the Patient

Sleep disturbance is often dismissed as being of little consequence. On the other hand, some patients attribute serious symptoms and signs to "lack of sleep" or "sleeping too much," thereby delaying help-seeking behavior. Abuse of sleeping medications is another problem that patients with sleep difficulties often develop. Certain patients become obsessed or frightened by especially vivid dreams which may be associated with a REM rebound phenomenon. A good night's sleep is very important for most patients for a sense of well-being and physiologic restoration. In a stressful environment like the hospital, sleep is especially important for the patient.

For the Physician

Sleep disturbance often indicates the presence of a medical or psychiatric pathology. In serious sleep disturbances, a comprehensive evaluation is necessary. Many *medications* affect sleep; some increase drowsiness and sleep through a depressant action on the central nervous system, others reduce sleep through stimulation of the central nervous system, and still others selectively affect REM (mostly by suppressing REM). It is important to consider the effect of the proposed medication on the patient's sleep and REM. The physician should be aware of the REM rebound phenomenon that can result in night-mares. Hypnotics should be judiciously, and only transiently, prescribed.

For the Community and Health Care System

Hospitals should provide an environment conducive for good sleep for patients. This includes reducing of noise and light levels and furnishing comfortable beds. Since painful conditions interfere with sleep, which may, in turn, produce physical discomfort, adequate *pain relief* should be provided for patients suffering from pain. Physicians should be educated concerning the need for adequate sleep and pain relief in medical patients. Many hypnotic agents are either ineffective, unsafe, or both. The public should be educated concerning the use of hypnotic agents, especially the dangers of abuse.

Recommended Reading

Biological Rhythms in Psychiatry and Medicine, Public Health Service publication 2088. Washington, DC, National Institute of Mental Health, 1970. Obtainable through the Superintendent of Documents, US Government Printing Office, Washington, DC 20402 at $1.75. This is a very comprehensive and easy-to-read summary of biological rhythms, including circadian rhythms, sleep and dreaming, and even sunspots and emotional rhythms. A little dated, but still a good background reading.

Freud S: *The Interpretation of Dreams.* This book, published first in German in 1900, has several translations. We would recommend the James Strachey translation, available in paperback (New York, Avon Books, 1965) or in the *Standard Edition of the Complete Psychological Works of Sigmund Freud* (London, Hogarth Press, 1973, vols 4 and 5). This is a landmark in understanding the meaning of remembered dreams. The psychoanalytic perspective concerning dreams and their interpretation is very lucidly and readably presented here. Dreams are seen as "wish fulfillment" through hallucination motivated by the need not to interrupt sleep. Many ideas discussed by Freud in this early work became the foundation of later psychoanalytic theory. Highly recommended.

Weitzman ED (ed): *Advances in Sleep Research.* New York, Spectrum Publications, 1974 and 1976, vols 1 and 2. These two volumes provide an extensive reference concerning the most current research findings about sleep. The chapters include, just to name a few, chemical anatomy of brain circuits in sleep and wakefulness, the phylogeny of sleep, the cellular basis of sleep cycle control, ultradian rhythms in sleep and wakefulness, maturation of sleep patterns of the newborn infant, sleep disturbances in catatonic patients, and biogenic amines. It is a multiauthored work. Volume 1 has topics of somewhat more general interest than volume 2.

References

Aserinsky E, Kleitman N: Reguarly occurring periods of eye mobility and concomitant phenomena during sleep. *Science* **118**:223–224, 1953.

Biological Rhythms in Psychiatry and Medicine, Public Health Service publication 2088, Washington, DC, National Institute of Mental Health, 1970.

Curtis GC: Psychosomatics and chronobiology: Possible implications of neuroendocrine rhythms: A review. *Psychosom Med* **34**:235–256, 1972.

Foulkes D: Dream reports from different stages of sleep. *J Abnorm Psychol* **65**:14–25, 1962.

Foulkes D, Vogel G: Mental activity at sleep onset. *J Abnorm Psychol* **70**:231–243, 1965.

Freud S: *The Interpretation of Dreams,* Strachey J (ed). New York, Avon Books, 1965. (Originally published, 1900.)

Friedman S, Fischer C: On the presence of a rhythmic, diurnal, oral instinctual drive cycle in man: A preliminary report. *J Am Psychoanal Assoc* **15**:317–342, 1967.

Guyton AC: *Textbook of Medical Physiology.* Philadelphia, WB Saunders, 1976, p. 734.

Hartmann E (ed): *Sleep and Dreaming.* Boston, Little Brown & Co, 1970, p. 408.

Hartmann E: *The Functions of Sleep.* New Haven, Yale University Press, 1973.

Hauri P: *The Sleep Disorders.* Kalamazoo, Mich., Upjohn, 1977.

Hobson JA: The sleep–dream cycle: A neurobiological rhythm, in Ioachim E (ed): *Pathobiology Annual.* New York, Appleton-Century-Crofts, 1975, pp 369–403.

Hobson JA: *The Sleep–Dream Cycle and the Single Neuron.* Nutley, NJ, Roche Laboratories, 1978.

Hobson JA, McCarley RW: The brain as a dream state generator: An activation–synthesis hypothesis of the dream process. *Am J Psychiatry* **134:**1335–1348, 1977.

Jacobs BL, McGinty DJ: Effects of food deprivation on sleep and wakefulness in the rat. *Exp Neurol* **30:**212–222, 1971.

Johnson LC: Psychological and physiological changes following total sleep deprivation, in Kales AA (ed): *Sleep: Physiology and Pathology.* Philadelphia, Lippincott, 1969, pp 206–220.

Jouvet M: Some monoaminergic mechanisms controlling sleep and waking, in Karczmar AG, Eccles JC (eds): *Brain and Human Behavior.* New York, Springer-Verlag, 1972, pp 131–161.

Jouvet M: The role of monoamines and acetylcholine-containing neurons in the regulation of the sleep–waking cycle, in *Ergehrisse der Physiologie,* vol 64, *Neurophysiology and Neurochemistry of Sleep and Wakefulness.* Berlin, Springer-Verlag, 1972, pp 166–308.

Kales A: Sleep and dreams. *Ann Intern Med* **68:**1078, 1968.

Kales A, Kales JD: Sleep disorders: Recent findings in the diagnosis and treatment of disturbed sleep. *N Engl J Med* **290:**487–499, 1974.

Kleitman N: *Sleep and Wakefulness.* Chicago, University of Chicago Press, 1965.

Morgane PJ, Stern WC: Chemical anatomy of brain circuits in relation to sleep and wakefulness, in Weitzman EE (ed): *Advances in Sleep Research.* New York, Spectrum Publications, 1974, vol. 1, pp 1–131.

Rechtschaffen A, Dement W: Narcolepsy and hypersomnia, in Kales A (ed): *Sleep: Physiology and Pathology.* Philadelphia, Lippincott, 1969, pp 119–130.

Rechtschaffen A, Kales A (eds): *A Manual of Standardized Terminology, Techniques and Scoring System for Sleep Stages of Human Subjects,* National Institutes of Health publication 204. Washington, DC, US Government Printing Office, 1968.

Sours JA, Frumken, P, Indermell RR: Somnambulism. *Arch Gen Psychiatry* **14:**595–604, 1966.

Van de Castle RL: Temporal patterns of dreams, in Hartmann E (ed): *Sleep and Dreaming.* Boston, Little Brown & Co, 1970, pp 171–181.

Vogel G, McAbee R, Barker K, *et al.:* REM pressure and improvement of endogenous depression, in Chase MH, Mitler MM, Walter PL (eds): *Sleep Research.* Los Angeles, University of California at Los Angeles, Brain Information Service/Brain Research Institute, 1976, vol 15.

PART III

ON ASSESSING A PATIENT
A Clinical Systems Approach

CHAPTER 9

Approach to Patients: The Systems–Contextual Framework and the Patient Evaluation Grid

1.   A 56-year-old man had a routine chest X ray as a part of his company's physical fitness program. The X ray revealed a coin lesion in the right lung, indicative of a tumor. When he was told that more medical workup was needed, he felt very perplexed and somewhat angry because he "felt so well." His wife, who was told of the possible implications of the X-ray shadow (cancer), became very anxious, which, in turn, made the patient more upset. Since he had always been a healthy, strong man, he attempted to dismiss the fact that there was a need for further medical tests and, in fact, did not keep his next appointment with the doctor. As the X ray had been done at the company's request, he was eventually told by his superiors that he had to report to the doctor, who, in turn, had to report to the manager. When the diagnosis of cancer was made, he was retired from work. A depressive syndrome ensued, his physical state deteriorated, and the cancer became symptomatic.

2.   A 7½-months-pregnant, 24-year-old black woman was admitted to the obstetrical ward because of toxemia of pregnancy. There had also been excessive weight gain. In the hospital, she was found eating white starch powder from a box. The intern learned that this was a common custom during pregnancy in some Southern subcultures.

3.   A 15-year-old girl was admitted to the surgical service for correction of tetralogy of Fallot (a form of congenital heart disease). In the hospital, she displayed excessive anxiety which was not controlled by diazepam (Valium). When the intern asked her detailed questions about her family, she found that the patient's parents had agreed to separate when their daugh-

ter's heart condition had been repaired. The patient was anxious about the impending separation of her parents!

4. A 45-year-old man had an operation for coronary artery disease. During the second postoperative day, he began to have frightening visual hallucinations. He was also tremulous and febrile. As the symptoms were very similar to delirium tremens, the astute medical student on the case asked the family about the patient's drinking habits. It turned out that he customarily drank at least half a dozen cocktails a day when he was working. In fact, even during his hospitalization, his wife had supplied him with several bottles of vodka which were "hidden" in his room. He lost access to alcohol only after the operation!

Once a person comes to the physician for medical care, it is the doctor's responsibility to carry out a comprehensive evaluation, to diagnose disease if present, and to treat the patient to the best of his or her ability. As noted in earlier chapters, the physician and health care pesonnel will, to a large degree, through their demeanor and behavior, determine how much cooperation the patient will give in the assessment and treatment process, and, further, what the patient's attitudes and expectations will be in future contacts with the health care system.

The Patient, His Components, and the Environment

To evaluate a diseased organ thoroughly, it is necessary to consider it in three broad perspectives that reflect the three levels of organization that are cogent to its function: (1) the function and state of the organ as a whole; (2) the function and state of components or subsystems of the organ, such as component cells and tissues, blood supply, and chemical subsystems; and (3) the function and state of of the larger system of which the organ is a part (e.g., the cardiovascular or digestive) and even its relationship with other organs (heart and kidney; liver and brain; etc.). For example, a thrombus in a coronary artery (part of the cardiovascular system) results in anoxia of myocardial tissues (chemical), leading to infarction (tissue), and thus reduces cardiac contractility (organ), resulting in congestive heart failure (system).

Similarly, in repairing an automobile, the mechanic must know the state of the engine, radiator, and other *components* of the automobile; the way the car is functioning as a *whole* (such as the maximum speed, handling characteristics, and how it looks); and the *interaction* of the automobile with factors outside (such as how the owner is maintaining it and whether it is habitually driven on particularly rough roads).

In approaching patients, a similar conceptual approach is useful—that is, a thorough evaluation of the patient that includes organizing data according to three dimensions: (1) the *biological dimension,* that is, the structural and functional state of physiochemical components and subsystems, including of course, healthy and possibly diseased organs; (2) the *personal dimension,* that is, the psychological state and behavior of the whole person (patient); and (3) the *environmental dimension,* that is, the environmental–interpersonal data, including interaction of the patient with the physical environment and with family, work, and the health care system, among others (Figure 27). Each of these levels or dimensions can be conceptualized as a *system,* with subsytems at each level and with interactions both within and across dimensions (see Chapter 20).

Disease, Illness, and Distress

A patient, by definition, is a person seeking help for experienced distress. The cause of the distress and the factors that contribute to it reside in and relate to the three dimensions discussed above, that is, the *biological,* the *personal,* and the *environmental–interpersonal.*

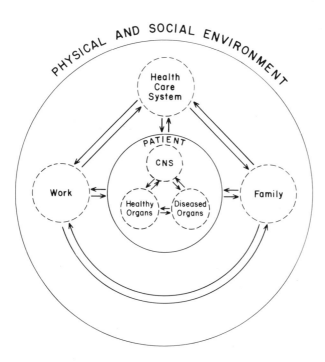

Figure 27. The patient, his components, and his environment.

The person experiences distress, such as anxiety, suffering, and depression (see Part II), which together with the symptoms emanating from the biological components constitute the *illness* (Feinstein, 1974), and these then interact with each other and with components of the environment.

Disease at the organ level often produces the experience of illness, but a disease process may exist without illness for extended periods (e.g., asymptomatic progression of a cancer, as in vignette 1), and a patient may experience an illness without evidence of disease (e.g., "psychogenic" pain; see Chapter 7). Factors at the personal level may contribute to the pathogenesis of disease, such as a habit of smoking or excessive drinking (vignette 4).

At the environmental level, interpersonal difficulties may result in the experience of anxiety, and in heterothetic (problems of living presenting as a symptom; see Chapter 1) help-seeking behaviors. Furthermore, help-seeking behavior is often prompted by family or friends of the patient. Environmental factors may also contribute to the pathogenesis of disease (Rahe, 1972), for example, environmental poisons, occupational toxins (e.g., heavy metals), and interpersonal loss (e.g., bereavement). Assessment of the environmental system is important also in the management of the patient, since treatment plans should take the patient's family and work situation into account.

The Systems–Contextual Approach

For a conceptualization of the three basic dimensions to be of practical help in the management of patients, a method is required for organizing the data into a form applicable to clinical care. For this purpose, we propose a *systems–contextual* method of approach which organizes information about the three dimensions according to three longitudinal *time contexts* organized with the patient's *help-seeking behavior* as the fixed point of time reference. These three time contexts we designate as (1) *current,* (2) *recent,* and (3) *background* contexts. They expand in scope and complexity with retrograde movement along the time from the present (current context) to the remote past (background context).

The *current context* refers to the cross-sectional *state* in each dimension at the time of help-seeking behavior. The *recent context* refers to *recent* changes and events in each system. This includes the appearance of symptoms and signs, as well as such stressful events as bereavement, retirement, recent hospitalization, and recent disease. The *background context* refers to traits, congenital and early childhood diseases, long-standing personality traits, and early environmental, interpersonal, and cultural influences. Early experience, heredity, constitution, personality style, family background, cultural heritage, etc., are included in the background context.

The Patient Evaluation Grid (PEG)

A three-by-three grid displaying the intersection of data regarding the three dimensions of organization (biological, personal, and environmental) with the three longitudinal time contexts (current, recent, and background) creates a nine-compartment grid which we have found useful in everyday clinical practice as well as in teaching and research. We call it the patient evaluation grid (PEG)* (see Figures 28 and 29).

In diagnosis, the PEG can serve as a useful guide in (1) taking a complete medical history, (2) performing the physical examination, and (3) planning further special diagnostic procedures (laboratory, etc.). For example, it is useful to have the PEG in mind while interviewing the patient and, eventually, to enter information into the squares with dates. To fill in relevant information in any empty square, the physician should ask questions of the patient and/or family about cultural and family expectations of the sick role, the meaning of illness, personality style, and other pertinent data (Leigh et al., 1980). In this chapter, we will discuss each of the elements of the PEG briefly in order to provide the reader with an overview. More detailed discussion of each of the contexts follows in subsequent chapters which will also illustrate its application in patient management.

What Goes into the PEG

Column A: Current Context. This column, which concerns the current state of the patient, has most immediacy for both the patient and doctor, since the information indicates the pressing needs of the patient as well as any constraints in therapeutic plans.

Biological Dimension. This square contains information about the patient's physical state, vital signs, and the classical data of the present illness, including physical symptoms and laboratory findings, which form the basis of clinical diagnosis and of many therapeutic decisions.

Personal Dimension. Data concerning the chief complaint, appearance, current psychological state, and anxiety level are contained here. The chief complaint relating to physical state belongs in both the biological and the personal dimensions to the extent that the patient is suffering from it. This

*The PEG was developed by H. Leigh, M.F. Reiser, and A.R. Feinstein in 1978.

Figure 28. Framework of the PEG.

DIMENSIONS	CONTEXTS		
	CURRENT (Current States)	RECENT (Recent Events and Changes)	BACKGROUND (Culture, Traits, Constitution)
BIOLOGICAL	Symptoms Physical Examination Vital signs Status of related organs Medications Disease	Age Recent bodily changes Injuries, operations Disease Drugs	Heredity Early nutrition Constitution Predisposition Early disease
PERSONAL	Chief Complaint Mental Status Expectations about illness and treatment	Recent illness, occurrence of symptoms Personality change Mood, thinking, behavior Adaptation — Defenses	Developmental factors Early experience Personality type Attitude to illness
ENVIRONMENTAL	Immediate physical and interpersonal environment Supportive figure, next of kin Effect of help-seeking	Recent physical and interpersonal environment Life changes Family, work, others Contact with ill persons Contact with doctor or hospital	Early physical environment Cultural and family environment Early Relations Cultural sick role expectation

Figure 29. PEG: Organization of relevant information. Biological dimension refers to the components of the patient, such as the organ systems, tissue, and chemical composition. Personal dimension refers to attributes of the whole person, including the psychological and behavioral aspects. This includes personal habits such as smoking and drinking. Environmental dimension refers to the psychosocial and physical environments surrounding the patient.

square also contains answers to questions such as the following: Is the patient coherent, confused, frightened, or depressed? What does the patient think about the symptoms? Does the patient expect hospitalization, a "shot," an operation, etc.? The information is valuable for an understanding of how the patient experiences illness and of his motivation in seeking help. Recognition of the patient's immediate need for help may consolidate the doctor–patient relationship and increase patient compliance.

Environmental Dimension. Examples of data that belong in this square are answers to the following questions: Who accompanied the patient? Who lives with the patient? Marital status? Who suggested seeing a doctor? Effects of the patient's illness on his family and occupation, etc.? The value of this square is its information about the patient's "significant others." At a very practical level, the next of kin, family, or friend is an important source of information, support, and, occasionally, consent.

Column B: Recent Context. This column contains highlights of *recent changes and events,* including symptoms, illness, and disease processes and their effects on the patient's life and family, as well as changes in long-standing patterns such as habits. This column also includes information about possible contributing, complicating, or precipitating factors of the illness and help-seeking behavior. "Recent" is used here as a relative term, its range being measured in days, weeks, and months—often as much as 6–12 months, seldom longer. All entries here should include the *date* or approximate *duration* of the event.

Biological Dimension. Recent physical change, weight gain or loss, injuries, discovery of hypertension, recent surgery, and medications are examples of data to be included here. Data found in this square provide information concerning early signs of current disease and possible contributing or antecedent factors, as well as physical effects of recent environmental and behavioral changes.

Personal Dimension. This square contains data concerning personality change, change in habits (e.g., increased drinking), mood change (e.g., depression), preoccupation with disease (e.g., conviction that he has cancer), etc. Mood and habit changes may contribute to disease (e.g., depression causing self-neglect and malnutrition and susceptibility to infection) or may be symptoms of a disease process (e.g., personality change in frontal lobe tumor).

Environmental Dimension. This section, which denotes possible environmental stressors causing disease or illness behavior (Mechanic, 1962; Rahe, 1972; McWhinney, 1972), is concerned with such data as change in residence or job, marriage, separation, divorce, bereavement, recent travel, exposure to doctors or hospitals, and recent illness in the family.

Column C: Background Context. The background factors indicate previous illnesses and medical experiences and predispositions to disease. They also set the tone and attitude of the patient toward illness and help-seeking behavior and adaptation to the sick role through personality, constitution, predisposition, and cultural experiences. The items appearing here represent relatively long-standing, stable characteristics of the patient and are usually resistant to change. This information is important in setting realistic goals for care as well as in understanding the patient's needs.

Biological Dimension. This square contains information concerning congenital conditions, constitutional vulnerability, predisposition, genetic endowment, and acquired tendency for specific diseases. Family history of hereditary disease and early injuries, diseases, and deformities also belong here, as do answers to such questions as history of functional disorders under stress and allergies.

Personal Dimension. Data such as the patient's personality type (see Chapter 15), habitual psychological defenses, and coping styles (see Chapter 5) belong here. They include answers to such questions as the following: Does the patient tend to deny the presence of symptoms and signs? Habitual complaining of minor symptoms? Tendency to be exacting and somewhat obsessive? Tendency to become overly dependent? The patient's habits (e.g., alcohol, smoking), hobbies, ambitions (e.g., always wanted to be a doctor), educational and intelligence level, etc., are also pertinent data here. How information is processed and interpreted by the patient, what current illness means to the patient, and how the patient may respond to planned therapuetic approaches may be determined by the factors found in this square.

Environmental Dimension. The patient's cultural background, early physical environment, ethnic origin, and religion are examples of data to be entered into this square. Answers to questions such as the following also belong here: Early exposure to illness in family? Cultural sick role expectations? Cultural myths about illness and treatment? Religious qualms about procedures? Early experiences with doctor or hospital? Information contained in this section may provide clues to the patient's current attitudes and expectations. Early contact with the physician or hospital may be related to unrealistic or irrational attitudes toward medical care.

The Significance of Contexts

By organizing longitudinal data into current, recent, and background contexts, the immediacy, novelty, or degree of habituation to a particular phenomenon becomes clear. For example, chest pain appearing in the recent context *de novo* has greater immediacy for the patient than chest pain that appeared in the background context column first. Although we are dealing here with chronological material along a time dimension, the material is seen from the vantage point of the patient's help-seeking behavior. Thus, the background, recent, and current contexts may affect one another bidirectionally. For example, if the patient is confused currently, he may not be able to give a complete or accurate past history.

The need for intervention or treatment and the ease with which this can be done increase in the order of background, recent, and current contexts. Although the background context information, in general, most often points to limiting factors in approaching the patient, certain background phenomena are amenable to change. For example, the patient's expectations and fantasies about a medical procedure may change if specifically discussed. In vignette 3, the congenital heart disease is a background context factor that is amenable to change. Also, the expectation that the parents would separate upon the girl's recovery could be discussed and coped with by counseling and possibly family therapy.

The Significance of Dimensions

The *biological dimension* provides information concerning the structure and status of the component parts of the person. Information referable to this dimension forms the basis of the diagnosis of disease. Data can be systematized most thoroughly at this level thanks to the expansion of our knowledge in this dimension through research in physiology, biochemistry, pathology, etc. Obviously, there are a number of subsystems or levels within the biological level. Thus, we can consider organs, tissues, cells, molecules, etc. Disease may involve alteration at any of these levels of organization within this dimension. In using the PEG, the entries in this dimension should include the important laboratory and physical findings as well as diagnosed and suspected diseases. In this dimension, as in others, the current context physical or physiologic state requires immediate attention and treatment. Information concerning the etiologic and predisposing biological factors is usually to be found in the recent and background contexts.

The *personal dimension* denotes qualities and characteristics ascribable to the totality of the patient, including the person's appearance, personality, disposition, habits, feelings, idiosyncrasies, fantasies, and prejudices. As the central nervous system, especially the brain, is the control center for the whole organism, the attributes of the personal dimension often represent the condition of the central nervous system, although they are not confined to it.

Background context personality or habits may be contributory to or markers of vulnerability to certain disease. For example, smoking contributes to lung cancer and coronary disease.

Recent context events or changes, such as personality change or mood change, may be secondary to disease (e.g., carcinoma of the tail of the pancreas) or an interpersonal event (e.g., bereavement), and, in turn, may give rise to a disease (e.g., depression resulting in malnutrition and infection) or to a change in behavior (e.g., increasing intake of alcohol resulting in problems at work and unemployment).

Current context information such as chief complaint (suffering), mental status, and behavior indicate the motivation for help-seeking behavior. Care must be directed toward the immediate need (relief from suffering that motivated the help-seeking behavior) if the patient is to receive satisfactory medical treatment, as he will be less motivated to comply with the physician's plans if the plans omit measures to relieve or ameliorate the specific current suffering. Relief of the immedate and specific suffering, such as overwhelming anxiety or pain, may be necessary before further evaluation can proceed (vignette 3). An important factor at the personal level is the patient's fantasies and expectations concerning the health care system. Elucidation of these is essential in any patient who has difficulties in complying with medical procedures or regimen, as simple direct reassurance or education may correct unrealistic fantasies and expectations.

The *environmental dimension* provides information concerning the physical and interpersonal environment in which the patient lives and functions. This environment, in the background context, helped shape the patient's personality and cultural aspirations and in a real sense, provided the patient with his constitutional endowment. Previous contact with the health care system and health care personnel provides information concerning the patient's sick role behavior. Changes in physical environment (e.g., getting a job in a chemical factory) may provide a clue to the cause of heavy-metal poisoning. Customs unique to subcultures may provide clues to unusual behavior (e.g., weight gain and unusual eating habit, as in vignette 2).

Recent life changes and life situations are the sources of the patient's current joys, sorrows, and concerns and may have provided contributing factors to illness (Rahe, 1972; Holmes and Rahe, 1968). The impetus to seek help at a particular time usually comes from a recent change or event, for example, interpersonal tension (McWhinney, 1972) or a relative falling ill with a similar disease.

The current interpersonal context provides information concerning the significant others involved with the patient. At a very practical level, the next of kin or friend who accompanied the patient to the physician or who is most readily available upon request is an important resource—a source of information concerning the patient and for obtaining consent for procedures when necessary.

Rational Patient Management

In formulating a rational patient management plan, consideration of the interrelationships among findings in the nine compartments of the PEG is useful. Although illness (the suffering or distress leading to help-seeking behavior) usually occurs in the presence of a disease, it does not always have a one-to-one correlation with it. For example, suffering (illness) may be present in the absence of disease (e.g., bereavement) and many result from the treatment of disease rather than the disease itself (e.g., pain caused by surgical operation to remove an asymptomatic malignant tumor of the breast). Problems of living presenting as a physical symptom are another example (McWhinney, 1972). The PEG will show, in each instance, the precipitating and contributing factors in one of the squares in the recent or current context. Events such as bereavement, unemployment, and psychological depression may be found in conjunction with biological changes leading to a disease, and such associations raise questions for research concerning the physiologic mechanisms involved. For example, in a patient with current streptococcal pharyngitis and recent bereavement, one may wonder about the possible role of the central nervous system state (induced by bereavement) in (1) lowering immunologic resistance and (2) influencing the likelihood of subsequent development of rheumatic fever or glomerulonephritis. On the other hand, the combination of the presence of systems and signs in the absence of identifiable disease and the absence of convincing evidence that illness behavior can be attributed to the personal and environmental–interpersonal dimensions may indicate the need for a further search into the possibility of a yet unidentified or incompletely understood disease.

In most situations, the PEG will identify the strains in the biological (disease), personal (illness), and environmental–interpersonal systems. It will also clarify the interrelations among these dimensions in the context of the patient's traits, recent events and changes, and current states. In many instances, the etiologic, precipitating, and influencing factors in the disease, illness, and interpersonal tensions will become clear. Rational care plans for the whole patient that emerge from this will, again, be three-dimensional, with priorities determined by the contexts and gravity. Gravity refers to the seriousness or degree of strain or potential strain, while priority refers to the temporal order of approach. Overwhelming anxiety, impending rejection by a loved one, or the presence of malignant cells are examples of gravity. Contextual factors such as traits, effect of recent events (change), and current states suggest the possible ease of intervention in increasing order. Although intervention at the level of etiology would be most effective, it is not always possible. Examples are many viral diseases, fracture, or pain without identifiable tissue damage. Even when etiologic treatment of a disease is indicated, its (timing) priority may be secondary to intervention at the personal level, for example, relief of anxiety so that hospitalization can take place, leading to etiologic treatment of the disease.

The priority of care or intervention is a matter of clinical judgment. For example, treatment of a grave disease may take priority over possible job loss due to prolonged hospitalization for a patient. On the other hand, relief from an anxiety state may take priority over discussing elective surgical treatment plans for a patient with a chronic disorder such as inguinal hernia. For a patient with a congenital heart disease (background context, biological dimension) who comes to the physician with vague symptoms and depressive affect (current context, personal dimension) and who had recently lost a spouse (recent context, environmental dimension), the priority may be, first, relief from the depression, which, in turn, may relieve the vague symptoms; second, interpersonal support; and third, possible treatment of the congenital heart disease. On the other hand, the priority for a chronically depressed patient (background context, personal dimension) who presents with exacerbated old or even new symptoms arising out of current problems of living would be to deal first with them, rather than with the chronic depression.

To operationalize the use of the PEG for patient care planning, the following steps may be taken:

1. Underline the factors that appear important
   a. in the patient's current suffering;
   b. in the pathogenesis of his disease;
   c. in his attitude and fantasies concerning his illness;
   d. in his perception and attitudes concerning the health care system.
2. Also underline major limiting factors in possible intervention and care, such as personality style, nature and quality of interpersonal relationships (supportive persons), and occupation.
3. On the basis of the PEG and, especially, the underlined factors, make a three-dimensional list of plans and assign priorities.

Summary

Comprehensive assessment of a patient must include evaluation of three levels of systems (dimensions): the biological (component) dimension, the personal (the whole patient) dimension, and the environmental–interpersonal dimension that surrounds the patient. *Disease* is a concept that implies a dysfunction in the biological dimension, while *illness* refers to the biological dysfunction plus the suffering and social problems attendant to the disease. Illness behavior, however, may be present in the absence of disease, and a disease need not produce an illness, especially in early stages.

From the vantage point of medical practice, it is useful to evaluate the three dimensions cited above in terms of three longitudinal time *contexts,* the current, recent, and background. This is the *systems–contextual* approach to patients. The three dimensions (biological–personal–environmental) intersected by the three contexts (current, recent, background) form the *patient evaluation grid* (PEG), which is the operational method by which information about a patient can be organized.

The PEG allows the clinician to anticipate problems relating to patient care and to assign priorities to management plans formulated in the three dimensions. In each dimension, the current context information represents the current state and pressing needs; the recent context information represents the contributing and precipitating factors; and the background context information represents the broad background factors from which the recent and current problems have emerged and which often are resistant to change and so may impose limits in constructing plans for management.

Implications

For the Patient

The patient brings with him three separate but interacting systems when he seeks help. Although the chief complaint may refer to distress (personal dimension) caused by a disease (biological dimension), the implications of hospitalization, the disease, and treatment plans inevitably involve his family, work, and physical surroundings. Factors in any of the dimensions may become an intervening variable influencing the patient's clinical course and behavior in the sick role.

For the Physician

By the use of the PEG and the systems– contextual framework in evaluating patients, the physician can approach or aspire to a comprehensive understanding of the patient. This understanding will complement a narrower medical model of disease that leads to the diagnosis and treatment of diseases rather than patients. Such an approach enables the physician to pay attention to (1) the pressing needs of the patient in the personal dimension (including felt distress; see Chapter 3), (2) the contributing and precipitating events, and (3) the factors that must be kept in mind as stable and limiting influences (e.g., the personality type of the patient and cultural sick role expectations) on the disease in the narrower sense.

For the Community and Health Care System

The need for a holistic, patient-centered perspective in medicine is increasing in urgency (Barondess, 1974). Such a perspective can be obtained by a general systems model of illness and health (Menninger, 1963; Engel, 1960, 1977). The systems–contextual approach we use is also based on a general systems model (Leigh and Reiser, 1977), but it is in practice closely linked with and complementary to the medical model through the use of the patient evaluation grid (Leigh *et al.*, 1980). We feel that this (or a similar) approach could be adopted with benefit especially in medical schools, where physicians of the future may, from the very beginning, learn the importance and interactions of the nine areas represented by the PEG. With this comprehensive framework, the science of medicine can develop side by side with the art of medicine.

Recommended Reading

Feinstein AR: *Clinical Judgment.* Huntington, NY, Robert E Krieger Publishing Co, 1974. This is an excellent and scholarly book on the science and art of clinical judgment in medicine. This includes the way physicians collect and use clinical data and the concepts of disease, illness, treatment, and response, among others. It has very interesting and thought-provoking chapters on diagnostic taxonomy, including how the concept of disease has changed throughout history. For example, some of the diseases in Hippocratic times were fever, cyanosis, consumption, and asthma. A highly recommended reading for students in medicine.

Leigh H, Reiser MF: Major trends in psychosomatic medicine: The psychiatrist's evolving role in medicine. *Ann Intern Med* **83**:233–239, 1977. In this article, we give an overview of the development of psychosomatic medicine. We show that the emphasis of psychosomatic medicine is the integration of biopsychosocial factors in the comprehensive management of patients. This is based on the emerging general systems model for all diseases in which the biological, personal, and environmental systems interact.

Menninger K: *The Vital Balance.* New York, Viking Press, 1963. This is a classic work by one of the most venerated psychiatrists in this country on a general systems model of psychiatric disorders. Although Menninger's taxonomy of emotional disorders (e.g., the "orders of dyscontrol") has not achieved wide acceptance, this represents an interesting alternative to the medical model of mental illness. There is extensive discussion on classifications in medicine as well as on the role of the physician in mental illness.

References

Barondess JA: Science in medicine: Some negative feedbacks. *Arch Intern Med* **134**:152–157, 1974.

Engel GL: A unified concept of health and disease. *Perspect Biol Med* **3**:459–485, 1960.

Engel GL: The need for a new medical model: A challenge to biomedicine. Science **196**:129–136, 1977.

Feinstein AR: *Clinical Judgment.* Huntington, NY, Robert E Krieger Publishing Co, 1974.

Holmes I, Rahe RH: The social readjustment rating scale. *J Psychosom Res* **1:**213–218, 1968.

Leigh H, Reiser MF: Major trends in psychosomatic medicine: The psychiatrist's evolving role in medicine. *Ann Intern Med* **83:**233–239, 1977.

Leigh H, Feinstein AR, Reiser MF: The patient evaluation grid. A systematic approach to comprehensive care. *Gen Hosp Psychiatry,* 1980 (in press).

McWhinney JR: Beyond diagnosis: An approach to the integration of behavioral science and clinical medicine. *N Engl J Med* **287:**384–387, 1972.

Mechanic D: The concept of illness behavior. *J Chronic Dis* **15:**189–194, 1962.

Menninger K: *The Vital Balance.* New York, Viking Press, 1963.

Rahe RH: Subject's recent life changes and their near future illness suspectibility. *Adv Psychosom Med* **83:**2–19, 1972.

CHAPTER 10

The Current Context of Help-Seeking Behavior

1. A 42-year-old man was brought to the emergency room of the general hospital by police officers who had found him lying on the street. The patient, unmarried, was identified as a known alcoholic who had been evicted from his room. The presumptive diagnosis after careful examination was alcoholic intoxication. After a few hours, he was alert and coherent, and his vital signs were stable. The emergency room physician felt that he could be discharged without any further treatment.

2. A 33-year-old married man carrying a paper bag containing a week-old sandwich came to see his doctor. He was obviously anxious and agitated. He told the doctor, "I am sure I am being poisoned by my wife. Please examine me and find out what poison she has been using. I brought this sandwich she made for me last week; I am sure that it is poisoned!" For several months the patient had suspected that his wife was having an affair and, recently, had been secretly following her to catch her with her lover. He was convinced that her lover was his boss. As evidence, he cited a recent raise he received in his salary. "Unless he has a guilty conscience, why would he give me a raise?" Although physical examinations and laboratory tests showed no evidence of poisoning, the patient refused to believe that he was not being poisoned. In fact, he accused the doctor of colluding with his wife.

3. A 45-year-old married woman was admitted to the psychiatric ward because of serious depressive symptoms, including suicidal ideation. On physical examination, her blood pressure was moderately elevated, and it was found that she had been taking a "blood pressure pill" for several weeks. A phone call to her internist by the psychiatrist revealed that the blood pressure pill was reserpine, a medication known to cause depression. The medication was discontinued.

In assessing patients, it is essential to understand the immediate current situation of the patient and its relation to his help-seeking behavior. In vignette 1, help was sought by the police for the patient because he was lying on the street drunk. Upon arrival in the emergency room, he was found to need no further acute medical treatment. For another patient, this would have been enough reason for discharge from the hospital, but this patient could not be sent home—he had no home to go to. The immediate *social* situation, in this case, dictated his being sent to a temporary shelter with referral to an alcoholic program.

In vignette 2, the help-seeking behavior was due to a *psychological state* (paranoid psychosis). In this psychotic state, no amount of reassurance by the physician would change the conviction; rather, the physician himself became an object of suspicion. In vignette 3, the psychiatric problem (depression) was probably due to the effects of the antihypertensive drug reserpine on the central nervous system. Here, the immediate *biological state* of the patient determined the nature of the illness that occasioned the help-seeking behavior. What is important to recognize here is that current social, psychological, and biological factors and states can and do participate and interact in influencing illness and help-seeking behavior.

The Current Context in the Biological Dimension

The biological state of the patient, that is, the state of the component systems, organs, and tissues, is, of course, most often the underlying basis of the patient's illness and help-seeking behavior. The diagnosis of the disease underlying the distress and symptoms often provides the physician with a logical approach to treatment of the *disease.* An understanding of the disease, combined with an understanding of the person and the environment of the patient, will lead to a rational management plan for the *patient.*

History, physical examination, and laboratory tests are the tools that provide information concerning the current biological state. In this dimension, one is concerned with bodily states—condition of tissues, organs, organ systems, etc. (e.g., is the heart enlarged because of overwork? If so, what is causing the overwork? Hyperthyroidism? How is the thyroid gland behaving? What is the plasma thyroid hormone level? etc.)

The Current Context in the Personal Dimension

At the level of the whole patient as a unit system, the psychological state and current behavior should be considered. Current behavior of the patient includes such observations as whether the patient is complaining of suffering such as pain or is experiencing anxiety related to symptoms such as grossly red (bloody?) urine. The concept of patient behavior (McWhinney, 1972) leading to doctor–patient contact is useful here (see Chapter 1). In addition to the current help-seeking behavior and chief complaints, other behaviors, such as manner of speech, tremor, perspiration, and gait, should be considered.

The psychological state of the patient can be ascertained by a mental-status examination and by direct observation of the patient's behavior. The significance of the current psychological state of the patient is that it colors the history that can be obtained from the patient, and it influences the efficacy or inefficacy of specific approaches to the patient for optimal management. For example, in the case of vignette 2, the patient's paranoid psychosis resulted in a definite distortion in history. The physician's reassurances only resulted in the breakdown of the doctor–patient relationship. Another example is the depressed patient whose history is often distorted systematically, that is, thoroughly permeated by a pessimistic, hopeless outlook and perspective as a result of the depressive syndrome. A confused patient will obviously give a confused history.

The mental status consists of the following components: (1) appearance; (2) levels of consciousness and orientation; (3) status of the communicative facilities (speech and movement); (4) cognitive processes (attention, concentration, comprehension, memory, perception, thinking logical thoughts, abstraction, judgment); and (5) affect (expression, experience, lability)—both subjective and objective.

Outline of the Mental-Status Examination

Appearance. Appearance is an excellent indicator of the sum total of a patient's mental status at a given point. Sloppy, disheveled appearance often signifies self-neglect or preoccupation and distraction. Flushed appearance and the smell of alcohol on the breath, combined with characteristic drunken behavior, point to the diagnosis of alcoholic intoxication. Pale, emaciated appearance accompanied by malodorous and sloppy dress may indicate the presence of depression or cachexia. Some patients with a lesion in some areas of the nondominant hemisphere of the brain may dress only one side of the body, completely oblivious to the presence of the other side. Such patients may pay attention only to one-half of the visual field.

Notations on appearance should include observations on the general impression made by the patient (sloppy, neat, emaciated, etc.), including any unusual features (completely shaved scalp, unusual bodily habitus, dress, etc.).

Levels of Consciousness and Orientation. Awareness of self and environment constitutes *consciousness* in the mental-status examination. Consciousness may be subdivided into *content* of consciousness and *arousal*. The sum total of mental functions, including the ability to *remember* and to *think*, comprises the content of the consciousness, while the appearance of wakefulness and response to stimuli form the bases of inference concerning arousal. The content of consciousness is largely a function of the cerebral hemispheres, while the state of arousal is largely a function of the reticular activating system in the brain stem (Plum and Posner, 1972) (see Figure 7).

Arousal. Levels of consciousness may be classified as follows.

• *Hyperalert* state—Increased state of arousal in which the patient is acutely aware of all sensory input. Anxiety and certain central nervous system stimulants can cause this state.

• *Alert* state—Normal degree of alertness.

• *Dullness* and *sleepiness*—May be due to fatigue and insomnia, as well as to sedating medications (either as primary effect or side effect). Metabolic derangements due to disease can also result in dullness and sleepiness, such as in uremia and hypercalcemia.

• *Clouding* of consciousness—A state of reduced wakefulness in which periods of excitability and irritability often alternate with periods of drowsiness. Illusions, especially visual, may occur, and the patient is often startled. Mild to moderate toxic states, withdrawal states, and metabolic derangements can cause this.

• *Confusional* states—In addition to clouding of consciousness, there is consistent misinterpretation of stimuli and shortened attention span. There is disorientation at least to time and often to place. Memory is often poor, and the patient appears perplexed. This is a more severe degree of clouding of consciousness.

• *Delirium*—When used to denote a particular and often fluctuating *level* of consciousness, delirium may include a florid state of agitation, disorientation, fear, misperception of sensory stimuli, and, often, visual hallucinations. The patients are often loud, talkative, and supicious and are sometimes completely out of contact with the environment. The degree of contact may vary. Delirium usually occurs in moderately severe toxic states and metabolic derangements of the central nervous system, including withdrawal from central nervous system depressants such as alcohol and barbiturates.

The term *"delirium"* is *sometimes* used to denote *all reversible organic brain syndromes* due to metabolic encephalopathy. When used in this sense, delirium is in contrast to dementia, which implies irreversible changes in the brain. Agitation and florid psychotic picture may be lacking in patients with delirium in this broader sense; that is, the patient with reversible confusion and disorientation may be placid and drowsy rather than agitated.

• *Stupor*—In this state, the patient is unresponsive to stimuli unless their application is very strong and repeated. Usually caused by diffuse cerebral dysfunction.

• *Coma*—Complete unresponsiveness to stimuli. Even strong and repeated stimuli cannot arouse the patient. This occurs in severe dysfunction of the brain, such as serious intoxication or severe head trauma.

Content of Consciousness. *Orientation* refers to the person's consciousness of the orienting markers, such as correct awareness of *time, place,* and *person.* Impairment of orientation results in *confusion.* The orientation of a patient is determined by asking questions such as, "What day of the week is it today?" "Where are you right now?" "What is your name?" In case of insufficiency in the cerebral cortical functions for any reason (most often due to metabolic derangement of the brain or neuronal destruction), orientation may be impaired to varying degrees. Impairment of orientation usually occurs in the order of time, place, and person. In hospitalized patients, disorientation as to date is not uncommon, perhaps due to the change in daily schedule following hospitalization, distractions by the medical procedures, etc. In the absence of cerebral insufficiency, however, most patients are oriented to the month and year if not to the exact date. Orientation as to person, especially to the patient himself, usually is not impaired until the very latest stage of cerebral insufficiency, although the patient may often forget the names of others, especially those persons encountered recently. Disorientation to the self in spite of relatively normal mental-status examination in other areas strongly suggests a dissociative disorder rather than cerebral insufficiency (organic brain syndrome).

Status of Communication Facilities (Speech and Movement). In assessing the communicative facilities of a patient, one should consider the integrity of the apparatuses, the effect of learning and psychological state, and the content of the communication.

Integrity of Apparatuses. The organs related to speech and movement should be assessed. Weakness of the tongue or facial muscles may produce dysarthria (difficulty in articulating words). Hemiplegia may cause the patient to gesticulate with only one hand. A painful lesion in the mouth may force the patient to be verbally noncommunicative. Deafness may result in nonresponse to a question.

Disorders of language *(aphasia)* caused by brain lesions may be present. Aphasia should be distinguished from dysarthria; the former is due to problems with language itself at the brain level, while the latter refers to difficulty in articulation. In aphasia, written language as well as verbal speech is affected. Aphasias may be roughly classified into *expressive* and *receptive* types. Expressive aphasia is related to lesions of the motor speech (Broca's) area in the dominant frontal lobe of the brain. The patient with expressive aphasia has major difficulties in translating thoughts to symbols; thus, what the patient wishes to express may come out in a distorted form or not at all. He is usually aware of this distortion or difficulty in his own speech and, for this reason, is usually reluctant to speak (or write). Receptive or sensory aphasia is due to lesions of the sensory speech (Wernicke's) area of the dominant temporal lobe. In this condition, the patient has difficulties in comprehending language, including his own speech. Thus, the patient's speech may be garbled, but he may *not* be aware of the problems with his speech. Unlike patients with expressive aphasia, those with the receptive form are usually fluent, although often incomprehensible to others. There are varying combinations and subtypes of aphasias, and for more complete discussion, the readers are referred to textbooks of neurology.

Effect of Learning and Psychological State. Given intact apparatuses for communication, the form of communication often depends on the psychological state of the patient and the effect of learning. The effect of learning determines the language in which the patient will express his feelings and thoughts as well as the fluency and facility of the language. For example, middle-class patients are more likely to use grammatically correct syntax and the elaborated code (see Chapter 3). Some patients may use dialects or culturally specific expressions. Current psychological state also determines speech and nonverbal communication. A euphoric patient is more likely to be effusive, verbose, and flamboyant; a depressed patient may be uncommunicative and withdrawn.

Content of Communication. What the patient is communicating forms the content of communication. Understanding the content of the patient's communication is essential for the physician to be helpful to the patient. This is more than just accepting the spoken language of the patient at face value; it involves an attempt to understand what the patient really *means* through his communication. For example, when a patient comes to the doctor and asks "Is there a cure for Hodgkin's disease?" much more may be involved than simple intellectual curiosity.

The content of communication often reveals the psychological state of the patient, for example, themes of hopelessness and death in depressed states, and bizarre contents in psychotic states. Extreme suspiciousness and ideas of persecution may indicate paranoid psychosis (as in vignette 2).

The content of communication includes the chief complaint, which is the perceived distress for which the patient is seeking help. For a further discussion of its significance, the reader is referred to Chapter 3. Pain is one of the most common chief complaints, and Chapter 7 should be referred to for a fuller discussion. The presence of delusions and paranoid thinking can also be determined by paying attention to the content of the communication (see below).

Cognitive Processes. These are the *processes* that determine the content of consciousness. The processes include attention, perception, memory, concentration, comprehension, abstraction, logical thinking, and judgment. Diminution in the function of any of these areas may indicate the presence of pathology in the cerebral cortex or limbic system. It should be noted, however, that what is important is a *decrease* in function *from the premorbid state* and not necessarily the absolute level of functioning, since the absolute level of abstract thinking, comprehension, etc., may be determined by background and by long-term variables such as constitutional endowment, educational level, and habitual functional level, as well as by illness. For example, cerebral pathology is more probably present in a college professor who cannot remember the names of the past five presidents than in a blue-collar worker with a tenth-grade education.

The cognitive processes can be tested both indirectly and directly. *Indirectly,* inferences can be made concerning the patient's memory, judgment, concentration, comprehension, etc., by asking the patient to describe the present illness and his personal history. Does the patient remember the dates (or years) of graduation from schools, marriage, etc.? Does the patient comprehend the nature of his illness and the proposed procedures? Does he remember what has been told him by the physicians? Does he seem to be aware of the possible risks and complications?

When there is any question concerning the patient's ability to concentrate, comprehend, or think in a logical fashion, a direct and formal testing of the cognitive functions may be necessary.

Direct Tests of Cognitive Processes. Before doing direct tests of cognitive processes, it is best to tell the patient the following: "Now, I would like to ask you to do some things that may seem a bit inappropriate, but they are part of evaluating memory and concentration and so forth. They can help us evaluate and adjust medications which may tend to make you feel drowsy or cause difficulty in concentrating," etc. This type of reassurance may put the patient at ease about possible errors he may make and gives the testing a medical context. In fact, sedating medications may need to be reduced if the patient is found to be too drowsy or if concentration is diminished.

1. Orientation. The significance of this was discussed above. When doing a direct cognitive testing, it is useful to ask questions concerning orientation first. The questions may be, "What day is today? What is the date (or day of the week)?" If the patient does not know, then, "What month is it now?" "What year?" may follow. Mild disorientation as to time (e.g., not knowing the date) is common even among normal persons, but severe disorientation (e.g.,

not knowing the month and year) is indicative of cerebral dysfunction. "Where are you right now? The name of this place?" These test orientation as to place. If the patient does not know, then, "Are you in a hospital, a hotel, or a supermarket?" The patient may know that he is in the hospital (or a doctor's office), but may not know the name of the hospital or clinic, which indicates a milder degree of dysfunction than not knowing the nature of the place or confusing it with somewhere else, such as a hotel room. The next question (orientation as to self) might be, "What is your name?" As discussed previously, dysfunction in orientation proceeds in an orderly manner from time to place to person. In fact, except in cases of very severe brain disease, orientation as to self is usually well preserved. Of course, delusional patients may have a distorted orientation as to self; for example, "I am Napoleon Bonaparte."

2. Memory, Attention, Concentration, Comprehension. Presidents: "Who is the President of the United States now?" If the patient answers correctly, "Yes; and before him?" etc., until four or five names have been given correctly. This tests recent memory and information of the patient. Most patients with average high-school education can remember four or five recent presidents.

Calculations: Asking the patient to do simple calculations can test the patient's ability to attend to and comprehend the physician's instructions and to concentrate and utilize immediate memory. "How much is 15 plus 17?" "25 minus 7?" If the patient has difficulty, an easier calculation involving single digits should be tried. Unlike additions and subtractions, simple multiplications, such as 4 times 6, are easier tasks, since they involve primarily long-term memory (which is resistant to decay) and comprehension of the instructions. Thus, if the patient can do 4 times 6 but not 15 plus 17, then one might wonder whether the patient has difficulties with concentration and immediate or recent memory but not with remote memory and comprehension (indicating possible brain dysfunction). On the other hand, if the patient has difficulties with both, low educational level or mental retardation might be suspected.

If there is reason to suspect difficulties on the basis of simple calculations, serial 7s and digit span might be done. *Serial 7s* are done by asking the patient to subtract 7 from 100 and to keep subtracting 7s from the result. This tests sustained attention and concentration as well as short-term memory. If serial 7s are too difficult for the patient, serial 5s or 2s may be tried. *Digit span* is tested by asking the patient to repeat a number of digits, such as 5–8–3–9–6–2. Digit span backward is tested by asking the patient to repeat in reverse order the numbers that you give him. For example, "If I say 1–2–3, please say '3–2–1.'" This tests primarily short-term memory and concentration. Most patients without brain dysfunction can do at least six digits forward and four digits backward.

Memory, especially recent memory, is very sensitive to dysfunction of the brain. There is some evidence that the limbic system structures, especially the hippocampus, are involved in the coding of recent memory into the long-term memory mechanisms (see Figures 4 and 5). Any metabolic derangement and structural damage to the limbic system (which is especially sensitive to anoxia) and the cerebral hemispheres can result in problems with memory.

When memory dysfunction is suspected, the physician can test the registration, retention, and recall of memory by the following steps: First, ask the patient if he remembers your name. If he does not, give him your name and ask him to repeat it (immediate memory: registration and immediate recall). Then, tell him that you would like him to remember the names of four objects, such as a pen, a telephone, a flashlight, and a book. Tell him to repeat the names of the four objects immediately. In about five minutes or so, ask the patient if he remembers your name; also, the names of the four objects (recent memory: retention and recall). The patient may be able to remember only one or two objects (diminished recent memory). If the patient cannot recall the names at all, ask the patient, "Please say 'yes' if any of the objects I name now is one of the objects I named before: pencil, pen, television, telephone, book," etc. (If the patient can identify the articles but could not remember them, it may indicate the presence of retention but difficulty with recall).

3. Abstraction. Similarities: This tests the ability of the patient to see similarities among objects and to categorize them on the basis of the similarities. For example, "What is the similarity between a cat and a dog?" The patient may answer, "They are both animals" (a good abstraction) or "They both have legs" (a concrete response). In case of the latter, you might ask, "Then how about a dog, a cat, and a snake?" At this point, the patient may be able to abstract and say, "They are all animals." Proverbs: For example, "What does the old saying, 'People who live in glass houses shouldn't throw stones' mean?" "Don't cry over spilt milk," etc.

In testing for abstraction, one should recognize that these are most subject to influences of educational level, cultural background, and language. For example, those from non-English-speaking cultures may have great difficulty in abstracting English-language proverbs.

A concrete response in tests for abstraction may indicate possible brain dysfunction, low educational level, low intelligence, or formal thought disorder, as in schizophrenia. An *idiosyncratic* or *bizarre* response may indicate an unusual way of thinking, as in psychosis. For example, "What is the similarity between a cat and a dog?" "They are both my enemies." "What does the proverb, 'People who live in glass houses shouldn't throw stones' mean?" "That means that even if you have enough money to buy a glass house, you should not throw away money. Stones are gems, you know, which cost a lot of money."

4. Logical Thinking and Judgment. Patients with brain dysfunction may

show varying degrees of difficulty with judgment. Judgment means the ability to act appropriately in social and emergency situations. Many questions concerning judgment also involve the ability to think logically. For example, "If you were in a crowded theater and happened to discover fire and smoke coming from the ceiling, what should you do?" A good answer would be, "I would tell the usher or manager." If the patient replies, "I would yell 'fire,' " the physician might ask, "If you yelled 'fire,' what would happen?" The patient with intact logical thinking may then say, "I guess that would cause panic . . . perhaps I should not yell fire.' " Other judgment questions include, "What would you do if you found an envelope with an address and a stamp on it on the street?"

Patients with personality disorders without organic brain dysfunction may give idiosyncratic or inappropriate responses to judgment questions. For example, an impulsive patient may say, "I would try to put out the fire by throwing my can of soda on it."

5. Perception. The patient's perception can be tested by first observing if the patient seems to be aware of the tester's presence and whether the patient seems to be responding to visual or auditory hallucinations (e.g., carrying on a conversation or touching). Then, the patient can be asked questions such as, "Have you ever had any experiences of hearing things or seeing things that weren't there?" "Any experience of things changing shape or becoming distorted?"

6. Delusions and Paranoid Thinking. A delusion is an idea firmly held by a patient which is not corroborated by reality. Delusions may be grandiose ("I am God"), persecutory ("Everybody is out to get me"), or depressive ("Worms are eating my brain out"). Some delusions involve diseases, such as, "I know I have cancer, no matter what the tests show." The term "paranoid" is often used to describe patients who have persecutory ideas or delusions.

The presence of delusions is usually manifested by the content of the patient's communications. Delusion formation is a process by which perceptions are put into some kind of perspective. Thus, strange bodily sensations, due to whatever cause, may be attributed to "poisoning" and continuing presence of anxiety to "people spying on me." Obviously, when cognitive processes are not functioning optimally, and when the anxiety level is high (such as in a hospitalized patient with preexisting cognitive difficulties due to poor blood supply to the brain), the risk of delusion formation is greater; it is easier to misperceive stimuli or attribute confusing stimuli to a cause unrelated to reality (e.g., "The doctors are trying to kill me so that they can give my kidneys to someone else").

In addition to indicating the possible presence of cognitive difficulties, delusions give clues concerning the emotional state of the patient. For example, persecutory delusions are associated with anxiety, grandiose delusions with euphoria, and depressive delusions with a depressive syndrome.

Affect and Mood. Affect refers to feeling and is synonymous with emotion, although the latter is sometimes used to denote the physiologic aspects of affect (e.g., emotional response; see Chapters 4 and 6). Mood refers to prevailing and relatively enduring emotional tone.

Affect can be documented by observation and direct questioning. By observation, one can see whether the patient's affect is *appropriate* or *inappropriate* relative to the topic of conversation (does the patient smile while talking of sad events?) and whether it is *stable* or *labile*. Labile affect, as manifested, for example, by laughing one minute and then crying the next, may be indicative of organic brain dysfunction, in which case, there will be additional signs of cognitive difficulties. *Flat affect* means the absence of any display of affect and is often associated with extreme use of isolation as a defense mechanism (Chapter 5) or with schizophrenia.

Direct questions about affect might be, "How do you feel right now?" "Do you feel anxious?" etc. Physiologic signs such as sweating, rapid heart rate, and facial expressions also reveal affective states.

Mood can be ascertained by asking the patient how he has been feeling recently, for the past week or two. Family, friends, and relatives of the patient may also provide useful information concerning the mood of the patient. Depression or chronic feelings of anger may contribute to illness and help-seeking behavior.

The Current Context in the Environmental Dimension

It is very useful to pay attention to the environment of the patient as he comes to the doctor for help. This includes observing who has accompanied the patient and at whose prodding or suggestion the patient decided to seek help, as well as who is available to help the patient should the need arise. For example, who might be able to sign a consent form for procedures in case the patient himself becomes incapable of doing so?

The patient's occupation and work environment are an important area of consideration in terms of possible expense of hospitalization and loss of wages due to illness, as well as in terms of possible toxins associated with certain types of work environments (e.g., heavy-metal poisoning in chemical factories).

The effect of the patient's assumption of the sick role on his family and work should also be considered. The physician may have to help the patient decide whether or not he should delegate his work to someone else during his hospitalization, on the basis of the expected incapacity, prognosis, and the necessity of the patient's personal involvement in work.

Interaction among the Current Context Dimensions

The psychological state of the patient (central nervous system), the biological state (state of the organs and tissues), and environmental factors are closely correlated and influence each other. For example, in anxiety states, there is often an elevation of blood pressure, pulse rate, and generalized sympathetic nervous system discharge, as well as increases in corticosteroid hormone levels. The anxiety related to hospitalization alone may result in increases in plasma levels of adrenocortical and, possibly, thyroid hormones. On the other hand, organ diseases and endogenous and exogenous toxins can influence the psychological state of the patient, including depression, anxiety, personality change, and even psychosis (see Table 8).

Table 8. Partial List of Organ Diseases
Often Associated with Psychiatric Syndromes

Anxiety

Hyperthyroidism
Pheochromocytoma
Carcinoid syndrome
Menopausal syndrome, premenstrual tension
Hyperinsulinism (including insulin overdose)
Withdrawal from a CNS-depressant drug (alcohol, narcotics, sedatives)

Depression

Carcinoma (especially tail of pancreas, but any occult cancer can cause depression)
Hypothyroidism
Hyperthyroidism
Diabetes mellitus
Cushing's syndrome
Addison's disease
Administration of ACTH
Antihypertensive therapy (especially reserpine, but also with methyldopa and propranolol)
Any electrolyte imbalance
Uremia

Euphoria/mania

Hyperthyroidism
Steroid psychosis
Multiple sclerosis (depression is also common in this syndrome)
Ingestion of a CNS stimulant (e.g., amphetamines)

Personality change

Frontal lobe lesion of the brain due to any cause, including metastases, diffuse encephalopathies,
    such as Alzheimer's disease, and focal lesions in lupus erythematosus

Table 8 *(continued)*

Paranoid psychosis

Steroid psychosis
Hyper- and hypothyroidism
Hypoglycemia
Amphetamine psychosis
Withdrawal from a CNS-depressant drug

Organic brain syndromes and toxic psychosis

Electrolyte imbalance
   Acid–base imbalance
   Sodium imbalance (especially hyponatremia)
   Potassium imbalance (especially hypokalemia)
   Magnesium imbalance (especially hypomagnesemia)
   Calcium imbalance

Drugs (withdrawal or intoxication)
   Alcohol withdrawal
   Barbiturate withdrawal
   Intoxication by any licit or illicit drug
Overmedication
   Tricyclic antidepressants
   Phenothiazines
      Anticholinergics
      Sedatives
      Analgesics (opiates, pentazocine)
   Digitalis
Undermedication
   Analgesics
Environmental toxins
   Heavy metals (lead, arsenic, copper, etc.)
   Organic phosphate compounds
Ventilation–perfusion problems
   Hypoxia (e.g., anemia, chronic obstructive lung disease)
   Congestive heart failure
   Hypovolemia (dehydration, hemorrhage, shock)
Neurologic diseases
   Cerebrovascular accidents (CVA)
   Tumor
   Infection
   Trauma
   Epilepsy
   Degenerative diseases (e.g., Alzheimer's disease)
Vascular diseases
   Arteriosclerosis
   Inflammatory disease of blood vessels (e.g., Systemic lupus erythematosus)
Endocrine diseases
   Thyroid (hyper- or hypo-)
   Parathyroid (hyper- or hypo-)

(continued)

Table 8 *(continued)*

Endocrine diseases *(continued)*
  Addison's disease
  Cushing's syndrome
Deficiency states
  General malnutrition
  Pernicious anemia (B_{12} deficiency)
  Thiamine
  Pyridoxine
  Pellagra (nicotinic acid deficiency)
Environmental factors
  Room location (noisy or too secluded)
  Lack of stimulation
  Poor lighting
Other
  Hypoglycemia
  Hepatic encephalopathy (ammonia intoxication)
  Uremia
  Fever
  Remote effects of malignancy
  Postanesthesia
  Porphyria
  Blood dyscrasias

An often frightening state in which a patient may present himself to the physician is the state of catatonia—the patient is mute, unresponsive, and rigid. When the physician changes the patient's posture by, for example, lifting up his arm, the arm remains in the new position ("waxy flexibility"). The vital signs are usually normal in this state. This *catatonic syndrome* has been regarded as typical of a form of schizophrenia. Many other conditions and diseases, however, can give rise to many features of the catatonic syndrome (as in Table 9). The presence of one or more features of the syndrome should not lead the physician to make the diagnosis of schizophrenia and forego further workup to rule out underlying medical or neurologic diseases.

As in the case of depression, the presence of any psychiatric syndrome should alert the physician to the possibility that it might be *secondary* to a disease in the biological dimension or to an environmental factor.

Summary

The current context of help-seeking behavior can be assessed at the environmental, personal, and biological levels. The *environmental* level information is important in understanding the patient's interpersonal resources,

Table 9. List of Conditions
Often Associated with the Catatonic Syndrome[a]

Psychiatric disorders
Schizophrenia
Affective disorders
Neuroses and related phenomena

Neurologic disorders
Basal ganglia (following bilateral surgical lesions of the globus pallidus)
Limbic system and temporal lobes
  Akinetic mutism
  Focal temporal abnormalities
Diencephalon
  Tumors and traumatic hemorrhage in the region of the third ventricle
  Focal lesions of the thalamus
Other brain lesions
  Frontal lobe tumors
  Focal frontal lobe lesions
  Anterior cerebral artery aneurysm
  Arterial malformation of the posterior circulation
  Diffuse brain trauma
  Diffuse encephalomalacia following closed head injury
  Petit mal status
  Postictal phase of epilepsy
  Wernicke's encephalopathy
  Tuberous sclerosis
  General paresis
  Narcolepsy
  Acute phase of encephalitis lethargica
  Cerebral macular degeneration

Metabolic conditions
Diabetic ketoacidosis
Hypercalcemia from parathyroid adenoma
Pellagra
Acute intermittent porphyria
Homocystinuria
Membranous glomerulonephritis
Hepatic encephalopathy

Toxic agents
Organic fluorides
Illuminating gas
Psychotomimetic drugs
Chronic amphetamine intoxication
Phencyclidine (PCP) intoxication

Pharmacologic agents
Aspirin intoxication
ACTH
High-potency antipsychotic agents

[a]After Gelenberg (1976). Reproduced with permission.

which, in turn, is helpful in planning rehabilitation and convalescence, among other things, and also in understanding possible contributory factors to illness, such as noxious environmental factors.

At the *personal* level, the current psychological state can be assessed by the mental-state examination. This information is important because it provides the physician with the immediate pressing needs and concerns of the patient as well as the immediate limitations (such as psychosis or confusion).

The current *biological* level information is the basis for the diagnosis of disease as well as often being the cause of the patient's distress. There are many biological disease processes and organ states that are associated with psychiatric syndromes. In many of these patients, the psychiatric syndrome (e.g., depression) may be the presenting complaint. Treatment of the underlying medical disease is essential for relief from the psychiatric syndrome in these patients.

Implications

For the Patient

The current context factors such as chief complaint, physical state, and interpersonal strain have the greatest urgency and immediacy for the patient, and help-seeking behavior is determined by, and directed toward, these factors. The immediate context variables may also limit the patient's ability to communicate (e.g., stuporous or psychotic state) or call for immediate intervention (e.g., state of hypotensive shock).

For the Physician

Understanding the patient's immediate needs, concerns, and limitations allows the physician to formulate immediate management plans. It is essential to understand the patient's immediate surroundings, including who accompanied the patient to the physician, as the family or friends can be invaluable as information sources and in health care planning. The physician should be aware that a number of organ states and *diseases,* such as occult carcinomas, can present with *psychiatric syndromes.* Thus, the presence of psychological abnormalities such as depression or psychosis should not be automatically taken as an indication that the patient is a "mental" patient whose problems are caused by factors at the environmental or personal level only. Even those psychiatric patients who have long-standing psychiatric illness may have, in addition, a medical disease.

For the Community and Health Care System

Medical education should place more emphasis on understanding patients in all three dimensions: the biological, personal, and environmental. Medical records should have provisions for documenting the factors at all three levels. Hospitals should pay attention to the immediate physical and social environments of patients and provide them with comfortable surroundings as well as a place for the family and friends accompanying patients. Hospital staff should be educated concerning the management of patients who are in altered states of consciousness, including stupor and psychosis. Since psychosis occurs in medical conditions requiring medical treatment, medical personnel should be trained to deal with such patients.

Recommended Reading

Alpers BH, Mancall EL: *Essentials of Neurological Examination.* Philadelphia, FA David, 1971. A concise and lucid manual for neurological examination which will complement the mental-status examination discussed in this chapter.
Harvey AM, Johns RJ, Owens AH Jr, *et al.: The Principles and Practice of Medicine,* ed 19. New York, Appleton-Century-Crofts, 1976, section 1 (The approach to the patient), pp 1–70. A good introduction to obtaining history, the diagnostic process, and approaches to management.
Plum F, Posner JB: *The Diagnosis of Stupor and Coma.* Philadelphia, FA David, 1972. This is an authoritative book on the evaluation of patients showing altered states of consciousness. A very good reference book.

References

Gelenberg AJ: The catatonic syndrome. Lancet **1**:1339–1341, 1976.
McWhinney JR: Beyond diagnosis: An approach to the integration of behavioral science and clinical medicine. *N Engl J Med* **287**:384–387, 1972.
Plum F, Posner JB: *The Diagnosis of Stupor and Coma.* Philadelphia, FA David, 1972.

CHAPTER 11

The Recent Context of Help-Seeking Behavior

1. A 50-year-old white married man, accompanied by his wife, comes to the psychiatrist's office with the chief complaint of severe depression which has become progressively worse over the past two months. The patient has trouble sleeping, has lost 20 pounds, and has difficulty concentrating. He has not gone to work for the last three days because "I feel so bad, I can't do anything." He has been constantly thinking about how worthless he is and has been contemplating suicide. On close questioning, the physician finds that three months ago, the patient was passed over for a promotion at work.

2. A 30-year-old single woman reports increasing asthmatic attacks which began about six months ago. History reveals that she had broken up with her fiance about seven months ago, after which her drinking increased. Incidentally, she has a cat in her apartment which was given to her by a friend about six months ago.

3. A 66-year-old widower is brought to the hospital by his neighbors because of his disruptive behavior. Lately, he has been observed walking around outside his apartment only half dressed and urinating in the street in full view of his neighbors. He also dumped his garbage in front of his neighbor's door. When the neighbor tried to speak to him, he was argumentative and assaultive. The neighbors could smell a strong stench coming from his apartment. Upon admission to the hospital (involuntarily, by commitment), he is found to have a tumor in the frontal lobe of the brain.

Also reread the vignettes in Chapter 9.

Recent changes and events in the patient's life often provide the physician with clues concerning the disease process and the factors contributing to it. In fact, illness itself is a recent change that causes help-seeking behavior. The changes may be a symptom of the disease process, as in vignette 3. Frontal lobe tumors often cause behavioral changes characterized by the loss of customary social behavior. In vignette 1, the loss of hoped-for promotion was responsible for the depressive syndrome. Either the acquisition of the cat or the loss of the relationship with the fiance, or the two together, may have been active in aggravation of the asthmatic syndrome in vignette 2.

The Recent Context in the Biological Dimension

Focusing on the events in this dimension in the recent context forms the *present illness* part of medical history. Recent changes and events in the biological dimension determine the present state and functioning of the organism. The precursors of disease and evidence of organ malfunction may be manifest in the recent past. Information concerning this may be obtained by careful history-taking. Such history should include specific questions about medications, including nonprescription and street drugs. Any history of recent visits to a doctor or hospitalization should be inquired into and information obtained from the physician or hospital.

Recent diseases, whatever the outcome, determine the level of resistance of the patient and the vulnerability to new disease processes. For example, the recent administration of a medication may have started an allergic reaction, setting the stage for a severe hypersensitivity reaction to subsequent intake of the same drug.

The Recent Context in the Personal Dimension

The psychological and behavioral aspects of the patient in the recent past comprise the recent context in this dimension. This includes changes in mood, interest, habits, and thoughts and other behavioral changes and events, for example, changes in smoking or drinking habits and changes in sleep patterns, appetite, and sexual activity.

Depression is an important recent context phenomenon that increases the risk of morbidity from any illness (see Chapter 6). For example, individuals who had an elevation of the depression scale on the Minnesota Multiphasic Personality Inventory (MMPI) were more likely to develop myocardial infarction without preexisting angina pectoris (Bruhn et al., 1969) and also had a poor prognosis once an infarction occurred. Depressed persons, of course, have a tendency to neglect personal hygiene and have poor dietary habits, which may contribute to increased likelihood of becoming ill. Fatigue, anxiety, and depressed mood may be manifestations of illnesses, such as in the case of hepatitis and infectious mononucleosis. Depression also often occurs secondary to cancer of the tail of the pancreas and other occult malignancies. The presence of depression in the recent context should draw the physician's attention to the possibility of an occult carcinoma and other medical disease that might cause depression (see Table 4).

Changes in personal habits such as drinking and smoking can directly contribute to pathogenesis of such diseases as coronary thrombosis, gastritis, pancreatitis, and liver failure. Increased drinking and smoking may be associated with strains in the environmental–interpersonal system, such as problems at work or with family.

Changes in interests may indicate changes in mood. For example, loss of interest in activities that usually provide the patient with gratification, such as hobbies and sex, is often associated with depression. On the other hand, getting involved in numerous activities and hypersexuality may be associated with a manic disorder. Certain drugs, such as amphetamines, and certain medical diseases, such as hyperthyroidism, can also cause hypomanic or manic behavior (see Chapter 6).

Another important area to be considered in the recent context at the personal level is the sleep pattern, which is an excellent example of the interrelationship among the biological, personal, and environmental dimensions (see Chapter 8).

The Recent Context in the Environmental Dimension

Changes in the *physical environment* of the patient can result in diseases associated with noxious agents. Such noxious influences include chemical poisons (e.g., lead and polyvinyls), infectious agents (e.g., the Legionnaire's bacilli), and changes in temperature, barometric pressure, noise level, etc., in the patient's living and working environment. History of foreign travel may explain an unusual infection in some patients.

Contact with street drugs and the drug culture is an important area to be evaluated, especially in relatively young patients. For example, a young man complaining of a peculiar sensation under his skin—that insects are crawling under the skin—may be suffering from the symptoms of cocaine intoxication ("cocaine bug"). In managing a young man admitted with multiple fractures after an automobile accident, ascertaining whether or not he has been using drugs, especially barbiturates, habitually, is important in order to prevent possible serious withdrawal reaction while in traction on the surgical intensive care unit. Barbiturates should never be withdrawn immediately from addicted patients, because convulsions and even deaths occur frequently during withdrawal. Information concerning drug use or exposure to drugs is often not volunteered. Direct questioning of the patients and friends or relatives is important.

Many heavy-metal poisonings, including lead and mercury poisoning, produce behavioral and neurologic manifestations and have to be differentiated from a psychiatric disorder.

The physical environment has effects not only in the biological system of the patient but also in the personal system *through psychological meanings.* A patient who has been accustomed to a large, single private office may become depressed or irritable in a crowded office after a change of job. Thus, environmental changes which may not, of themselves, be sufficient to cause disease directly may nevertheless cause an illness through perception of the change at the personal level.

Changes in the interpersonal–social environment have an important effect on help-seeking behavior in two ways: First, interpersonal strain may increase help-seeking behavior (Mechanic, 1962) (see Chapter 1); second, certain changes in the interpersonal environment may contribute to illness or disease through mechanisms not as yet clearly understood (see Chapters 4 and 6). For example, persons with a past history of residential or job mobility have higher rates of coronary disease than persons who have not had such mobility (Syme *et al.,* 1965; Jenkins, 1976). Significantly increased mortality and morbidity rates were found for bereaved first-degree relatives within the first year of bereavement (Parkes, 1972; Jacobs and Ostfeld, 1977; Rees and Lutkins, 1967). Increased blood pressure was found in persons who were experiencing job loss (Kasl and Cobb, 1970).

Holmes and Rahe (1968) developed the concept of "life change units" (LCUs) and the relative degree of necessary adjustment required to common life changes such as marriage and divorce. The relative weights were determined on the basis of questionnaires given to a large number of subjects. According to this scale, called the Social Readjustment Rating Scale, death of spouse has a value of 100 LCUs; divorce, 73; marriage, 50; all the way down to minor violations of the law, 11 (see Table 10). Rahe and his colleagues found that those who had fewer than 150 LCUs for a given year reported good health for the following year, and of those who had between 150 and 300 LCUs, about half reported illness in the following year (Rahe, 1972). Seventy percent of those who had more than 300 LCUs during the year had illnesses in the following year. A number of retrospective and prospective studies showed a significant relationship between mounting life changes and the occurrence of sudden cardiac death, myocardial infarction, accidents, athletic injuries, tuberculosis, leukemia, multiple sclerosis, diabetes, etc. (Rabkin and Struening, 1976). The presence of social support systems may have a protective effect

Table 10. Life Change Events and Life Change Units[a]

	LCU values
Family	
Death of spouse	100
Divorce	73
Marital separation	65
Death of close family member	63
Marriage	50
Marital reconciliation	45
Major change in health of family	44
Pregnancy	40
Addition of new family member	39
Major change in arguments with wife	35
Son or daughter leaving home	29
In-law troubles	29
Wife starting or ending work	26
Major change in family get-togethers	15
Personal	
Detention in jail	63
Major personal injury or illness	53
Sexual difficulties	39
Death of a close friend	37
Outstanding personal achievement	28
Start or end of formal schooling	26
Major change in living conditions	25
Major revision of personal habits	24
Changing to a new school	20
Change in residence	20
Major change in recreation	19
Major change in church activities	19
Major change in social activities	18
Major change in sleeping habits	16
Major change in eating habits	15
Vacation	13
Christmas	12
Minor violations of the law	11
Work	
Being fired from work	47
Retirement from work	45
Major business adjustment	39
Changing to different line of work	36
Major change in work responsibilities	29
Trouble with boss	23
Major change in working conditions	20
Financial	
Major change in financial state	38
Mortgage or loan over $10,000	31
Mortgage foreclosure	30
Mortgage or loan less than $10,000	17

[a]From Gunderson and Rahe (1974). Reproduced with permission from Charles C Thomas.

against the occurrence of illness in spite of high LCUs (Dean and Lin, 1977). Thus, an understanding of the nature of and changes in the interpersonal environment of the patient is an important part of a comprehensive evaluation of the patient.

To elicit the data related to the recent context in the environmental dimension, the physician should ask *specific questions* in addition to obtaining a chronological history of the present illness. The specific questions include the following: Has there been any change in residence in the past five years or so? Any changes in your job? Any changes in your family such as divorce, separation, remarriage, death of a family member, etc.? Did you go on a vacation, and, if so, where? Do you have any difficulties at work? Have you had any trouble with the law? Have you known anyone who became ill recently or who had an operation or an accident?

Summary

The recent context of help-seeking behavior consists of recent events and changes in the environmental, personal, and biological dimensions. In the environmental dimension, exposure to physical toxins and changes in interpersonal systems (such as bereavement and job changes) should be considered. At the personal level, changes in personal habits, attitudes, and mood are important factors. Depression has been shown to be associated with increased morbidity. The recent context in the biological dimension includes recent diseases, surgical procedures, and medications. It also includes biological rhythms, which are influenced by factors in the environmental and personal dimensions, and which, in turn, have far-reaching effects in all dimensions.

Implications

For the Patient

The recent context events and changes are frequently the sources of current concerns, joys, and sorrows of the patient. Examples include recent diagnosis of a disease, marriage, or bereavement. Many events and plans occurring in contact with the health care system will be interpreted by the patient in relation to the recent context variables. For example, a patient whose friend recently obtained good relief from back pain by surgical procedures would expect surgical procedures if he develops back pain himself. A patient who is newly married may be more concerned about long-term health and more inclined to engage in help-seeking. On the other hand, a patient who has been depressed recently is likely to neglect personal hygiene and not seek medical help in spite of obvious symptoms and signs. Certain life changes and recent changes may increase the likelihood of the patient's becoming ill.

For the Physician

Understanding the recent events and changes in the patient's bodily functions, behavior and mood, and environment often provides the physician with clues concerning the contributing and precipitating factors of current illness and possible associated conditions that must be considered in managing the patient. They include changes in habits, such as increased drinking or smoking that may contribute to liver and respiratory disease. Environmental changes such as trips or changes in working conditions may be responsible for a rare infection or poisoning. Mood changes such as depression may need to be treated in addition to the disease at hand. Changes in sleep patterns and other biological rhythms often provide the physician with important information.

For the Community and Health Care System

In developing a health care system centered around the patient rather than merely the disease, medical education should emphasize the recent events in the patient's life and environment which have an important impact on the patient's current feelings and attitudes. Understanding of the recent context information should lead to preventive measures and improvement of the overall quality of the patient's life by managing aspects of the patient's recent experiences that are amenable to intervention. This includes teaching better coping skills.

Recommended Reading

Gunderson EKE, Rahe RH (eds): *Life Stress and Illness*. Springfield, Ill, Charles C Thomas, 1974. A symposium on the topic of life stress and illness. Multiauthored, multifaceted discussion on the role of life changes, especially in heart disease and depression.

Jacobs S, Ostfeld A: An epidemiological review of the mortality of bereavement. *Psychosom Med* **39**:344–357, 1977. This is a succinct and comprehensive review of literature concerning the increased risk of morbidity and mortality following bereavement. A critique of the methodologies used in the studies as well as a discussion of possible mediating factors in the increased morbidity can be found in this article.

Jenkins CD: Recent evidence supporting psychologic and social risk factors for coronary disease, Parts 1 and 2. *N Engl J Med* **294**:987–993, 1033–1938, 1976. This is a comprehensive review of the psychosocial risk factors in coronary disease, the commonest cause of death in the United States. Many recent context factors, such as anxiety, depression, and interpersonal problems, seem to be precursors of angina pectoris. Sleep disturbance is shown to herald all presentations of coronary disease. Jenkins also discusses the association between coronary disease and certain background context risk factors, such as status incongruity, dietary habits, and the type A personality pattern. Highly recommended.

References

Bruhn JG, Chandler B,Wolf S: A psychological study of survivors and nonsurvivors of myocardial infarction. *Psychosom Med* **31**:8– 19, 1969.

Dean A, Lin N: The stress-buffering role of social support. *J Nerv Ment Dis* **165**:403– 417, 1977.

Gunderson EKE, Rahe RH (eds): *Life Stress and Illness*. Springfield, Ill, Charles C Thomas, 1974.

Holmes I, Rahe RH: The social adjustment rating scale. *J Psychosom Res* **11**:213– 218, 1968.

Jacobs S, Ostfeld A: An epidemiological review of the mortality of bereavement. *Psychosom Med* **39**:344– 357, 1977.

Jenkins CD: Recent evidence supporting psychologic and social risk factors for coronary disease, Parts 1 and 2. *N Engl J Med* **294**:987– 994, 1033– 1038, 1976.

Kasl SV, Cobb S: Blood pressure changes in man undergoing job loss. A preliminary report. *Psychosom Med* **32**:19– 38, 1970.

Mechanic D: The concept of illness behavior. *J Chronic Dis* **15**:189– 194, 1962.

Parkes CM: *Bereavement: Studies of Grief in Adult Life*. New York, International Universities Press, 1972.

Rabkin JG, Struening EL: Life events, stress, and illness. *Science* **194**:1013– 1020, 1976.

Rahe RH: Subjects' recent life changes and their near future illness susceptability, in Lipowski ZJ (ed): *Advances in Psychosomatic Medicine*. Vol 8: *Psychosocial Aspects of Physical Illness*. Basel, Karger, 1972, pp 2– 19.

Rees WD, Lutkins SG: Mortality of bereavement. *Br Med J* **4**:13– 16, 1967.

Syme SL, Hyman MM, Enterline PE: Cultural mobility and the occurrence of coronary heart disease. *J Health Hum Behav* **6**:178– 189, 1965.

CHAPTER 12

The Background Context of Help-Seeking Behavior

1. An 18-year-old single white man was admitted to the hospital for an open-heart procedure. He was a thin young man who appeared anxious and sickly. From an early age, he was diagnosed as having a congenital heart defect (tetralogy of Fallot). His mother was observed by the staff to be hovering over him always and generally overprotective. The patient was considered by the staff to be immature and impulsive.

2. A 19-year-old single white man, John, has just graduated from high school with honors. This was a source of deep satisfaction for his family physician, because John has superior intelligence in spite of phenylketonuria, a hereditary disease that can cause severe mental deficiency if it is not diagnosed and treated early. In John's case, the condition was diagnosed at birth and treated with a specific diet (phenylalanine-free diet). His family, with the help of the doctor, has successfully prevented the mental deficiency.

3. When the first exposure after hatching of certain birds, such as mallard ducks, is to a human, they will follow that person and for the rest of their lives behave toward him as if he were their mother. This phenomenon, called "imprinting," occurs only during a limited period in early life, that is, roughly between 16 and 32 hours after hatching.

4. A 43-year-old married black man was admitted to the hospital with bronchial pneumonia. Upon admission, he was considered by the staff to be guarded and suspicious. History revealed that as a child who grew up in the South, he had spent an entire year in a hospital. The prolonged stay was due to chronic recurrent complications following surgery, and the child and his family had felt somewhat mistreated.

Constitution (genetic plus early experiential factors); congenital conditions; perinatal, infantile, and early childhood environment; physical and personality development and familial influences; and broad cultural factors constitute the background context of help-seeking behavior. Some of the factors are biologically programmed, for example, genetic factors and possibly imprinting phenomena similar to those observed in animals (vignette 3). Generally, traits reflecting background context factors are relatively stable and not easily modified by the time the patient seeks help. Certain congenital anomalies, however, may be amenable to curative intervention at any time in one's life, as in vignette 1.

The physician should recognize that alleviation of a disability of long-standing duration may require major psychological adaptation by the patients and family. For example, some patients who have been blind for a long time due to cataracts may paradoxically become psychotically depressed or paranoid after an operation which is successful in restoring vision.

The Background Context in the Biological Dimension

The background context factors in the biological dimension include the genetic endowment and other constitutional factors of the patient. The latter include nonhereditary congenital anomalies, such as the sequelae of rubella infection of the mother during the first trimester of pregnancy.

A genetic abnormality does not necessarily result in phenotypic expression. For example, in phenylketonuria, proper diet can completely prevent the mental retardation (vignette 2).

Certain physical and laboratory findings may serve as "genetic markers" of an abnormality or a predisposition to a disease. For example, long fingers and toes in conjunction with high arched palate indicate Marfan's syndrome. Persons with Marfan's syndrome are particularly predisposed to develop serious vascular disease (dissecting aneurysm) due to connective tissue abnormality. Elevated serum pepsinogen level (which is a genetic trait) is also a marker of those individuals who are at risk for developing duodenal peptic ulcer disease. Interestingly, elevated serum pepsinogen is associated with certain psychological characteristics common in duodenal peptic ulcer patients (Weiner et al., 1957). This suggests that the psychological characteristics may result from complex interactions among the effects of infant behavior, the genes causing elevated serum pepsinogen, and the behavior of the mother during the child's development. For example, Mirsky (1958) postulated that infants with this genetic trait may have a higher than normal need for nurturance and loving contact, thus setting the stage for frustration of these needs if extra amounts of such care are not provided. This may lead to development of the psychological characteristics that result from conflict over dependency wishes. Background context data at the biological level should include family history of diseases and illnesses, including alcoholism, substance abuse, psychiatric illnesses, and suicide.

The Background Context in the Personal Dimension

The relatively stable (trait) characteristics of the patient as a whole constitute the background context in this dimension. They include the personality type, intelligence, general outlook and tendencies, attitudes, habits, and habitual psychological defense mechanisms and coping styles in the face of illness. The patient's personality type and his habitual defense mechanisms are important in his adaptation to the sick role (see also Chapters 5 and 15). The background context personality factors generally represent stable *"givens"* that the physician and the health care system must respect and work with, rather than "problems" to be treated. This is especially true in short-term treatment situations such as brief hospitalizations.

Information concerning the patient's *habits* may be helpful both in shedding light on the diagnostic process and in suggesting management approaches. Personal habits include drinking and smoking, drugs, personal hygiene, exercise, sleeping, and diet. Specific questions should be asked about habit patterns. For example, "How much do you drink? Every night?" "How long have you been smoking?" "Have you been smoking more or less recently, say, in the past month?" A history of excessive drinking in a jaundiced man suggests a diagnosis of alcoholic cirrhosis, and hemoptysis in a middle-aged man who is a heavy smoker suggests possible lung cancer. A patient who has a history of heavy drinking is at risk for developing delirium tremens if an acute medical condition prevents him from drinking. Sedatives such as benzodiazepines may need to be given prophylactically to such a patient who may be in the hospital for an acute medical condition unrelated to alcoholism.

Attitude toward illness is usually long-standing and determines the patient's illness behavior as well as sick role performance. It is influenced by many factors, including the patient's socioeconomic status, religion, other cultural expectations, and the personality.

The *coping styles* in the face of illness is a concept described by Lipowski (1970). The concept is closely related to the personality type of the patient (Chapter 15) and defense mechanisms (Chapter 5). In the presence of the specific threatening situation of illness, many patients tend to show one of the following two *cognitive* coping styles: *minimization* and *vigilant* focusing. Patients who minimize tend to use selective inattention—not hearing, not seeing, not understanding, or ignoring the facts or the significance of the illness and/or its consequences. Obviously, this type of cognitive coping tends to occur in conjunction with the psychological defense mechanisms of *denial, repression,* and *rationalization.*

Vigilant focusing is characterized by hypervigilance and is often associated with the orderly, exacting personality. The patient copes with the threat by paying sharp attention to the problem and attempting to know everything associated with it. There is often a constriction of awareness so that matters not relevant to the problem at hand may be ignored. *Isolation of affect* and *intellectualization* are defense mechanisms that are frequently used in conjunction with this cognitive coping style.

Personality as a Factor in Pathogenesis of Disease

Some specific personality types and conflicts have been considered to be especially associated with certain specific medical diseases (Alexander, 1950). For example, peptic ulcer patients were observed to show exaggerated aggressive, ambitious, and independent attitudes as an overcompensation for repressed dependency needs and longing for love. Such a psychological conflict (between dependency needs and inhibition of them because of personal and social expectations) was considered to contribute importantly to the etiology of the *"psychosomatic" diseases.* Although there is often an association between patterns of psychological conflicts and certain medical diseases, such association is no longer considered to be etiological (although "core conflicts" may be related to vulnerability to disease, and their activation may play some role in precipitation of disease states) (Leigh and Reiser, 1977).

More recently, overt behavior patterns such as the *type A behavior* described by Friedman and Rosenman (1974), characterized by ambitiousness, competitiveness, and a sense of time urgency, have been associated with an increased risk of coronary disease, especially in younger individuals, but it is still unclear whether (or, if so, in what way) this behavior pattern may be causally related to the development of coronary artery disease.

Theoretical concepts have been changing rapidly in response to constant accumulation of new research data (see Reiser, 1975, for a fuller discussion of this topic).

The Background Context in the Environmental Dimension

Broad cultural influences, including the patient's ethnic origin, socioeconomic status of his family during childhood, the region or country in which he spent his childhood, native language (or bilinguality), religious background, and the size of the family (e.g., number of siblings, presence or absence of extended family), are among the factors comprising the background context in the environmental dimension.

As already discussed in Chapter 3, *language* is often associated with the socioeconomic status of the patient as well as with early cultural background. Whorf postulates that language actually shapes the way experiences are perceived and processed (Whorf, 1956). For example, the Hopi Indians do not have words that denote time as an entity. Thus, time is perceived as continuous and flowing, without the familiar sense of the *amount* of time and *division* of time (such as "two days ago" or "three years from now"). The Indo-European language (which includes most of the Western languages, including English) has a tendency to divide events into nouns, adjectives, verbs, and adverbs. This analytic mode of thinking is also the basis of scientific thought. However, there is a tendency to equate the word with an entity; that is, if a word exists, there is a tendency for us to assume that it also has a body and substance *(reification)*. Creating a word for a condition or disease also gives a sense of control over it—thus, the desire of patients to know the name of the disease.

The Whorfian hypothesis of language determining thought is controversial; for example, Chomsky has shown that the "deep structures" of language, which are ultimately reflected in thought processes, may be universal across cultures, while the "surface structure," the actual syntactical arrangement and use of words, may be culture bound (Chomsky, 1972).

Religion plays a role in personality development and in the patient's relationship to illness. Durkheim, in his classic book, *Le Suicide* (1897/1966). postulated that the higher suicide rate among the Protestants in Europe in comparison to the Catholics was related to the spirit of free inquiry, desire for knowledge, and weakening of the communal bond in Protestantism. This was called egoistic suicide—suicide due to exaggerated individualism in which life becomes empty and loses its meaning; the other types of suicides described by Durkheim are "anomic suicide," due to the lack of regulation in activity, as in achievement and times of financial well-being, and altruistic suicide, in which the social bonding is so strong that cultural goals are found beyond individual existence (see Chapter 6). Members of certain fundamentalist sects and of some Catholic households may see illness as an act of God and take a fatalistic attitude toward it and, consequently, may be less likely to seek medical help. Some medical procedures may come into conflict with the patient's religious background, such as abortion in Catholics and blood transfusion in Jehovah's Witnesses.

It is important to recognize that patients have *varying degrees* of religiosity and also that the childhood religion or parental religion is *not* necessarily identical to the patient's. Thus, some patients derive great comfort from seeing a minister or priest in the hospital, while others feel upset or angry when visited by the clergy. It is necessary to *ask* the patient about religious matters and the desirability of involvement with the clergy. Some patients assume that the involvement of the clergy necessarily means that their illness is terminal.

Early family environment is probably the single most important factor in the background context in the environmental dimension. This includes physical aspects, such as nurturance, dietary provisions, and contact behavior. For example, in the treatment of phenylketonuria (vignette 2), it is essential to provide the child with a phenylalanine-free diet. Parental cooperation is obviously essential and, in turn, is determined by their involvement with the child, whether the child was planned and wanted or not, and the quality of the marital relationship. Experiments with monkeys by Harlow and his associates show that *tactile sensation* is an important element of attachment behavior (Harlow and Harlow, 1966a,b). They showed that if infant monkeys were given inanimate dummies with apparatus for the provision of milk as mother surrogates, they invariably chose the soft terry-cloth-clad surrogates ("terry-cloth mothers") as opposed to "wire mothers." In fact, even if the terry-cloth mothers did not provide nurturance, the infants clung to them rather than to the tactilely unsatisfying wire mothers. The monkeys who were reared by such artificial mothers had difficulties in social and sexual behavior in adulthood, but some of the adverse effects were neutralized by exposure to peers in childhood.

In mice, early isolation results in relatively lower blood pressure in adulthood, but if the isolated mice are exposed to intense psychosocial stimuli through situations of dominance challenge, their blood pressure rises to a significantly greater extent than that of nonisolated controls (Henry *et al.*, 1975). Thus, early experiences of a social interactional nature may determine the reactivity to situations in later life.

Family interactions play an important role in generating predisposition to psychiatric illness. For example, Lidz and associates found that the families of adolescent schizophrenic patients were often characterized by marital schism or marital skew. In the *schismatic families,* each spouse was caught up in his or her own personality difficulties with a chronic failure to achieve complementarity of purpose or role reciprocity. In the *skewed families,* the psychopathology of one marital partner dominated the home so that often very bizarre and distorted ideas and behaviors were taken as the norm in the families (Lidz *et al.*, 1965).

Intersystems Interaction in the Background Context—Development

The process of the ontogeny of the patient *(development)* occurs through time by the interaction of the three systems—biological, personal, and environmental. The process of physical maturation itself is genetically programmed, including the development of secondary sexual characteristics. The development of the person, including the personality characteristics and assumption of social roles, is a result of complex interactions of factors at all levels of organization. A detailed discussion on development is beyond the scope of this book, so the reader is referred to a standard textbook of child development (e.g., Lewis, 1971).

In this section, we will briefly and schematically review the stages of libido development as originally described and conceptualized by Freud* and the developmental schemata of Erikson and Piaget. All of these theories are *epigenetic;* that is, a later development stage is built upon the foundation of the preceding stage, so that difficulties in any stage may result in difficulties in the next stage. On the other hand, successful overcoming of a difficulty in any given stage can help to resolve difficulties carried over from a previous stage.

Freud

Freud's major developmental theory is based on the "libido theory," that is, the vicissitudes of the sexual drive. He postulated that the primary erogenous zones of the sexual libido were concentrated in the mouth during the first year of life—the *oral stage*. In other words, the mouth is the organ predominantly involved in the experience of pleasure during this period. The pleasure may be in sucking and, later, in biting. Initially, during this stage, the object of attachment or love is considered to be the self (autoerotic); that is, pleasure is derived from the self in the act of sensual sucking. Later in the same stage, the infant comes to recognize that the mother provides him with the food, the breast, and comfort. Thus, his mother becomes the love object. Passive longings and dependency are thought to be associated with this stage.

The second stage of development according to Freud is the *anal stage,* which occurs during the second year of life simultaneously with toilet training. During this stage, the child's major bodily concern shifts to the anus and its control—which provides a sense of mastery. The act of excretion itself, as well as retention of feces, can be pleasurable. Sadistic impulses and concerns over control and mastery are associated with this stage. The oral and anal stages are considered to be *pregenital* stages as compared to the next stage of development, the phallic or Oedipal stage.

The *phallic* or *Oedipal* stage takes place between the ages of approximately 3 and 6 and is ushered in with the discovery of the genitals by the child. In this stage, erotic sensation concentrates in the genital organs, and the child experiences strong love directed toward a parent. Freud postulated that boys

---

*This omits later additions to psychoanalytic theories concerning the psychology of the ego and its development.

and girls differ in experiencing this stage. For both boys and girls, the mother is the initial object of love. During this stage, the boy feels an intense desire to possess his mother and replace his father as her primary lover. This incestuous wish, however, results in the fear of retaliation by the father in the form of castration *("castration anxiety")*. The boy gradually relinquishes his incestuous wishes and, instead, identifies with his father—to become like him, so that in the distant future, he would possess a woman like his mother. Thus, the boy's interest, for the time being, turns away from love and sex, and a period called "latency" sets in. Freud thought that the discovery by the boy that girls do not have a penis was a major factor confirming the fear that castration could actually occur.

In the case of a girl, Freud postulated, the discovery that she does not have a penis results in a serious disappointment in her mother, her initial love object. Thus, according to Freud, she feels defective and becomes envious for a penis *(penis envy)*. Because of this feeling of having been castrated, the girl turns her love from the mother toward the father, the person who, unlike the mother, has a penis. Freud postulated that the girl thus has the fantasy of obtaining a penis from her father, which becomes transformed into a wish to have a baby, a penis substitute. In the girl, too, latency occurs because of the fear of complete loss of love from her mother—which produces an identification with the mother.

The phenomenon of little boys and girls experiencing an intense love toward the parent of the opposite sex is called the *Oedipus complex,* after the Sophocles tragedy *Oedipus Rex.* Psychoanalytic theory postulates that unsuccessful resolution of the Oedipus complex is the cornerstone of the development of certain types of neurosis.

If the child has difficulties in progressing from one stage to another because of severe frustrations or excessive gratification, psychoanalytic theory postulates that there may be a *fixation* at that developmental stage; that is, the characteristics of the stage may persist throughout life. Thus, conflicts over dependency or over control and mastery may be the result of fixation at the oral or anal stage, respectively. Problems with sexuality and love often arise as a result of difficulties in resolving the Oedipal situation successfully. When a person encounters difficulties, there may be a tendency for him to return to the behavioral and psychological patterns of an earlier developmental stage in which more gratifications were experienced or a sense of mastery occurred. This phenomenon is called *regression* and is considered to be an important mechanism in psychopathology. Regression may be responsible for secondary enuresis in a child who feels jealous of a newly arrived sibling. (Regression may also be adaptive; see Chapter 5.)

The period of *latency* lasts from about age 7 until adolescence. During this period, children relinquish intense sexual interest and tend to play with playmates of the same sex.

With the onset of adolescence, there is a resurgence of heterosexual interest. The true *genital stage* sets in as the person finds a spouse and is involved in a mature love relationship.

Although the phenomena of infantile sexuality and Oedipus complex are well established, the concept of penis envy has undergone modifications. Thus, the girl's penis envy may be more related to the culturally inferior expectations of girls in the past rather than to the anatomical difference per se. In the boy, a wish to fuse or identify with the mother and a wish to be able to bear children may also have important consequences in development.

Erikson

Erik Erikson described eight developmental stages in humans on the basis of *developmental tasks* (Erikson, 1963). Erikson, who is himself a psychoanalyst, has paid special attention to the relationship of the developing individual to the demands of society and culture. His stages are as follows:

1. Basic Trust vs. Basic Mistrust. This stage is essentially identical to the Freudian oral stage, in which the infant, through the experience of a trusting relationship with the society (family) in the form of feeding, comfort, etc., learns to develop a sense of basic trust and confidence. Unsuccessful outcome results in a basic sense of mistrust.

2. Autonomy vs. Shame and Doubt. This stage roughly parallels the Freudian anal stage, in which a sense of regulation or control develops. "Holding" and "letting go" are the two social modalities the child *experiments* with. Successful outcome results in a sense of autonomy, a sense of self-control without loss of self-esteem. Difficulties with the developmental task result in a pervading sense of shame and doubt.

3. Initiative vs. Guilt. This stage is parallel to the Freudian stage of the Oedipus complex (phallic stage). During this stage, the child is more energetic, more loving, brighter in his judgment, and, at the same time, more relaxed. There is a quality of planning and "attacking" a task. During this stage, as a result of regulation between inner drives and internalized inhibitions (due to a developing conscience), the child gradually develops a sense of moral responsibility and unconflicted initiative. Difficulties in this period result in complete repression of initiative or in overcompensatory "showing off."

4. Industry vs. Inferiority. Paralleling the Freudian latency period, the child learns to win recognition by learning and producing things. Children receive systematic instruction during this stage and acquire the basic skills (such as the three Rs—reading, 'riting, and 'rithmetic) required for work. Unsuccessful outcome results in a sense of inadequacy and inferiority.

5. Identity vs. Role Confusion. Erikson considers the period of adolescence to be of great importance in the development of the sense of identity. This is the period in which the person develops a sense of inner sameness and continuity, a sense of direction and self. Career choices are also made during this stage. The danger in this stage is "role confusion."

6. *Intimacy vs. Isolation.* This covers the period of young adulthood, in which the person is ready and eager to fuse his identity with those of others. This involves commitment to concrete affiliations and partnerships with others. Mature love relationships, colleagueships, and friendships develop. Difficulty in achieving this developmental task results in a sense of isolation and self-absorption.

7. *Generativity vs. Stagnation.* This is the stage of middle adulthood, in which the primary concern is the establishment and guidance of the next generation. Generativity includes the concepts of creativity and productivity. Childbearing and childrearing are common generative activities. Failure to participate in generative tasks often results in a sense of stagnation and personal impoverishment. Erikson states that such individuals may regress to an obsessive need for pseudointimacy and indulge themselves as if they were their own or one another's only child. Early invalidism may become a vehicle of self-concern.

8. *Ego Integrity vs. Despair.* In old age, acceptance of the individual's life with satisfaction is reflected in "ego integrity," a sense of assurance of order and meaning for humankind. The lack of this integrity is signified, according to Erikson, by fear of death and despair that the time is now too short to attempt to "start another life or try out alternative roads to integrity."

It will be noted that the Eriksonian developmental stages are comparable to the Freudian ones except that the Freudian stages are based on sexual drives, while the Eriksonian stages are based on "ego tasks," and that Erikson's stages span the whole life cycle, while Freud's stages stop with the development of mature genitality.

Piaget

Jean Piaget, a Swiss psychologist, studied the development of intelligence in children. Piaget's developmental stages, then, are based on the structure of intelligent thinking, rather than on love relationships, as in Freud, or on social tasks, as in Erikson. According to Piaget, one can distinguish three periods of intellectual development: (1) the sensorimotor period (birth to 2 years); (2) the period of representative intelligence and concrete operations (2 to 11 years); and (3) the period of formal operations (past 12 years through adulthood).

1. *The Sensorimotor Period.* During the first 18 months to 2 years of life, the infant learns through repetition—initially, from blind imitative repetition to

repetitions in anticipation of results and invention of new methods through combinations of previous experiences. Response—feedback loops called "circular reactions" form an important part of the experience.

2. *The Period of Representative Intelligence and Concrete Operations.* This stage may be subdivided into the preoperational phase (ages 2 to 7 years) and the phase of concrete operations (ages 7 to 11 years).

   a. Preoperational Phase (2 to 7 years). During the period of 2 to 4 years of age, the child begins to use symbols; that is, he begins to use a word or an object to stand for or represent something else that is not immediately present. Symbolic play (e.g., making believe that a piece of cloth is a pillow) and language soon develop.

   b. Phase of Concrete Operations (7 to 11 years). When the child develops the notion of conservation (of volume or weight), he is in the period of concrete operations. Now the child knows that the same amount of clay can look as if there were more clay if divided into a number of smaller balls. The child also has a clear notion of hierarchical classifications, especially if concrete objects are involved. For example, he can answer correctly the question "Which would make a bigger bunch, one of all the primulas or one of all the yellow primulas?" (Ginsburg and Opper, 1969).

3. *The Period of Formal Operations.* As the child reaches adolescence, his thought processes move from concrete operations to a more flexible, abstract mode. The thought transcends here and now. With adolescence, the person begins formal, propositional thinking, in which logical thinking and hypothesis-testing are prominent features.

Piaget's developmental stages are based primarily on normal children and his theory does not form the basis of a psychopathologic understanding. However, it emphasizes the process of "discovery learning"—derivation of a higher level of intellectual functioning by the incorporation of experience.

Summary

The background context includes hereditary, constitutional, personality, and early environmental factors such as language, religion, and family interactions. Early physical environment may also play a major role in the present state of the patient.

At the personal level, personal habits, including drinking and smoking, personality and coping styles, and behavior patterns should be evaluated. Genetic givens and laboratory findings often provide clues to constitutional vulnerabilities to illness.

Development is a complex intersystems event. Freud formulated developmental stages on the basis of sexual drives, with emphasis on the love relationships in children. Erikson formulated developmental stages on the basis of social tasks, and the whole life cycle is seen as having period-specific tasks. Piaget studied the intellectual development of children.

Implications

For the Patient

The factors in the background context determine the patient's stable expectations of himself, the environment, and the health care system. They also determine his skills, talents, and limitations. Often, patients are not aware of the specific ways in which the background context factors determine their current attitudes and feelings.

For the Physician

Understanding the patient's background context factors in all three dimensions is essential in arriving at rational management plans. The physician should also consider what background factors tend to reinforce, and what factors tend to conflict with, the patient's recent and current context factors. For example, a patient whose depression followed a therapeutic abortion may be influenced by the background context factor of childhood religion, although she may no longer profess Catholicism. In this instance, recognition of the source of guilt feelings in childhood may aid in alleviating present depression. Early experience of mistreatment may determine present perception of the health care system, as in vignette 4. The physician should ask specific questions concerning early family environment, socioeconomic status, and residence; parents' occupations; ethnicity; religion; etc.; when obtaining a family history and past history.

For the Community and Health Care System

Medical education should include an understanding of the role of background environment and habits in the pathogenesis of illness. Educational programs concerning smoking and excessive drinking can have major preventive effects. More research is needed in order to understand optimal environment and childrearing techniques.

Recommended Reading

Erikson EH: *Identity, Youth and Crisis.* New York, WW Norton & Co, 1968. This contains discussion on the identity problem of adolescence and a review of Erikson's ideas concerning the developmental stages throughout the life cycle. This work and Erikson's *Childhood and Society* are very important in understanding the social–cultural influences in the personality system.

Freud S: *The Complete Introductory Lectures on Psychoanalysis,* Strachey, T (ed). New York, Norton, 1966. A lucid and easy-to-read exposition of Freud's basic ideas. Highly recommended for an understanding of Freud's early developmental theory and psychoanalysis.

Ginsburg H, Opper S: *Piaget's Theory of Intellectual Development: An Introduction.* Englewood Cliffs, NJ, Prentice-Hall, 1969. This is a very readable and substantive review of Piaget's contributions in understanding intellectual development in children. It describes the major experiments done by Piaget with good discussions of the implications.

Lewis M: *Clinical Aspects of Child Development.* Philadelphia, Lea and Febiger, 1971. This is a concise and readable textbook on child development. It is an overview of development from the prenatal period to early adolescence. It also contains a chapter on psychological reactions to bodily stresses such as acute illness, birth defects, and surgery. Highly recommended.

Reiser MF: Changing theoretical concepts in psychosomatic medicine, in Reiser MF (ed): *American Handbook of Psychiatry,* ed 2. New York, Basic Books, 1975, vol 4, pp. 477–500. A comprehensive and historically oriented review of theoretical concepts in psychosomatic medicine.

Shapiro D: *Neurotic Styles.* New York, Basic Books, 1965. For a very vivid description of some personality styles.

References

Alexander F: *Psychosomatic Medicine.* New York, WW Norton, 1950.

Chromsky N: *Language and Mind.* New York, Harcourt Brace Jovanovich, New York, 1972.

Durkheim E: *Suicide,* Simpson G (ed). New York, The Free Press, 1966. (Originally published in French, 1897.

Erikson EH: *Childhood and Society,* ed 2. New York, WW Norton & Co. 1963.

Friedman M, Rosenman RH: *Type A Behavior and Your Heart.* New York, Alfred A Knopf, 1974.

Ginsburg H, Opper S: *Piaget's Theory of Intellectual Development: An Introduction.* Englewood Cliffs, Prentice-Hall, 1969.

Harlow M, Harlow H: Affection in primates. *Discovery* **27**:11–17, 1966a.

Harlow H, Harlow M: Learning to love. *Am Sci* **54**:244–272, 1966b.

Henry JP, Stephens PM, Axelrod J, et al.: Effect of psychosocial stimulation on the enzymes involved in the biosynthesis and metabolism of noradrenaline and adrenaline. *Psychosom Med* **37**:227–237, 1975.

Leigh H, Reiser MF: Major trends in psychosomatic medicine: The psychiatrist's evolving role in medicine. *Ann Intern Med* **87**:233–239, 1977.

Lewis M: *Clinical Aspects of Child Development.* Philadelphia, Lea and Febiger, 1971.

Lidz T, Fleck S, Cornelison AR: *Schizophrenia and the Family.* New York, International Universities Press, 1965.

Lipowski ZJ: Physical illness, the individual and the coping process. *Psychiatry Med* **1**:91–102, 1970.

Mirsky LA: Physiologic, psychologic, and social determinants in the etiology of duodenal ulcer. *Am J Dig Dis* **3**:285–314, 1958.

Reiser MF: Changing theoretical concepts in psychosomatic medicine, in Reiser MF (ed): *American Handbook of Psychiatry,* ed 2. New York, Basic Books, 1975, vol 4, pp 477–500.

Slobin DI: *Psycholinguistics.* Glenview, Ill, Scott Foresman & Co. 1971.

Weiner H, Thaler M, Reiser MF, *et al.:* Etiology of duodenal ulcer: I. Relation of specific psychological characteristics to rate of gastric secretion (serum pepsinogen). *Psychosom Med* **19:**1–10, 1957.

Whorf BL: *Language, Thought, and Reality,* Carroll JB (ed). New York, Technology Press and Wiley, 1956.

PART IV

ON MANAGING A PATIENT

CHAPTER 13

The Case of the "Sick Tarzan": A Challenging Case History

The following case is presented in some detail in order that the reader may use a systems–contextual framework in analyzing the history. Rational and comprehensive management plans should emerge from the data arranged according to the patient evaluation grid (PEG).

A 59-year-old married executive of a small company was admitted to the intensive care unit with nausea and severe chest pain radiating to the left arm which had developed suddenly in the morning following a hot bath. He immediately called his wife and asked her to call for an ambulance. Electrocardiograms (EKGs) and enzyme studies upon admission confirmed the diagnosis of massive myocardial infarction (MI). This was the patient's first admission to a hospital, and there was no past history of serious illness. Family history was not significant except that his father had died from MI at age 72. His mother had died from pulmonary edema at age 75.

Upon admission to the intensive care unit, absolute bed rest was prescribed, and continuous monitoring of the EKG was instituted. Orders were written for administration of diazepam (Valium), 5 mg four times a day, and meperidine (Demerol), 50 mg every four hours for pain. Procainamide, 500 mg intramuscularly every six hours, was prescribed when he developed bursts of paroxysmal ventricular contractions (PVCs), an irregularity of the heartbeat which is common after MI and indicates hyperirritability of the heart muscle.

On the day of admission, he posed no problem for the doctors and nurses. His complaints were confined to the "gas pain" in his upper abdomen. On the second day, however, he was found sitting up in a chair beside the bed, in spite of the doctor's orders to stay in bed. He appeared agitated at night and asked for large doses of Valium to make him relax. The nurse wrote, "Patient is very arrogant but easily subdued with firmness.'' On the fourth day after admission, he became agitated and refused to have his blood drawn for laboratory tests. He screamed to the nurses that he wanted to sign out on the same day and was found exerting himself trying to lift up his bed. He was reproached by the nurse with no effect. He refused to cooperate in measuring his fluid intake and output and poured urine on the floor. The next day, he said to the nurse, "My doctor thinks I had a heart attack. All I need is to get back my strength, which I lost from being in here too long.'' He was again observed lifting up his bed. He told the nurse that he wanted to exercise by lifting up his bed 40 times a day. He was flushed and sweaty, and multiple PVCs occurred. Finally, the nurses persuaded the cardiologist to ask for psychiatric consultation.

The following are transcribed segments of the tape-recorded interview with the psychiatrist:

DOCTOR: Could you tell me something about how you came to be in the hospital?

PATIENT: Doc, when I came here, I was sick. . . . I admit I was sick and I wanted to be helped. Now after the first stages are over, I get impatient. I can stay in bed for a certain amount of time. You know, the first day I was here, I was jumping out of the bed every two seconds—I didn't know why, but I'm accustomed to sleeping on a flat board, and the bed was at an angle and my back just broke on me. I couldn't sleep. The second night, they gave me sleeping pills so I was able to take it. Do you understand?

DOCTOR: Yes. I think so. Let's backtrack a little bit. Could you tell me what happened in the first place, that brought you to the hospital?

PATIENT: You mean the heart attack? You want me to tell you something? I laid my wife that morning—let's be frank. And instead of resting a minute, I jumped into a hot tub of water, boiling hot water. I didn't give my heart a chance to rest, and it was a little too much for me. If I had rested just one minute, you know, lay alongside her and relaxed a minute, nothing woulda happened. In the beginning, I came downstairs, and I sorta felt sorta squeamish, so I said to myself, "You know, I oughta stand in front of the open window and breathe deeply.'' I've got a *big* chest so I can take in a lot of air. Then, I had a drink of pineapple juice. You know, I don't drink small amounts of anything! I guzzled that, I am telling you, and when I guzzled that, all of a sudden, she gave me a bang in the heart. And I knew right away I had a heart attack.

DOCTOR: I see. It must have been frightening to you.

PATIENT: No, I don't get frightened at nothing—nothing scares me. All I did was holler up to my wife. I've got a bull voice—you know what I mean, I can't help myself. You understand, I got a powerful chest so it comes out strong. So, she came down, and I says, "Call the doctor, tell him I had a heart attack." As I said, in the hospital, I got uncomfortable staying in bed. They had my bed raised, and I couldn't sleep. So I got up and walked around.

DOCTOR: What kinds of thoughts were you thinking as you got up and walked about?

PATIENT: You want to know something, Doc? *Nothing bothers me.* I am just telling you. I am an impatient guy. I don't let nothing bother me. I found that a long time ago, that if you don't let nothing bother you, you're the happiest guy in the world. Let them call you a dope, let them call you anything, but you got *peace of mind.*

DOCTOR: Could you tell me more about that? You learned a long time ago. . . .

PATIENT: At age 37, I had pains in my head, and I had diarrhea for years, and my family, every one of my aunts and uncles died of cancer, and I took an X ray and I figured, "Gee, I got cancer, too." Let's be frank. I had a cousin at 31 die of cancer, too. He died of leukemia, so I figure it was me. But when they told me it was all from nerves, I says, "You see this book. It's open right now. This book is closed. If you ever see me get excited again, you can insult me from morning to night, you can call me anything you want, and I will look at you and I don't give a damn." And you wanta know something—from that day on, I don't give a damn about anything. I learned one thing. If you got a calm mind, nothing is gonna hurt you. You know, a lot of doctors don't realize it.

After more discussion about past history, the doctor asks about the patient's wife.

PATIENT: My wife? In earlier years, we used to fight like hell. Now, I love her so much I could kiss her. And she knows it. And I let her do what she wants. She likes folk dancing, I let her folk dance. She wants me to stay home with her on Saturdays, I stay home with her.

DOCTOR: How has she reacted to your being in the hospital?

PATIENT: Oh, she was very shocked. The thought of me, *me* being sick. She couldn't take it, you know. I'm imperishable. That's the way she looks at me. You want to know why? Because I look at myself that way. I looked at myself as imperishable. In other words, nothing could hurt me.

DOCTOR: Could you tell me some more about your being imperishable?

PATIENT: In my youth, I was so strong that in order to get any satisfaction, I had to wrestle with four or five fellows at one time. I used to wade into a gang of fellows, 14, 15 fellows, just for the excitement of a little exercise. I had muscles like this here; I had two calves under here, like watermelons. I was what they called a natural strong man . . . but today I feel sorta weak—not full of pep, if you know what I mean.

DOCTOR: You're feeling weak?

PATIENT: I think it's because they don't let me move my blood in the hospital.

DOCTOR: Move your blood?

PATIENT: Yeah. I'll explain it another way. Do you remember, years ago, they had a couple of operations in the African veldt? Now, these operations that they had in the fields, everyone survived, yet the ones they had in the hospital, those guys died. You want to know why? Those guys had to get off the bed and pull themselves along to get home. They moved their blood. I am convinced that moving the blood is the most important thing to stay alive. Once you start laying in bed without moving and letting your blood move, you might as well bury yourself. That's how I feel. I tell you the honest truth, doctor. And, someday, you fellas are going to come to the same conclusion—that moving the blood is the most important thing of all.

The case of the sick Tarzan constituted a medical emergency. In the early phase of MI, maximal myocardial rest is essential. His insistence on lifting the bed to "move his blood" was seriously jeopardizing his life. In fact, there were increasing signs of myocardial distress, as evidenced by increasing cardiac arrhythmia. To consider rational management plans for this patient,* however, we must first consider certain important factors in the management of patients in general.

*Discussed in Chapter 19.

CHAPTER 14

The Doctor–Patient Relationship

1. *"A pint of blood was extracted from his right arm, and a half-pint from his left shoulder, followed by an emetic, two physics, and an enema comprising fifteen substances; the royal head was then shaved and a blister raised; then a sneezing powder, more emetics, and bleeding, soothing potions, a plaster of pitch and pigeon dung on his feet, potions containing ten different substances, chiefly herbs, finally forty drops of extract of human skull, and the application of benzoar stone; after which his majesty died."*

The foregoing is a description of a heroic treatment of King Charles II (Van Dyke, 1947*).

2. *A 35-year-old woman suddenly developed a toxic megacolon and was admitted to the hospital on an emergency basis. She is known to have ulcerative colitis, which has been under control until now. Her physician had left the country on vacation two days prior to this acute exacerbation.*

The history of medical therapeutics until about 100 to 150 years ago is largely that of the doctor–patient relationship and the "placebo effect." Most ministrations by physicians would have been more harmful than beneficial to the patient, but for the natural recuperative powers of the human organism supported by the beneficial effects of the doctor–patient relationship. Four of the most famous medications used by physicians until about the 18th century were unicorn's horn, used to detect and protect against poisons in wines; benzoar stones, as antidotes for all kinds of poisons; theriac, as a universal antidote; and powdered Egyptian mummy, as a universal remedy, including wound healing (Shapiro, 1960). The unicorn's horn usually came from the ivory of the narwhal or elephant, according to Shapiro. Doctors were dangerous to pa-

---

*As quoted by Shapiro (1960). Reprinted with permission.

tients! What is surprising, however, is that, in spite of such noxious treatments, many patients, in fact, got better or even completely recovered.

The benefits of the placebo effect are psychologically determined by *expectations* and *hopes* shared by the patient and the doctor. Action, ritual, faith, and enthusiasm are important ingredients (Findley, 1953). The physiologic mechanism and pathways by which these effects are mediated are largely unknown, but at least one has been clarified in recent experiments (Levin *et al.*, 1978) which have demonstrated the physiologic mechanism underlying one important type of placebo effect, that is, relief of *dental* pain by injection of a pharmacologically inactive (placebo) solution. Patients with dental pain who responded to placebo injection (placebo responders) and a matched sample of control patients with dental pain who did not (placebo nonresponders) were given placebo injections plus naloxone, a drug which blocks opiate receptor sites in the brain. Naloxone blocked the pain relief in the placebo responders but had no effect upon the pain in control patients. These findings strongly suggest that placebo responders experience relief from pain by secreting endorphins, which are known to relieve pain by activating opiate receptor sites (see Chapter 7). Hypnotic relief of pain, on the other hand, does not work by this mechanism—it is *not* blocked by naloxone (Goldstein, 1976).

Balint (1964) calls the doctor "the most frequently prescribed drug." In this context, the doctor–patient relationship exerts major therapeutic influence. Sometimes this may be dramatically demonstrated when a patient, suddenly realizing that his trusted physician is not available, has an acute exacerbation of disease. This is especially true when the physician "covering" for the absent doctor is new to the patient and does not have an ongoing relationship with the patient (vignette 2).

The doctor–patient relationship involves, in addition to expectation of help, some specific therapeutic elements. *First,* an ongoing supportive relationship with a respected and competent professional may serve as a buffer against excessive anxiety and strain for the patient as he attempts to cope with illness. *Second,* as we will see in Chapter 17, many of the physician's activities (as in taking the medical and personal history and in performing the physical examination) may in themselves have intrinsic psychotherapeutic effects and serve to consolidate the supportive, trusting aspects of the relationship. *Third,* by providing the patient with an opportunity to share life problems, the physician may relieve the sense of helplessness and hopelessness that goes with feeling alone in the face of vexing, threatening, and sometimes overwhelming conflictual situations and feelings. *Fourth,* the physician as an objective observer may serve as a source of information (education) and counseling which help the patient to cope with his problems. *Fifth,* we know that the patient brings to the relationship with the doctor preexistent unconscious feelings, attitudes, and expectations. The latter are reactivated feelings, attitudes, and expectations that the patient originally experienced as a child toward caretaking adults, most often parents and older members of the nuclear family, and often, too, the family physician or pediatrician who cared for the patient in childhood. The reexperiencing of these reactivated inner (memory) feelings, attitudes, and expectations *as current responses belonging to the physician* is called "transference." The phenomenon of transference may exert a powerful influence on the patient's mental and emotional state, and the concomitant physiologic events may then influence pathophysiologic processes (see Chapter 4). A "positive" (i.e., trusting, loving, respectful) transference component in the doctor–patient relationship may help to modulate stress responses, induce relaxation, permit recuperative forces to take hold, and so serve to augment beneficial effects of medications and other therapeutic measures. These phenomena will be further discussed in Chapter 17.

Of course, the physician also brings unconscious attitudes, feelings, and expectations to the relationship and should be alert to elements in his own makeup which may intrude into his relationship with particular patients.

Obviously, a good ongoing doctor–patient relationship makes it easier for the physician to recognize heterothetic help-seeking behavior and to deal with it appropriately. And the physician who "knows" his patient and family and takes the opportunity to stay abreast of these aspects of the patient's life on the occasion of regular physical checkups, etc., will be optimally situated to help his patient when trouble of any sort develops. In a good doctor–patient relationship, the patient feels that the physician will be available to answer questions, listen to life problems, provide helpful information and counsel. Reentering a trusting relationship with the physician may recreate the physiologic and psychological states associated with comfort and healing (Adler and Hammet, 1973).

Clarification and education are important aspects of the modern doctor–patient relationship. Participation in a shared belief system, by rendering anxiety-producing symptoms comprehensible, may in itself exert beneficial effects through reduction of anxiety and associated physiologic processes. In the past and in other cultures, symbolic manipulation as practiced by shamans in rituals has been shown to be effective in healing certain medical conditions (Levi-Strauss, 1963). Clarification and education allow the patient to understand and share the assumptions upon which the physician bases his treatment plan. To achieve this, the physician must first understand the patient's ideas and concepts about the illness and how it may be managed. Kleinman *et al.* (1978) suggest the following line of inquiry to elicit the patient's ideas about the illness.

1. What do you think has caused your problem?
2. Why do you think it started when it did?
3. What do you think your sickness does to you?
4. How severe is your sickness?
5. What kind of treatment do you think you should receive?
6. What are the most important results you hope to receive from this treatment?
7. What are the chief problems your sickness has caused for you?
8. What do you fear most about your sickness?

Once the patient's model is understood, the doctor is in a position to discuss with the patient the *discrepancies* in their respective models and to share his own understanding of the illness. Some *compromise* may be necessary if elements of the patient's model, although medically incorrect, have such preemptive importance for the patient that he cannot give them up, for example, in the case of the sick Tarzan (Chapter 13), the idea of "moving blood" as being so important in treatment.

The educational activities of the physician need not and should not be confined just to the illness at hand but should include education concerning prevention of disease and hygienic principles of living and should be ongoing in nature.

The modern doctor–patient relationship is rooted in magic and primitive superstitions (e.g., of the shaman), and it exploits placebo phenomena when and as appropriate. *But* it has developed into *much more than that* and more, too, than simply the "art of medicine" as practiced by intuitive, empathic, and humane physicians. It now also includes implicit psychotherapeutic elements and explicit specific technical procedures that can be understood as applications of basic principles of human behavior and of mental phenomena to the practice of medicine. Properly managed, its effects can articulate synergistically with those of other therapeutic procedures, such as use of drugs and corrective surgery. The patient's expectation that the doctor will help is based, then, not only on magical beliefs but also on the scientific principles of modern medical biology and behavioral science (see Chapter 17).

Open and comfortable communication between the patient and the doctor is essential for this synergistic linkage to occur. In its absence, patients may fail to comply with the doctor's prescriptions, otherwise effective medications may turn out to be less than optimally effective, and valid surgical procedures may have unexpected adverse side effects because of the patient's anxiety and mistrust. Conversely, some patients may engage in scientifically unsound treatment methods (e.g., Laetrile) administered by the equivalent of modern-day shamans rather than seek help from a competent physician.

Summary

In spite of ineffective and often harmful methods, prescientific medicine was often effective, probably because of the effects of placebo phenomena and nonspecific supportive aspects of doctor–patient relationship.

Current understanding of the doctor–patient relationship regards it as rooted in shamanistic magic and placebo effects, but specific psychotherapeutic elements are now included which link it effectively and understandably to the effects of conventional medical procedures. An ongoing, open channel of communication between the physician and the patient is essential in order for an effective doctor–patient relationship to develop. In addition, the physician must understand the patient's own ideas and models of illness and educate the patient in order that he and the patient can ultimately share common belief systems and common goals for the treatment.

Implications

For the Patient

The patient's ideas about illness and the pattern of his participation in the doctor–patient relationship are based upon his past experiences and cultural expectations. *Discrepancy* between the patient's and the doctor's models of illness may interfere with development of an optimal doctor–patient relationship because a shared belief system—an important ingredient of a good doctor–patient relationship—does not exist. A patient's *lack of compliance* or *cooperation* with the medical regimen may be a sign of a poor doctor–patient relationship or deterioration of a previously good one.

For the Physician

An understanding of the patient's ideas and models about illness and health care is essential for an optimal doctor–patient relationship. *Specific questions* are necessary to elicit this information. The patient's cultural background and his family's attitude toward illness are important data in this regard. The physician may judiciously utilize the powerful doctor–patient relationship as a *therapeutic tool* and should pay attention to it in his work with patients.

For the Community and Health Care System

Education of the general public concerning illness and health care is important, since shared expectations play an important role in fostering good doctor–patient relationships. Medical education should inform students about the therapeutic significance and use of the doctor–patient relationship in addition to the technical aspects of treatment in the practice of scientific and effective medicine.

Recommended Reading

Balint M: *The Doctor, His Patient, and the Illness.* New York, International Universities, Press, 1964. This is a classic, describing the discussions between Dr. Balint, a psychoanalytically oriented psychiatrist, and a number of general practitioners in England about their patients. A good discussion on the relationship between the doctor and the patient and also on psychological understanding of patients. Has interesting vignettes and case histories.

Kleinman A, Eisenberg L, Good B: Culture, illness, and care: Clinical lessons from anthropologic and cross-cultural research. *Ann Intern Med* **88:**251–258, 1978. A good discussion on the cultural patterning of sickness and care, with emphasis on understanding the patient's models concerning illness.

Levi-Strauss C: *Structural Anthropology.* New York, Basic Books, 1963. A classic. Contains very interesting and vivid description of symbolic manipulation of shamans. Fascinating reading.

References

Adler HM, Hammet VBO: The doctor–patient relationship revisted: An analysis of the placebo effect. *Ann Intern Med* **78:**595–598, 1973.

Balint M: *The Doctor, His Patient, and the Illness.* New York, International Universities Press, 1964.

Findley T: The placebo and the physician. *Med Clin North Am* **37:**1821–1826, 1953.

Goldstein A: Opioid peptides (endorphins) in pituitary and brain. *Science* **193:**1081–1086, 1976.

Kleinman A, Eisenberg L, Good B: Culture, illness, and care: Clinical lessons from anthropologic and cross-cultural research. *Ann Intern Med* **88:**251–258, 1978.

Levine JD, Gordon NC, Fields HL: The mechanism of placebo analgesia. *Lancet* **2:**654–657, 1978.

Levi-Strauss C: *Structural Anthropology.* New York, Basic Books, 1963.

Shapiro AK: A contribution to a history of the placebo effect. *Behav Sci* **5:**109–135, 1960.

Van Dyke HB: The weapons of panacea. *Sci Mon* 64–322, 1947. (As quoted by Shapiro AK: A contribution to a history of the placebo effect. *Behav Sci* **5:**109–135, 1960.)

CHAPTER 15

The Patient's Personality

1. A 67-year-old man was admitted to the hospital for evaluation of fainting episodes. Upon admission, he started complaining about the "sloppy service," wanted to have food specially brought in from a restaurant every day, and called the office of the president of the hospital to complain about the delay in the nurses' responding to his calls. History revealed that he was a self-made man who was still active as the chairman of the board of a large corporation. Soon the patient was considered by the doctors and nurses to be a "pain in the neck" and a "crank," and they tried to avoid dealing with him as much as possible. This resulted in further delays in medications and responses to his calls.

2. The doctor asked, "Do you have any pains in your chest?" The patient replied, "Yes, doctor, I have so much pain in my chest—like constant pressure and pins and needles, and then I have these terrible aches and pains in my stomach, I have indigestion and constipation, and pains in my spine. My head hurts, too, and all my joints."

"It sounds like you are suffering a lot."

"I suffer all the time, what with my pain and my luck . . . you know, when I had my operation for my back, the wound would not heal, then I had an abscess which was treated with penicillin—then I had this reaction to penicillin so they had to stop it. My husband left me while I was still in bed from the operation, and the house burned down. That's when my arthritis flared up, and my headaches started. My old doctor gave me aspirin for it, which caused my stomach ulcers . . . when they started bleeding and I had to have an emergency operation. . . ."

Personality and Character

How an individual reacts to illness, and the willingness with which he assumes the sick role, are determined in large measure by his personality. *"Personality"*

253

is a broad general term which refers to *characteristic patterns of thought, behavior, and feelings* of an individual. It includes, among other things, cognitive style, temperament, tolerance for anxiety, and patterns of defense and coping. In its broadest sense, personality includes the concepts of character and "neurotic styles," the latter referring to habitual symptomatic ways in which a person perceives and thinks (Shapiro, 1965). The term "character" is often incorrectly used as a synonym for personality.

Character was used in a special sense by Wilhelm Reich, who regarded it as a "defensive armour," an aggregate of characteristic psychological defenses (see Chapter 5) utilized so often by the person that it functioned as a "structure" always in a state of readiness, in preparation to react to anxiety-provoking situations (Reich, 1949). Seen in this special light, character has a primarily defensive function and can be regarded as one component of personality.

The Concept of Personality Types in Patients

Although each individual has his own unique personality, it is sometimes useful in the context of medical care to classify patients according to arbitrary but loosely defined "personality types." Identification of the personality type or style of a patient does not necessarily imply a need for changing it through treatment. Its value lies rather in the fact that assessment of the personality type helps us to understand the meaning of illness for the given patient and, in turn, its influence upon sick role performance. This understanding can then provide the rationale for developing optimal ways of interacting with the patient. Without it, an impasse can develop between a "difficult" patient and health care personnel.

Habitual ways (e.g., neurotic styles) of dealing with stressful situations often become exaggerated when a person is ill, particularly when he finds himself in the strange environment of the hospital (see Chapter 16). Thus, a person who has a tendency to be precise and controlling may become even more precise and controlling in the hospital, even to the extent that his personality may come into conflict with the sick role expectation of allowing himself to become dependent upon the hospital personnel.

The meanings of illness, of hospitalization, and of medical procedures to a patient are congruent with his personality type, and the ways in which patients and physicians relate to one another are influenced by the interaction of their personalities. Kahana and Bibring (1964) described seven personality types often encountered in the general hospital and discussed how illnesses might have differential meaning according to differences in personality styles and how different management approaches might be used depending on the personality style of the patient. The ten personality types we present here are modifications and expansions based on their work.

Personality Types and the Sick Role

Patients may be categorized by personality types as follows*:

1. Dependent, demanding patients
2. Orderly, controlling (obsessive compulsive) patients
3. Dramatizing, emotional (histrionic) patients
4. Long-suffering, self-sacrificing (masochistic) patients
5. Guarded, suspicious (paranoid) patients
6. Superior and special (narcissistic) patients
7. Seclusive, aloof (schizoid) patients
8. Impulsive patients with a tendency to act out
9. Patients with mood swings (cyclothymic)
10. Patients with chronic memory deficits and a tendency to confusion (chronic organic brain syndrome)

Dependent, Demanding Patients

It is said that one can detect this type of personality by noting the amount of luggage the patient brings to the hospital. An exaggerated caricature form of this personality is indeed seen in the patient who comes into the hospital as if he were prepared to stay for months, if not years. Patients of this type have a need for a great deal of reassurance and often want special attention from health care personnel. They tend to become dependent upon the doctor and others who are involved in their care and often make frequent, inappropriately urgent calls to nurses and doctors. When their (excessive) demands are not met fully, they tend to feel angry and rejected.

The underlying dynamic for this type of personality is considered to be a regressive wish to be cared for as if by an idealized, nurturant mother. The fear of being rejected, left out in the cold, and neglected tends to exaggerate the *need for reassurance and care*. The *sick role* may be considered to be a temptation for these individuals to return to a state of infantile dependency, and they may consider the *illness* to be a result of a lack of protection and concern by others. This *regressive, dependent behavior* is congruent with some aspects of Parsons' description of the sick role except for the third and fourth elements, that is, considering the sick role as an undesirable state of being and cooperating with the doctor in becoming well again (Chapter 2).

The incessant demands of a patient of this type, coupled with relative comfort in the dependent position, may be regarded by others, especially doctors and nurses, as "enjoying" being sick. Hostile behavior, when excessive demands for attention are not met, provokes anger and conflict. The nurses, for

---

*The terms in parentheses are "psychiatric" terms denoting extreme forms of the personality characteristics (patterns).

example, may feel that the patient wants too much attention, while the patient feels that the nurses are cold and uncaring.

There is an opposite side to this coin as well. A patient of this type was referred to the psychiatrist by an alarmed surgeon because he too eagerly consented to an amputation the first time it was discussed as a possibility. In this instance, it was learned that the doctor had been overly indulgent with the patient, allowing special privileges and giving an inordinate amount of care and attention. The patient, before long, regarded the doctor as an omnipotent, mothering figure and wanted to go along with anything that the doctor suggested might be good for him.

Orderly, Controlling Patients

Such patients tend *not* to show feelings and generally experience illness without outward signals of emotional reaction. Their descriptions of symptoms are complete, precise, and dispassionate. (Isolation is often used as a defense mechanism by these patients; see Chapter 5.)

This personality style is motivated by a *desire to control* external as well as internal states. Behind the desire to control may be *fear of loss of control—of being helpless.*

The *sick role* is obviously a difficult pill for patients with these personality characteristics to swallow. Removal from normal responsibilities and daily routine may be experienced as disruptive. Being unable or not permitted to "help themselves" may be an alien experience for them. Needing to seek advice and help from a professional may generate concerns about who will control whom, and they may feel deeply threatened by the control that doctors and nurses must assume over their lives and bodies in order to administer necessary medical care.

In response to these threats, they may become contentious, complaining, and accusatory. Usually quite conscious of time and details, for example, medication schedules, they may become incensed and critical if the nurse brings a pill a few minutes late.

Such patients do *not* respond favorably to blanket reassurances. They are likely to wonder if the physician is competent when reassurances are given without firm foundation in facts. The doctor's explanation of one hopeful laboratory finding may be far more reassuring to this type of patient than many impressionistic but unsupported optimistic statements.

A rule of thumb in dealing with this type of personality is to attempt to recruit the patient to be a part of a therapeutic team effort against the illness. This enables him to feel that the physician respects his autonomy enough to ask him to cooperate in the common endeavor. Detailed explanations of the diagnosis, the physical and laboratory findings, and treatment plans are helpful, especially for more educated patients. Sometimes it is useful to the patients to help the treatment team by keeping a diary of symptoms or by recording some of their clinical data, such as volume of water drunk and urine voided.

> A chemistry technician with diabetes mellitus was admitted for treatment of leg ulcers. Within days after admission, he complained of the "sloppiness" of the doctors and nurses, their lack of punctuality in bringing him medications, etc. Successful management involved the physician's acknowledging the patient as someone related to the medical profession. ("As a chemist, you would understand the mechanism of diabetes mellitus. Now, we want to treat this with diet and insulin, and we will follow the course with urine tests for sugar. It means so and so, etc.") In addition to giving the patient credit for his knowledge of chemistry, the doctor taught him to change his own medicated dressings (he could do it "much better than any nurse") and to keep track of his medications to be sure that they were taken on time.

Dramatizing, Emotional Patients

Patients with this personality type tend to come across as being rather charming and fun to talk with. They have a certain dramatic flair when giving accounts of their lives and often are quite amusing. Their histories tend to be more *impressionistic* and diffuse than precise. They may be overtly *seductive:* female patients wearing provocative negligees and "parading around" in the hospital; male patients making sexually seductive comments to nurses and female physicians. There is a tendency for these patients to consider their relationship with the doctor as special, with sexual overtones. The medical staff often finds itself split around these patients, some liking them very much and others feeling angry with them. The patients themselves have usually unwittingly provoked these split reactions.

A major concern underlying such behavior is the need to be *attractive and desirable* to others, to prove their *"masculinity"* or *"femininity"* over and over again and to gain care and support. An *underlying fear* that they might not be found attractive and desirable is, of course, accentuated by illness, with its threat to the integrity of the body. As patients, persons of this type have an exaggerated need to be reassured that they are still attractive and will not be deserted.

The *sick role* may or may not be compatible with this type of personality. On the one hand, the dependency and social perquisites inherent in the sick role afford some of these patients an acceptable opportunity to exhibit and "flirt" with authority figures in a situation which sets limits. Patients with extreme forms of this personality, in spite of their overtly sexually provocative behavior, tend to be rather inhibited in actual sexual encounters. For them, the hospital and medical treatment may be exactly the type of setting they find most comfortable for seductive behavior without danger of actual sexual activity. On the other hand, some patients become extremely frustrated by the confinement and limitations of the sick role, especially if they had been accustomed to active, exhibitionistic, and gratifying life-styles. For example, a man who had been accustomed to a "Don Juan" life-style may find the restriction of sexual activity in the hospital most unbearable.

These patients respond best if the doctor responds, within set boundaries and limits, a certain amount to their needs to engage him. However, this should not be overdone, as these patients also tend to be frightened if their characterological seductiveness seems to lead to unexpected intimacy. Showing some *warmth and personal concern* is usually all that is needed. When there seems to be a split in staff feelings, these should be openly discussed and resolved in staff meetings. It may also be necessary to set *firm limits* with the patient, at the same time indicating concern and willingness to continue to take care of the patient. *Repeated reassurances* are often necessary. With this group of patients, unlike the orderly, controlling personalities, the doctor's personal manner and attitudes are relatively more important in providing reassurance then factual content, that is, discussion of objective findings and test results.

Long-Suffering, Self-Sacrificing Patients

Some experienced physicians say that this personality type can be diagnosed by the pitch and tone of the patient's first utterance in the doctor's office. Such patients often speak in a wailing, complaining voice, and usually the history involves a long list of *hard luck and disasters:* surgical operations followed by complications, trusted persons turning out to be untrustworthy, promised cures for a symptom bringing on more symptoms and side effects than relief, etc. They almost always have endured protracted pain and suffering, and this "present illness" represents an additional suffering for a patient who seems to have been "born to suffer" (vignette 2).

When listening to patients with this type of personality, one usually finds that they have taken care of someone else despite all their own suffering and misery. They take much pride in relating how this feat was achieved in the presence of so much suffering and so many misfortunes. Often, that someone else is a child, a spouse, or a parent.

A major underlying dynamic in these patients is considered to involve strong feelings of guilt which do not allow them to enjoy life for themselves. With a "need" to suffer in order to expiate the guilt feelings, *altruistic activities* (such as caring for others) in the presence of physical or emotional pain may allow them some covert gratification (claim to happiness). Thus, these patients appear as if they are "exhibiting" their misfortunes, sufferings, and altruistic acts.

Another underlying dynamic in such patients is the use of *pain and suffering as a life-style, as a means of maintaining interpersonal relationships.* These are patients who might be *"addicted" to the sick role.* The sick role is taken on from time to time throughout their lifetime, although they also feel proud of having taken care of others despite the sick role restrictions. A closer scrutiny reveals that the sick role is assumed as a way of meeting their needs indirectly through suffering and through ongoing contact with the physician. Many patients diagnosed as "hypochondriacs" have this personality type.

Patients with this type of personality often become severe problems for health care personnel. Typically, they tent to *react negatively to reassurances,* totally frustrating the doctors. When the physician prescribes a medication with reassurance, for example, that it should relieve pain, the patient is likely to return complaining of more rather than less pain, which may now be felt in areas which were previously free of pain! In addition, he may have nausea and dizziness. He may even overtly blame the physician for the added troubles, but most often this is attributed to bad luck. The physician, nevertheless, is often *made to feel guilty* by these patients. This frequently results in a *rejection* of the patient by the physician, which adds to the patient's feeling of being mistreated. Thus, these patients commonly have a history of repeated rejection or transfer from doctor to doctor. The long-suffering, self-sacrificing patients, although asserting belief in Parsons' third and fourth sick role expectations, actually refute them in their behavior. Those who become addicted to the sick role fail to fulfill the sick role expectations of "considering the ill state as being undesirable" and "attempting to get well as soon as possible by cooperating with the physician."

Patients with this personality type are best managed when the physician gives *"credit"* to their suffering and expresses appreciation for their courage and perseverance in the face of protracted pain and hardship. It is a mistake to promise such patients complete relief from pain and suffering. In fact, since they need to expiate guilt and maintain relationships, such a promise may provide a powerful reason for the patients' "refusal to improve." Taking away the symptoms and suffering would leave them exposed and helpless, without any means of relating to others.

Recognition of this pattern will also help the physician to recognize the necessity to accept and set limited goals for the treatment in order to avoid later frustration, feelings of helplessness, and reactive anger. This can prevent or postpone the development of disruptive tension in the relationship with the patient. It is often helpful for the physician to approach this type of patient with some degree of pessimism, such as, "Although we cannot take away the pain completely, this medication may take the edge off the pain somewhat."

Attempts to mobilize altruistic tendencies may also be helpful. For example, a female patient may be persuaded to seek proper treatment to alleviate crippling pain so that she might be better able to care for her children.

One has to differentiate this type of personality from patients who experience protracted suffering due to actual complications from treatment. Patients suffering from chronic illnesses without this character style do not show the self-sacrificing element, and although they may feel rather cynical about the prolonged illness, they do not show the tendency to "refuse to improve."

Guarded, Suspicious Patients

Patients with this personality type are always *watchful* and concerned about the possibility that harm might be done to them, intentionally or unintentionally. They are quite fearful of being exploited or taken advantage of. They are quite sensitive to the possibility of criticism. They are prone to wonder about ulterior motives or any suggestions or remarks made by the health care personnel, especially if they are ambiguous. These patients are also apt to misinterpret statements and actions and read something ominous or threatening into them. This is especially true in the presence of great anxiety, as in being hospitalized, and in states of reduced cerebral function that impair the integration of sensory input.

Such patients also tend to *blame others for their illness.* For example, a patient may claim that he developed a heart attack because the employer did not provide air conditioning for his work area and "poisoned the air" with carbon dioxide exhaled by so many others.

These patients, obviously, do not enjoy being in the *sick role.* The dependency upon the health care personnel increases their feelings of vulnerability, and with that comes the fear that persons in positions will do things to them that might take advantage of them. Although they see the ill state as an undesirable one, they cannot *trust* the physicians enough to cooperate fully.

A good strategy for *management* of these patients is the assumption of a relatively neutral attitude concerning their suspicions, criticisms, etc., without becoming provoked by them or arguing with them. A helpful statement is, "I understand how you feel under the circumstances." Identifying their suspiciousness as "sensitivity" is also helpful, as these patients like to feel that they are not "fools." Occasionally, agreeing with the patients about their inconveniences about which they are suspicious and then putting the blame on impersonal things like hospital regulations can diffuse their feelings of anger from being directed toward the health care personnel.

Above all, providing as little cause for suspicions as possible is important. This involves *consistency* on the part of the health care personnel in terms of information imparted. It is also necessary to explain, in as much detail as feasible, the nature of the patient's illness and plans for treatment. This will tend not only to minimize the suspiciousness but also to reduce the likelihood of litigation in case of complications, as this type of patient is likely to be litigious as well. When a procedure is recommended to the patient, it is best to present it as objectively as possible, not to arouse the suspicion that the doctor is trying to "manipulate" the patient for ulterior motives.

Superior and Special Patients

These are patients who behave like VIPs, whether or not they have such designation in actuality. Such patients have a tendency to appear snobbish, self-confident, and sometimes grandiose (vignette 1). They are often quite *proud* of their bodies and their physical abilities. This basic style might be partially covered up by exaggerated, artificial humility. There is a sense of arrogance and disdain when they are in contact with other people. Though these patients may seek the most prestigious medical centers and the most eminent physicians when ill, there is often an air of tentativeness when the physician explains anything to them. They may display an arrogant attitude, especially toward persons on the lower strata of the hospital hierarchy, such as house officers, student clerks, and nurse's aides. They are likely to threaten to notify the chief of service or the director of the hospital of any inconveniences they suffer. They also use "name-dropping" to try to impress the health care personnel.

Many patients with this personality style have *idealized body images,* and *illness* represents a threat to the maintenance of this body image. Many neurotic patients with overvaluation of physical prowess, stamina, and fitness were found to have developed the neurosis after illness or injury, often of a minor nature (the "athlete's neurosis"; Little, 1969).

The patients with superiority feelings naturally do not find the *sick role* agreeable. Their need to see themselves as being perfect and invulnerable is contradictory to the notion that they "cannot help themselves" and are in need of more competent help. Although they may submit to this unpleasant situation, they often attempt to find weaknesses and faults in the physicians, as if to reduce them down to size in order to still feel superior to them.

Needless to say, health care personnel often resent this type of attitude. The result is often a battle between the caretaking persons and the patient, each attempting to cut the other down!

Successful *management* of these patients involves a certain degree of magnanimity on the part of the health care personnel, allowing the patient to boast of his strengths. When this is done, the patient may feel secure enough to identify the caring persons with himself—as being almost perfect. It is, however, a mistake to be unnecessarily humble in relation to these patients. An attitude of security about one's professional competence, while recognizing the worth of the patient, is important to ward off insecure feelings on the patient's part that he might not be in the best hands, after all.

Seclusive, Aloof (Schizoid) Patients

This is the type of patient who seems to be remote, detached, and not in need of any interpersonal contact. They usually prefer to be in private rooms and seldom speak or relate to other patients or staff. They like to be involved in solitary activities, such as reading or listening to music. They appear shy and uninvolved. Nurses are sometimes so disturbed by the aloofness and lack of personal response that they suspect depression and bring the patient to the attention of the physician. Some patients with this personality might also appear to be eccentric, with affinities for activities associated with the countercultures, such as health foods and quasireligious sects.

The main concern of these patients is a *desire not to be intruded upon by others;* they wish to maintain a sense of tranquility by being absorbed in themselves and things familiar to them. Any attempt at socialization by others may be seen as an intrusion threatening their fragile tranquility.

Illness is seen as a threat to this self-absorption and tranquility. These patients, therefore, have difficulty in adjusting to the *sick role,* with its expectation of dependency upon and cooperation with the health care personnel. The patients come to terms with the role expectations through *noninvolvement* at a personal level while allowing the medical process to go on. Thus, a patient with this personality may appear to be strikingly unconcerned about illnesses and procedures which would normally be expected to arouse much anxiety. Of course, many patients with this personality *delay seeking help* because of their aversion to the intrusion into their privacy which is necessary in receiving medical care. On the other hand, some patients with this personality may find the sick role as an excuse to find interpersonal relationships without true intimacy.

In *managing* such patients, it is important to recognize and respect the need for privacy. Although socialization and sharing are important to most people, these patients need to protect their privacy and tranquility. Some of these patients, however, may be able to form some relationship with one or two members of the hospital staff. These members can then serve as "translators" for these aloof patients.

Impulsive Patients with a Tendency to Act Out

These are the patients who keep on doing things they did not "mean" to do, usually on the basis of some impulse. These patients may appear to be rational and well controlled, until an impulsive action occurs. Usually, however, they have a history of being involved in interpersonal or legal difficulties because of some maladaptive acting-out behavior. The characteristic feature is a *lack of deliberation,* with decisions being reached on the spur of the moment. Patients with this character style seem to lack tolerance for sustained thinking and for frustration. They often say that they acted "without thinking" or "could not help" what they did and often are quite remorseful after the action. In the health care system, these impulsive actions usually involve some aggressive acts against the health care personnel or ill-advised decisions such as *signing out against medical advice* despite having a serious illness.

These patients seem to feel an overwhelming sense of impotence in the presence of relatively minor frustrationss and appear to be *unable to delay gratification* or to feel gratified by anticipatory cognitive processes such as planning.

The patient with an impulsive personality style is likely to seek help for relatively minor symptoms based on the immediate pain or discomfort experienced, and he is likely to demand *immediate relief* from the discomfort. If immediate relief is not produced, the person is prone to act out by such aggressive acts as cursing at the physician or kicking an article of equipment in the treatment room. Such patients, although wanting immediate relief from symptoms, often have difficulty in tolerating the treatment process, especially when it also involves some discomfort, such as swallowing a gastric tube. Although the patient may appear to have understood the necessity of such a procedure, he is as likely to curse and attempt to sign out in the midst of the procedure when discomfort occurs. Thus, cooperation with the physician (a *sick role* expectation) is a difficult achievement for these patients.

Medical professionals, trained to be always deliberate and objective, tend to dislike patients with this personality type. They see these patients as being defective and childish. In fact, this style may be a manifestation of a *defect in the integrative functions of the brain* rather than a primarily developmental personality style. It is important, therefore, for the health care personnel to deal with it as a defect, just as they have to recognize and deal with a diabetic patient's metabolic defect. The *management* strategy, thus, would involve preventing situations in which the defect would be of major consequence and making compensations for it when it is avoidable.

For example, tranquilizers may be utilized more freely for these patients as a partial preventive measure against outbursts of aggression. Pain should be treated especially vigorously. Firm limit-setting is also necessary to establish some external control over their acting-out behavior. In fact, these patients feel reassured by firm limit-setting, which also gives them a sense of external control and caring. Whenever possible, persons familiar to the patient, such as friends and relatives, should be mobilized to support and control the patient.

Patients with Mood Swings

These are patients who characteristically have "ups and downs," that is, periods of relative euphoria and hyperactivity followed by periods of depressed feelings and lack of energy. Although most people have some periods characterized by euphoric or depressive moods, persons who have this personality trait exhibit such mood swings consistently. During the "up" periods, they feel optimistic, ambitious, and usually physically well. During the "down" periods, feelings of pessimism and a sense of malaise predominate. If these changes are exaggerated so as to cause major problems in function, the psychiatric diagnosis of bipolar depressive disorder may be made (see Chapter 6).

The importance in recognizing this personality trait lies in that depending upon the period in which the person finds himself, the reaction to illness and to the medical treatment may be different. When an illness occurs during an up period, the patient may not even recognize the presence of the symptoms, or even if he recognizes them, he may brush them aside as being of no consequence. If he happens to be in a down phase, however, he may feel quite pessimistic about the symptoms and attach all kinds of grave implications to them. In fact, he may be convinced that he has a terminal illness for which there is no hope by the time he sees the physician. In addition, because of the feelings of malaise and lack of energy experienced during the down phase, these patients may experience exaggerated discomfort which may be caused by minor dysfunctions.

Patients with this personality trait might be more prone to develop severe depression in the presence of major stress such as a serious medical illness. If a patient who has this pattern develops evidence of serious depression, including feelings of hopelessness, guilt, and lowered self-esteem, coupled with weight loss, anorexia, sleep disturbances, and, perhaps, suicidal thoughts, referral to a psychiatrist should be made for definitive treatment. This is also true for any other patients who show similar evidence of depression (see Chapter 6).

Patients with Chronic Memory Deficits and a Tendency to Confusion (Chronic Organic Brain Syndrome)

Chronic organic brain syndrome (dementia) is a medical condition rather than a personality type, but a discussion of such patients is warranted in view of the frequency with which they are encountered in the medical setting and because many patients with these characteristics have a tendency to continue to show them over some periods consistently and become management problems.

These patients are usually relatively advanced in *age* and tend to have difficulties with memory, especially of *recent information* and events, and to develop *confusion* and *irascible behavior* in *unfamiliar surroundings.*

This condition is caused by an *irreversible change in the brain* due to loss of neurons, most commonly because of chronic cerebral ischemia. Other causes include such chronic metabolic disorders as diabetes mellitus and neurologic disorders such as stroke. This condition should be differentiated from the acute organic brain syndromes. Acute organic brain syndromes (delirium) are caused by *reversible* metabolic changes in the brain, such as those associated with delirium tremens, anoxemia, and intoxications. Acute organic brain syndrome is a reversible state, not a personality trait, and its treatment should be directed at the etiology (see Chapter 10). While mental manifestations of chronic organic brain syndrome and acute organic brain syndrome may overlap to a large degree, in acute organic brain syndrome, there is usually a *demonstrable metabolic abnormality with which the recent onset of memory difficulties and confusion coincides.*

In *chronic organic brain syndrome,* the defects have been present for a considerable time, and a careful *mental-status examination* (see Chapter 10) will reveal cognitive difficulties in one or more of the following areas: attention, concentration, calculation, abstraction, judgment, and orientation. *Affect* also tends to be labile, that is, changeable. Thus, the patient may be laughing one moment, crying the next. Their narrative accounts tend to be *circumstantial,* that is, wandering around, in a rambling manner, although they will usually make the intended point eventually. They often show the so-called *"sundowning syndrome"* —worsening of agitation and confusion toward the evening and night. This is thought to be caused by the diminution in sensory input and orienting cues during the night.

The patients may manifest *inappropriate and impulsive behaviors* due to loss of inhibitory functions of the cerebral cortex. Often, there is an exaggeration of preexisting personality traits, such that a patient who had been guarded and suspicious may become even more paranoid, with delusion formation. *Delusions* and *paranoid ideations* are especially apt to occur, since integrative functions of the brain are diminished.

Illness in the presence of chronic memory deficits and a tendency to confusion presents an added complication. In the first place, even if the patient decides to seek help, his *memory* might be so faulty that he may forget his doctor's appointment. Once in the hospital, he may become *confused* in the *unfamiliar surroundings,* so that he might be found wandering about the hospital trying to go to the kitchen, etc. *Such a patient is unlikely to be able to remember the explanations* the physician gave him concerning the illness and procedures, and he may feel subjected to a puzzling indignity at a procedure like a sigmoidoscopy, for example, even if the procedure and its need had been explained to him previously. Sometimes the patient is aware of his loss of mental functions, and when confronted with a deficit (e.g., if he cannot answer a question asked by a physician), he may become panic-stricken and disorganized (the *"catastrophic reaction"*; Goldstein, 1975).

In *managing* these patients, it is important to provide them with a *familiar environment* to reduce confusion. This involves bringing familiar objects to the hospital, such as pictures of family, and encouraging family and friends to visit and spend time with the patient. As the patient's main defect is with recent memory, it is important for the health care personnel to introduce themselves repeatedly and to explain what they are up to before starting any procedure with the patient. They should also repeatedly *orient* the patient, that is, tell him what day it is and what the names of the hospital, the ward, and his physician are at every available opportunity. In order to prevent confusion, it is also important to provide a calendar and a radio or television for such patients. A night-light is helpful to prevent confusion at night if the patient awakens.

Since the brain function of such patients is compromised, drugs that tend to depress central nervous system function should be avoided, if possible. These include most minor tranquilizers, such as diazepam (Valium) (see Chapter 18).

As outpatients, their memories concerning *medication schedules* should not be trusted especially with potent medications. Many deaths have resulted from patients with memory deficits taking multiple doses of medication (many times the prescribed doses) because they had forgotten that they had already taken the medicine that day. Such medicine should be given to a member of the family who can then dispense it.

In planning the medical management of such patients, it is essential to mobilize the *support of the family* or, where necessary, community and social support systems.

From Types to Individuals

As should be clear from our discussion so far, the various characteristics of personality types are not mutually exclusive but tend to coexist in varying combinations. One of our most gratifying experiences is to hear our students complain to us, after a discussion of personality types, that they could not actually categorize a single living patient neatly into any single type. The personality types described here are like caricatures. In real life, it is the rule rather than the exception to see patients with characteristics belonging to several personality types. For example, one patient may be orderly and controlling *and* guarded *and* suspicious, or another may be dependent and demanding *and* also have mood swings. Any of these personalities may develop chronic memory deficit. Once an individual is recognized as being unique, with certain characteristics from several different personality types, then the management of such a patient can be truly individualized.

Summary

How an individual reacts to illness, and the willingness with which he assumes the sick role, are determined by his personality. Ten personality types often encountered in medical settings are discussed: (1) dependent, demanding; (2) orderly, controlling; (3) dramatizing, emotional; (4) long-suffering, self-sacrificing; (5) guarded, suspicious; (6) superior and special; (7) seclusive, aloof; (8) impulsive; (9) those with mood swings; and (10) those with chronic memory deficits and a tendency to confusion. *Illness* and *hospitalization* tend to have different *meanings* depending upon the personality type of the patient.

Management strategy should take into account the personality style of the patient, since an effective approach with one type of patient may induce noncooperation in another type. For example, detailed explanation of contemplated procedures may win the confidence and cooperation of an orderly, controlling type of patient but may frighten a patient who has the dramatizing, emotional personality. Because of the heightened anxiety, such a patient may not be able to understand the explanation, and a general reassuring attitude with a general, undetailed explanation may be more helpful for him. An orderly, controlling person often has difficulty in accepting the *sick role* expectations of dependency, while a long-suffering, self-sacrificing type of person may be "addicted" to certain aspects of the sick role.

Although an understanding of the prominent features of a patient's personality can help the health care personnel in planning effective approaches, most patients do not fall into one or the other personality "type." Familiarity with the commonly encountered personality types and the meaning of illness to them should help the health care personnel to *individualize* their approach to individual patients.

Implications

For the Patient

Illness interacts with the individual's personality system and determines his help-seeking behavior (including whether or not he will seek medical advice), adaptation to the expectations of being a patient (sick role), and performance as a patient. Depending upon the personality characteristics, *illness, hospitalization,* and *medical care have different meanings to patients.* A patient is usually unaware of his personality characteristics and of the relationship of these characteristics to his feelings about being a patient. Thus, any conflict or contradiction arising between the personality needs and the sick role expectations has a tendency to be seen by both the patient and the physician as a specific conflict arising from specific situations; that is, the patients have a tendency to blame a specific doctor or nurse for not understanding them or not caring for them (or for being incompetent, neglecting, etc.).

For the Physician

Understanding the patient's personality style can help the physician formulate an *optimal approach* to the patient. Physicians should also be aware that their own personalities influence how they treat their patients, and a particular mix of the physician's and patient's personalities may bring about a *conflict* in the medical setting. For example, an orderly, controlling type of physician may find himself feeling challenged and unrespected while treating a patient who also has an extremely orderly, controlling personality. Taking some distance from the situation emotionally when such conflicts arise and understanding the personality needs of patients can help the physician avoid becoming entangled in unnecessary personality conflicts (e.g., "power struggle") and meet the patient's needs. Physicians should also be aware that conflicts arising between patients and other health care personnel may reflect a lack of understanding on the part of the health care personnel about the personality needs of the patients. The physician can then educate others in how to approach patients while taking into account their personality characteristics.

For the Community and Health Care System

Training for physicians and health care personnel should include the skills for assessing patients' personality types and their interaction with illness and sick role behavior. The health care system should recognize that a patient brings into the medical setting an exaggeration of his premorbid personality characteristics in addition to being a person defined by the presence of the particular illness which made him a patient.

For preventive medicine to be effective, methods should be devised to induce persons with personality types that tend to avoid assuming the sick role to seek help when needed. Health care personnel should be educated to recognize those patients whose main motivation for being patients is perpetuation of certain aspects of the sick role. Then, the treatment for them can be more effective by avoiding the pitfalls of premature removal of the legitimacy of the sick role or unnecessary laboratory tests or surgical procedures.

Recommended Reading

Kahana R, Bibring G: Personality types in medical management, in Zinberg N (ed): *Psychiatry and Medical Practice in a General Hospital*. New York, International Universities Press, 1964, pp 108–123. This is the classic description of the personality types often seen in medical settings. The reader will find somewhat more detailed discussion of the psychodynamics and possible evolution of the personality types, as well as management approaches with examples.

Shapiro D: *Neurotic Styles*. New York, Basic Books, 1965. (Also available in paperback.) The author describes the cognitive characteristics of the major "neurotic" (or "personality," in less exaggerated form) styles, such as hysterical, obsessive–compulsive, and paranoid styles. An important book for understanding the influence of personality styles on how individuals perceive the world and how they think.

References

Goldstein K: Functional disturbances in brain damage, in Reiser MF (ed): *American Handbook of Psychiatry,* ed 2, vol 4: *Organic Disorders and Psychosomatic Medicine*. New York, Basic Books, 1975, pp 182–207.

Kanaha R, Bibring G: Personality types in medical management, in Zinberg N (ed): *Psychiatry and Medical Practice in a General Hospital*. New York, International Universities Press, 1964, pp 108–123.

Little CJ: The athlete's neurosis: A deprivation crisis. *Acta Psychiatr Scand* **45**:197, 1969.

Reich W: *Character Analysis*. New York, Orgone Institute Press, 1949.

Shapiro D: *Neurotic Styles*. New York, Basic Books, 1965.

CHAPTER 16

The Hospitalized Patient

1. A 42-year-old married woman was admitted to the hospital for an elective gallbladder operation. Her attending physician greeted her upon her arrival at the hospital, and she was assigned a private room and a private-duty nurse. The hospitalization was not going to be as bad as she thought; the large donation her husband had made to the hospital last year had been very well advised.

2. The nurse phoned the intern on call at 3:00 A.M.

Nurse: *Doctor X, I am sorry to call you at this time, but Mrs. Smith's i.v. infiltrated, and she needs her i.v. antibiotic. . . .*

Intern: *Oh, hell! Why don't you go ahead and restart the i.v.? I know that you can do it as well as I.*

Nurse: *I am sorry, Dr. X. I'm not allowed to restart an i.v. unless I am in the ICU.*

Intern: *Come on! I saw you starting an i.v. on Mr. Jones only this morning.*

Nurse: *Yes, but that was in the ICU. Remember, I sometimes work two shifts. I will get into trouble if I start an i.v. on a regular ward. Rules are rules.*

Intern: *Oh, OK. I am wide awake now anyway. There should be a hospital rule that says i.v.'s are not allowed to infiltrate after midnight!*

3. During the first few days of hospitalization in a typical teaching hospital a typical patient with low back pain has the privilege of meeting the following persons:

    1. The receptionist and admitting office personnel
    2. The ward secretary
    3. The head nurse and one or two additional nurses (take vital signs)

4. *The intern (does a history and physical exam)*
5. *The medical student doing clerkship (may be more than one) (history and physical exam)*
6. *The resident (history and physical exam)*
7. *The attending physician (brief history and physical exam)*
8. *The dietician*
9. *The maid*
10. *The nurse's aide*
11. *The lab technician—blood team*
12. *The radiologist and technician when X rays (at least routine, probably more) are taken*
13. *Consultants: Usually, at least one or two consultations are given each patient. For example, in this case, the consultation may be with an orthopedic or neurosurgeon; with a psychiatrist if the patient seems to be anxious; and, finally, with an anesthesiologist if an operation is being considered.*
14. *Possibly a social worker or the clergy*
15. *Other patients on the same ward*

> *During the hospitalization, the patient may have to make the acquaintance of a whole new set of medical students, interns, residents, and even attendings as they rotate off the particular service. The same is true of the consulting teams, which, in turn, consist of residents, attendings, and students.*

The hospital is a microcosm with which most of us have intimate contact. Most of us were born in a hospital, have some contact with one during our lifetime (if we do not actually work in it), and usually can expect to die in a hospital. Hospitals are seen by the society in many different ways—as a necessity, a frightening place, a source of community pride or shame, an important industry, an employer, etc.

Many of those who are ill either are already in the hospital or will be admitted to one sooner or later. We will consider the hospital as a social system and then, the environment of the hospital as it pertains to the patient.

The Hospital as a Social System

Kinds of Hospitals

Hospitals can be classified on the basis of the length of stay of the patients, the kinds of services provided, and the type of management. Thus, we can consider short-term vs. long-term, general vs. special, and community vs. noncommunity hospitals. The most common type of hospital in the United States is the short-term general hospital (see Figures 30 and 31).

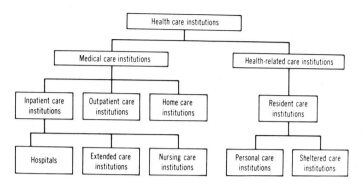

Figure 30. Classification of health care institutions by function. (From Freeman *et al.*, 1972. Copyright 1972 by Prentice-Hall. Reproduced with permission.)

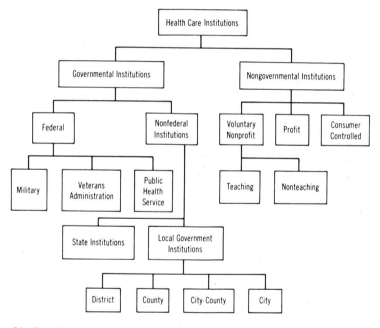

Figure 31. Classification of health care institutions by control. (From Freeman *et al.*, 1972. Copyright 1972 by Prentice-Hall. Reproduced with permission.)

The People in a Hospital

The hospital is an open system and is influenced by the culture of the greater society and community of which it is a part. The social status of the people in the hospital, to a large extent, reflects that of the larger society, although there is also a hierarchical social structure within the hospital. This is so because, to a great degree, the hierarchy in the hospital is parallel to that of the larger society. Those high up in the hospital hierarchy are also likely to have high status outside.

One possible exception here is the patient. In terms of the hospital hierarchy, the patients find themselves at the bottom rung—they are the least familiar with the ethos and culture of the hospital. And, as transients, they are more likely to "put up with" inconveniences and occasional mistreatments than to make an issue of them. But here, again, the social status of the patient in the larger community plays a role. The VIPs are more likely to insist on, and receive, better personalized service than the "charity patients." Patients with high social status, patients who have professional ties to the health community, and those who had families who were willing and able to intercede for them with the health professionals have been shown to receive the kind of care that meets their expressed needs (Roth and Eddy, 1967; Scott, 1969) (vignette 1). The differentiation between the charity patient and the paying private patient is rapidly disappearing, thanks largely to the widespread family insurance coverage of the working population. Psychiatric patients, however, still tend to receive different diagnoses and treatments and assignments to different types of hospitals (state hospital vs. private hospital) depending on social class (Hollingshead and Redlich, 1958; Myers and Bean, 1968). Psychiatric patients from the higher classes have lower hospitalization rates and, once hospitalized, tend to be discharged earlier.

Patients in hospitals also may be informally classified according to their attractiveness and interest value for the staff. Thus, there are the "fascinomas," that is, the most interesting patients, on the one hand; and the "crocks," that is, the most undesirable patients, on the other. The degree of attention, sympathy, and support the patient receives often varies in accordance with this informal classification.

The personnel in the hospital are formally organized in a hierarchy. The general hospital's hierarchical structure is often very complex, with competing lines of authority and priority. Figure 32 shows a typical administrative organization. An important feature of the organization is that there are *two lines of authority,* as in Figure 32. The physicians are organized in a collegial fashion, although there is a stratification according to the specialty and status of the physicians into attendings, residents, interns, and students. This collegial organization of physicians is an outgrowth of the historical position of the physician as "visitor" or "guest" in the hospital (Coe, 1970). Of course, without these guests, the hospital cannot function. All other employees of the hospital are organized along another administrative line.

This dual line of authority is very different from almost any other kind of organization. In the customary single-line-authority organizations, like busi-

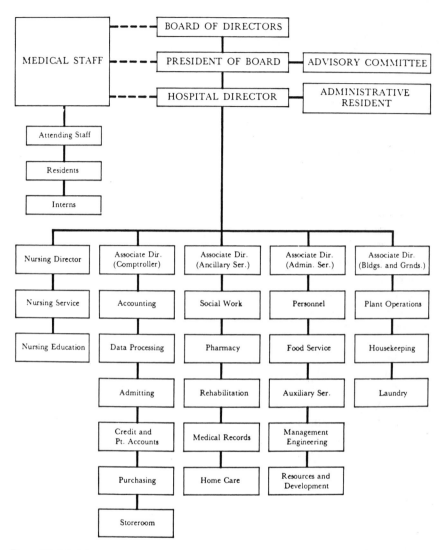

Figure 32. Administrative organization of a general hospital. (From Coe, 1970. Copyright 1970 by McGraw-Hill. Reproduced with permission.)

ness, government, and the military, decision-making powers rest in the offices of the managers who direct the activities of the workers. In the hospital setting, however, the administrative managers have little authority concerning patient care, while the members of the medical staff, who are akin to consultants in single-line-authority systems, actually make decisions. The administrators' authority is often restricted to matters concerning providing the means by which the doctors' orders may be successfully carried out (Coe, 1970). A potential conflict arises from the different sets of values: For the administrators, the primary concern is money, while for the physicians, it is patient care and sometimes teaching and clinical research as well.

The dual-authority system can have major consequences in regard to *nursing*. Unlike physicians, nurses are directly responsible to the administrative structure of the hospital. However, in terms of professional activity, they are the recipients of the doctors' orders and share with the physicians a primary commitment to the patient. On occasion, this results in a "double bind," a conflict between a nurse's professional role and her role as a hired employee of the hospital subject to the rules and regulations of an employee (vignette 2).

The hospital system is also characterized by an *extreme division of labor*. The professional, administrative, and nonprofessional staffs have clearly distinguishable and separate tasks, orientations, and loyalties. The stratification of occupational levels is rigid, and there is a *"blocked mobility"* in each level (Smith, 1955). Personnel cannot be promoted from one occupational level to another in the hospital without first resigning from their present position and obtaining further education. For example, without further schooling, a nurse's aide cannot be promoted to a registered nurse, and a janitor cannot be promoted to a hospital administration post. However, the physicians can and do become promoted to a higher rank, for example, from intern to resident to attending physician, without further formal schooling. A floor nurse can advance to being a head nurse but not to being a physician.

This blocked mobility often results in the formation of cliques and special interest groups which are organized along occupational lines. Thus, nurses are more likely to talk with nurses most of the time, and physicians with physicians. One study showed, for example, that a doctor is three times more likely to speak with another physician than with a nurse and that his interaction with personnel in other occupational groups is minimal. The frequency of conversational interaction of a nurse with other nurses was twice that of a nurse with other occupational workers (Wessen, 1958).

This same phenomenon is observed with respect to speciality lines even among physicians. Thus, a surgeon is more likely to talk with another surgeon than with a dermatologist, and a psychiatrist probably interacts with other psychiatrists most of the time. An obvious side effect of this *group formation* along occupational and specialty lines is the development of communicational barriers between occupations and specialties, and these can give rise to misunderstandings and mutual suspicions. This problem is especially acute if communication between nursing staff and physicians is blocked. It may take days for the nurse to communicate to the physician that his patient has been ruminating about depressive topics and not eating, even though other nurses may have known it all along. For example, in the case of the "sick Tarzan," the doctors were not informed directly by the nurse about his agitation and attempting to lift up the bed until the fifth day of hospitalization.

Another characteristic of the hospital organization is that it is *authoritarian* in nature. This is especially so concerning matters of patient care. The administrative authority is of the rational–legal type, based on the power residing in a particular office and concentrated at the top of the hierarchy. The nature of the physician's authority is more prestige-oriented and charismatic, related to the heavy responsibility of "saving people's lives," than rational–legal, related to the primary goal of the hospital–patient care. The dual line of authority, however, results in conflicts between the lines, the most common type being between the physicians and administrators.

This type of conflict may become especially pronounced when planning for changes or renovations of a hospital. A study in England on four general hospitals asked the patients, staff, and administrators, "What is most important to alter in this hospital from a patient's point of view?" Each group had differing ideas about what was of primary importance. The administration emphasized physical change of the hospital, such as the provision of dayrooms; the doctors and nurses wanted to improve patient care, for example, by increasing the number of nurses; while the patients wanted to improve the quality of life in the hospital by improving the food, providing television sets, etc. (Raphael, 1965).

A more complicated authority relationship exists, especially among the medical staff, in a teaching hospital. The attending staff may be subdivided into the elite, university-affiliated professor types and the private practitioners in the community. Some hospitals have separate units, one for the academicians and another for the private physicians. Members of the academic attending staff are subject to dual roles, that of the clinician in the *hospital* and that of the teacher–researcher in the *university,* each of which has its own reward (promotion) systems based on different criteria. In some teaching hospitals, the house staff (interns and residents) may have conflicts in dealing simultaneously with the community attending physicians who are their patients' primary physicians and with the academic attending physicians to whom they are also responsible.

An interesting feature of the hospital as a hierarchical system is that, somewhat like in the military, one can *identify* the *status* and *rank* of a person by *dress, speech,* and, to a lesser extent, habits and manner. Usually, the least neatly dressed, most disheveled people are the patients, and the most well-dressed and well-groomed people are the attending physicians and hospital administrators. Physicians are often recognizable by the lab coats and uniforms (including the rank—e.g., attendings wear suits or long lab coats, while residents' and interns' costumes are usually different, as are the nurses'). Registered nurses wear uniforms different from those of practical nurses or nurse's aides. Some patients and outsiders take advantage of this and may "pass" for a doctor or nurse with appropriate dress and manner in the hospital, either to leave without permission or even to steal drugs or equipment.

The Organization of an Inpatient Unit

A typical inpatient unit of a general hospital consists of the following: beds, patients, nursing staff, ancillary staff, supporting staff, and physicians. Usually, all but the physicians and patients are more or less permanent; patients are transient, and the physicians generally rotate on and off inpatient units.

The number of beds usually determines the number of nursing staff to which the unit is entitled. Beds may be subdivided into private, semiprivate, and ward beds.

The *nursing staff* usually consists of a head nurse, an assistant head nurse, registered nurses, licensed practical nurses, and nurse's aides. Depending upon the hospital, several nurses may be jointly responsible for the care of a number of patients ("team nursing"), or one nurse may primarily care for one patient ("primary nursing"), with the help of other nurses. The licensed practical nurses and nurse's aides assist the registered nurse. They are all responsible to the head nurse, who, in turn, is responsible to the nursing supervisor of the division of nursing (e.g., medical or surgical) or to the director of nursing of the hospital. The head nurse and the registered nurses are also the recipients of the doctors' orders and are professionally required to carry them out competently. Nursing care, however, is not confined to carrying out the physicians' orders—it also includes interaction with the patients and providing comfort and evaluating distress when it occurs. It is obvious that good communication is essential between the nurse and the physician if the nursing care is to be coordinated with the therapeutic management plans of the physician.

The *ancillary staff* consists of the professionals related to patient care in a specialized area, such as dieticians, social workers, clergy, and the administrator (or the administrative intern) of the ward. They have liaison relationships with the nursing staff and sometimes with the physicians.

The *supporting staff* consists of the ward secretary or unit manager, who answers the telephones, makes sure that all the forms are in stock, etc., and the maintenance staff, including the janitors. Members of the supporting staff are usually responsible to a separate hierarchical administrative structure.

The physicians usually found on an inpatient service are the attending physician(s), the residents and interns (house staff), and the medical students. In teaching hospitals, the house staff is usually in charge of the patient, supervised by the attending and aided by the medical student. The physicians usually form a team around the patient, the team consisting of an attending physician, a resident, an intern, and a medical student. However, if the attending physician is not a full-time hospital or university physician, the house staff may have divided loyalties between the community-based attending and the full-time university-based physician supervisor to whom the house staff report as well.

Another socially complicating characteristic of the young physicians, particularly the house staff, is that they wield much power even though they are transient and relatively inexperienced members of the unit. Many members of the nursing staff on the unit may have been there for as long as 10 or 20 years and may be more knowledgeable about procedures and medical problems encountered on the ward than are the house staff, who change every few weeks or months. The mobility of the house staff may be envied by the less mobile staff members.

For a ward unit to function optimally, it is necessary that (1) each staff member has defined, unambiguous, and unchallenged roles, (2) there is effective leadership and cooperation among disciplines, (3) there are smooth and open channels of communication between and among all the persons involved—including the patient, and (4) there is a spirit of commitment to cooperative efforts for good patient care.

To ensure the smooth running of this complex organization, many hospitals now assign *liaison psychiatrists* to inpatient services. The liaison psychiatrist, as a physician who is knowledgeable in psychosocial aspects of patient care and in organizational dynamics as well as biological aspects of illness, is often in a position to understand the dynamics of a ward and the complex interactive relationships between the medical and psychological aspects of patients and the ward problems. He may be in a position to improve and foster good communication between all concerned and to integrate multiple and fragmented observations for the primary physician. He is optimally situated to serve as a catalyst in opening up communications since, *unlike* everyone else on the ward, he does not report to any administrative authority who might take unfavorable action against a member of the ward, such as the nursing supervisor or the chairman of the department of medicine. The liaison psychiatrist may be an independent agent or may himself be a psychiatric resident, reporting to the department of psychiatry. The liaison psychiatrist is often assisted effectively by a *liaison nurse,* a psychiatric nurse with advanced training in liaison psychiatry, who may run liaison meetings with the nursing staff and act as a communicative link between the nurses and the physicians.

The liaison psychiatrist functions best when he forms a team with the primary physician (house staff or attending), the head nurse, and the social worker, in cooperation with the liaison nurse.

In most hospitals, the liaison psychiatrist also does psychiatric consultations on the patients in the unit. These involve evaluation and treatment of emotional or behavioral disorders of patients in the general hospital. Depression, suicidal attempts, confusion, delirium, personality difficulties, drug-related problems, and intention to sign out against medical advice are common reasons for referral of patients to the psychiatrist. The liaison psychiatrist often finds that an aberrant behavior of a patient reflects division and conflict among the staff. For example, a patient who receives conflicting information and advice concerning his illness from his attending physician and intern may be understandably confused and may wish to sign out. The liaison psychiatrist may arrange a meeting between the patient, the intern, and the attending to clarify the conflicting information.

The Hospital and Outside Organizations

Many organizations interdigitate with the hospital in personnel, patients, and material. Others have major impact on the policy decisions of a hospital. Financial support for the hospital may come primarily from the government (federal or local), charities, businesses, or, rarely, from profits.

Laws and regulations at all levels directly influence hospital practices. Examples include the legislative acts requiring nondiscrimination because of race and the formation of professional standards review organizations (PSROs). Insurance companies' policies and practices, such as what procedures are covered, for what types of illness, and for how long, also influence hospitalization patterns and length of stay of patients.

Educational institutions, especially *medical schools,* have major direct influences on the hospitals. Many full-time physicians in hospitals are also faculty members in medical schools and are influenced by the values and practices of the medical school. The prestige of the hospital is often directly related to the degree of affiliation with, and the prestige of, the medical school. This, in turn, affects the quality of the hospital personnel. (The more prestigious institutions can attract better qualified staff.)

Religion and moral standards of the community have an effect on the hospital in influencing the types of patients admitted. (E.g., Catholic hospitals have more Catholic patients and are unlikely to have many elective abortions.)

The quality of patient care and physical and personnel adequacy of the hospital are scrutinized by such organizations as PSROs, the Joint Commission on Accreditation of Hospitals, and the American Medical Association.

Hospitals generally have intimate relationship with other hospitals, and each may refer patients to the others. Chronic care hospitals and psychiatric hospitals often receive patients from general hospitals. Clinics and the offices of private practitioners in the community often refer patients to the general hospital for admission.

The Hospital Environment

When a patient is admitted to a hospital, he finds himself in a strange environment and an alien culture. He is usually apprehensive, because he has a condition considered too serious to be treated in the doctor's office. The intensity of his apprehension increases with his uncertainty about what to expect in the hospital. Much of what will happen in the hospital depends upon tests and procedures to be done there; for example, laboratory test results may indicate the need for an exploratory operation. Depending on what is found at operation, there may be a need for radical surgery, chemotherapy, or no treatment—possibly the difference between life and death. *Uncertainty reigns.*

The *physical environment* of the hospital is not of much help in alleviating admission apprehension and anxiety. Cold, impersonal architectural styles, dark, gloomy rooms, and busy, business-like, and forbidding staff characterize many traditional, especially older, hospitals. Patients often feel like unwelcome guests who nonetheless have to stay for, and in fear of, their lives.

Once in a hospital room, particularly multiple-bed rooms, the patient may be confronted with almost total *lack of privacy.* Conversations can be overheard, and many of the most private functions such as elimination now become public—often patients do not have *control* over when to bathe, urinate, or defecate—sponge baths are given by nurses, intimate parts of the body can be poked, observed, photographed, X rayed, opened, or even cut with little advance warning and, it seems to the patient, by almost anyone wearing a uniform. There even is little control over what the patient can eat or drink.

The *language* spoken by the "people who count" in the hospital, the doctors and nurses, often sounds foreign to the patients—somehow distant and professional. They feel too stupid to ask questions—besides, the staff members seem to be so busy. The patients also may be in terror of offending the doctors and nurses—after all, their lives *literally* depend on them.

An interesting situation occurs at the time of *doctors' rounds.* The history of the patient, often including rather personal and confidential material, is presented to the attending while other patients, their visitors, and other staff (possibly the janitor and the maid) are looking on. Then, the patient may be undressed to varying degrees to be examined by a number of persons including the medical students. Heated debates concerning the diagnosis and treatment plans may take place among the house staff members and the medical students. The intern or resident who had the closest relationship with the patient may be humiliated by the attending for his lack of knowledge or for (horrors!) stupid proposals about treatment. Occasionally, discussion concerning a patient whom the doctors have already finished seeing continues in front of the next patient's bed. Of course, the patient before whose bed the discussion takes place assumes that the discussion is about him! Thus, sometimes patients get entirely erroneous ideas about their conditions and treatment plans at the time of medical rounds.

Most patients' personal habit patterns must undergo change in the hospital. Their activities change and so do their habits concerning food, routine, and personal hygiene. Patients who like to play golf or work every day may have to, instead, read or watch television. Patients who are accustomed to sleeping alone may find it hard to fall asleep in a multiple-bed room and annoying to be awakened in the middle of the night for the check on vital signs (blood pressure, pulse rate, temperature, and respiration). One patient's groaning, snoring, or moaning may keep other patients awake. Sedating medications, on the other hand, may keep patients constantly in a daze.

Many patients lose track of time in the hospital, and those who have the vulnerability become confused. Even if the elderly patient with cerebral arteriosclerosis had not been confused at home in his usual habitat, in the absence of normal cues to help orient themselves, many such patients become disoriented, confused, and agitated in the hospital, especially toward the evening when fewer cues are available (sundowning syndrome).

It should be understood that patients may become very *self-centered* in the hospital, partially as a function of the anxiety concerning the self and also partially due to the regression fostered by the hospital environment (see Chapter 5). When this happens, a patient may develop a tendency to think that almost anything he sees or hears is somehow related to him. Patients commonly think that conversation overheard between the doctors or nurses in the corridor concerns them; even conversations between other patients may be misinterpreted. The implication of this is that the staff should refrain from saying things within hearing of any patient (especially in the corridors or in the same room as the patient behind drawn curtains) which might be misconstrued in any way.

Certain specialized units in the general hospital present particular problems due to the physical and interpersonal environment. They include the intensive care unit, recovery room, operating room, hemodialysis unit, isolation unit, and cancer ward.

The *intensive care unit,* including the coronary care unit, has been thought to be contributory to a psychiatric syndrome called the "ICU psychosis." This is usually characterized by confusion, agitation, and a florid paranoid psychosis. ICU psychosis is most often considered to be an organic psychosis due to sensory deprivation (monotony), electrolyte imbalance, and multiple medications that are often administered in the ICU. Drug-induced psychosis, especially by meperidine (Demerol) and by antiarrhythmic agents such as atropine, lidocaine, and procaine is also common in the ICU.

The physical setting of the coronary care unit seems to have an impact on the general feeling tone of patients. Leigh *et al.* (1972) studied two types of coronary care units in the same hospital: an open, four-bed type and closed private cubicles. They found that patients were freer to express hostility, were concerned about possible shame, and manifested more anxiety concerning mutilation in the "open" unit, whereas patients in the cubicles were unable to express hostility directly but tended to deny and displace hostility or direct it inward and were more concerned about loneliness and separation. In the coronary care units studied, patients who showed high levels of hostility directed inward, low levels of overt hostility, and high levels of separation anxiety had a higher risk of developing cardiac arrhythmias.

Hackett and his colleagues (1968) showed that patients who were able to deny anxiety effectively in the coronary care unit had a better prognosis than those who were unable to deny their anxiety. Witnessing other patients' distress and death is another hazard of being in an ICU. Most patients are able to deny these events effectively, but the next time, they tend to state a preference to be in single rooms (Hackett *et al.,* 1968). Although most patients deny being apprehensive in the coronary care unit, they nonetheless think about rather sad events, such as the death of loved ones in the past. An implication of this is that the physician need not feel constrained to inquire of these patients whether they are thinking upsetting or sad thoughts, lest he "suggest" such thoughts to them.

Psychological preparation is important in transferring patients out of the coronary care unit. Klein *et al.* (1968) found that patients had emotional reactions and more frequent cardiovascular complications (accompanied by an increase in urinary catecholamines) if they were transferred out of a coronary care unit without preparation. On the other hand, when the patients were psychologically prepared beforehand about the transfer, and when the primary nurse actually accompanied the patients to the new ward and introduced them to the new nurse, there were fewer complications after the transfer and less increase in urinary catecholamines.

The (surgical) *recovery room,* like the ICU, is a very confusing environment. Here, there is a curious and intense mixture of sensory overload and sensory monotony. There is always activity and usually no night–day difference because of artificial lighting and absence of windows. In addition, the patients are, as a rule, heavily sedated and in the process of recovering from anesthesia. Organic brain syndrome due to central nervous system depression brought on by anoxia (operative), medications, electrolyte imbalance, etc., is common. Severe pain can contribute to the disorientation.

Some patients in the surgical recovery room are also unable to talk because of tracheostomies or soreness due to endotracheal tubes. This often results in severe frustration and fear on the patients' part, as well as agitation. For these patients, provision of a pencil and paper is often extremely welcome.

A rather frequent cause of agitation and psychosis during the postoperative phase is withdrawal from alcohol and other central nervous system depressants (see vignette 4, Chapter 9). Patients' drug and alcohol histories should be carefully obtained at the time of hospitalization to prevent such withdrawal reactions from complicating the postoperative picture. Many alcoholic patients secretly bring alcoholic beverages into the hospital. Thus, delirium tremens can occur three days postoperatively, even though the patient may have been in the hospital for many days prior to the surgery.

A special form of psychosis, called *postcardiotomy* delirium, has been reported after open-heart surgery. Typically, the picture, consisting of illusions, visual hallucinations, and paranoid delusions, occurs after a lucid period of three to four days following the operation. The sensory monotony, sensory overload, amount of time on the artificial pump, and sleep deprivation in the surgical recovery unit have been suspected as contributing factors. The personality of the patient also seems to contribute to the development of postcardiotomy delirium—those individuals scoring high on the dominance scale on Cattel and Weber's 16 Personality Factor Questionnaire have a greater tendency to develop it (Kornfeld et al., 1972). The delirium usually clears within 24–48 hours after the patient is transferred to a standard hospital environment (Kornfeld et al., 1972). This postcardiotomy delirium can be distinguished from the organic brain syndrome some patients have after open-heart surgery in that in the latter, the confusion is demonstrable immediately after the surgery, without any intervening lucid period.

The *operating room* is an environment in which patients often hear more than they see. In the course of the induction of anesthesia, hearing is the last sensory modality to become anesthetized and the first one to return. Even when the patient seems to be unconscious, he may still be able to hear. Conversations before an "unconscious" anesthetized patient, therefore, should be cautious and judicious. Thoughtless joking about the patient or discussions about the serious nature of his disease should be avoided. Special psychotherapeutic measures such as ventilation under hypnosis may sometimes be necessary to work through anxiety and depression resulting from the effects of conversation overheard during anesthesia (Cheek, 1959).

The *hemodialysis unit* provides life support for many patients with chronic renal failure. Being dependent upon the machine for life creates a number of psychological problems, including a sense of lack of control and of being dependent upon external control. Some patients do not comply with the restriction in salt and fluid intake, and the suicidal rate is greatly increased. Electrolyte imbalance and uremia often produce organic brain syndromes and depression. Here, again, successful use of denial has been associated with good prognosis.

Isolation rooms are provided in the hospital for patients with infectious diseases or when reverse isolation (guarding against exposure to infection) is necessary, such as in immunodeficiency diseases. The patients are in individual rooms, and everyone entering may have to wear a mask and a gown. There is a reduction in the number of visitors. In extreme cases, the patient may be in a plastic "bubble," totally insulated from the outside, only touched through plastic gloves at the end of plastic arms built into the walls. Sometimes, individuals dressed in "space suits," wearing gloves, of course, may touch the patient. In this type of environment, the most significant complaint by patients is their inability to touch or be touched by another human being (Holland *et al.,* 1970). The significance of touching in development has already been discussed in Chapter 12.

The *cancer ward* increases anxiety and defensiveness on the part of both the patients and the staff. Patients are especially attuned to the doctors' attitudes—for signs of hope or evidence of rejection. Although patients usually do not ask the physicians directly about the prognosis of advancing cancer, they tend to consider the physicians' continuing interest almost as a commitment to cure. The physicians, on the other hand, tend to use the defense mechanisms of denial, isolation, and intellectualization vis à vis the patients, concentrating on the laboratory results and tissue findings. It is easier for the physician not to confront the patient's approaching death and the doctor's impotence in the face of this inevitability (Leigh, 1973).

Doctors, therefore, have a tendency to minimize their contact with patients, leaving this up to the nurses. The nurses often feel unhappy and angry about having to be the only persons left to deal with the patients at a personal, emotional level. Opening up communications between the nurses and doctors, and showing doctors that their continuing interest is essential for the patients' maintenance of hope, can alleviate this situation. A liaison psychiatrist can contribute to this by being the catalyst for such communication (Klagsburn *et al.,* 1973).

The hospital environment, in general, is a strange and anxiety-provoking environment for the patient. In the face of such anxiety, the patient responds with an exaggeration of his personality style, habitual coping mechanisms, and defenses. In the case of the sick Tarzan (Chapter 13), we see that he was in the coronary care unit, where his anxiety level was increased by the sensory monotony and need for lying in bed. During the interview, his personality style of exaggerated showing off, dramatizing tendencies, as well as the need to be in control was clearly demonstrated. One also sees evidence of major denial ("Nothing bothers me"), which augers well for the patient in terms of prognosis, if only it would be modulated and he would stay in bed.

Summary

The hospital is a *complex social system,* influenced by various factors in the larger society. The formal hierarchical organization of the hospital personnel has *two lines of authority:* the physicians and all of the other employees. Nurses, unlike physicians, are directly responsible to the hospital administration and at the same time, are responsible to physicians in terms of patient care. Across occupations in the general hospital, there is a *"blocked mobility";* that is, one cannot be promoted from one occupational level to another without further schooling.

Physicians often have *dual loyalties:* patient care and academic, especially in teaching institutions.

The typical *inpatient unit* in a general hospital is the functional unit in patient care, consisting of the beds, patients, nursing staff, ancillary staff, supporting staff, and physicians. Liaison psychiatrists and liaison nurses can play an important role in the smooth function of such a unit.

The hospital environment, in general, is characterized by *uncertainty* and lack of control from the patient's point of view. Certain special areas of the hospital, such as the intensive care unit, have their own special environments and attendant problems.

Implications

For the Patient

The hospital environment is a highly anxiety-provoking one in which the patient is threatened with the loss of autonomy and, possibly, life. *Privacy* is often disregarded, and patients feel too stupid to ask questions or make requests. There are particular problems associated with special areas of the hospital. Patients should be *prepared,* if possible, about what to expect in the hospital, including whom to ask for information, etc.

For the Physician

For obvious reasons, physicians feel quite at home in the hospital. They therefore tend to feel that the patients should share their feeling of ease and familiarity in the hospital. Physicians should recognize how frightening and strange the hospital environment is for the patients. Physicians should make deliberate attempts to *ask* patients about their reactions to the physical and interpersonal environments of the hospital and encourage them to *communicate* their thoughts and feelings. Physicians should also recognize that cooperation among the professions and occupations in the hospital, including nurses and other workers, is essential for good patient care. Doctors should encourage the *nurses to report* any new observations concerning patients and to communicate openly about difficulties or dissatisfactions. Doctors should also recognize the *"double bind"* nurses often feel in having dual lines of authority to which they are responsible.

For the Community and Health Care System

Hospitals should be constructed *aesthetically* and *functionally*. Every room should have paintings, calendars, and television or radio. Educational programs should be designed for patients and potential patients about where to get information in the hospital and where to "gripe," and the hospital administration and the medical establishment should encourage communication and cooperation among different occupational groups in the hospital. Medical education should emphasize respect for a patient's *privacy* and the importance of not embarrassing patients (or the medical student, for that matter) on walk rounds. Hospitals should provide *liaison psychiatrists* for patient care units to foster cooperation and communication among different groups and also to prevent and manage behavioral and emotional problems of patients.

Recommended Reading

Coe RM: *Sociology of Medicine*. New York, McGraw-Hill, 1970. A lucid and concise textbook of medical sociology. Has a good chapter on the hospital as a social system, as well as on the development of the modern hospital.
Kornfeld DS: The hospital environment: Its impact on the patient. *Adv Psychosom Med* 8:252–270, 1972. A good review paper on the hospital environment's impact on the patient. Good list of references for interested readers.

References

Cheek DS: Unconscious perception of meaningful sounds during surgical anesthesia as revealed under hypnosis. *Am J Clin Med* 1:101, 1959.
Coe RM: *Sociology of Medicine*. New York, McGraw-Hill, 1970, pp 270–271.
Freeman HE, Levine S, Reeder LG: *Handbook of Medical Sociology*. Englewood Cliffs, NJ, Prentice-Hall, 1972, pp 276–277.
Hackett TP, Gassem NY, Wishnie HA: The coronary care unit: An appraisal of its psychologic hazards. *N Engl J Med* **279**:1365–1370, 1968.

Holland J, Harris S, Plumb M, *et al.*: Psychological aspects of physical barrier isolation: Observation of acute leukemia patients in germ-free units. *Proc Int Congr Hematol*, 1970.

Hollingshead AB, Redlich FC: *Social Class and Mental Illness.* New York, John Wiley & Sons, 1958.

Klagsburn S: Cancer, emotions and nurses, *Am J Psychiatry* **126**: 1227–1244, 1970.

Klein RF, Kliner VS, Zipes DP, *et al.*: Transfer from a coronary care unit. *Arch Intern Med* **122**:104–108, 1968.

Kornfeld DS, Heller SS, Frank KA, *et al.*: Personality and psychololgical factors in postcardiotomy delirium. *Arch Gen Psychiatry* **31**:249–253, 1974.

Leigh H: Psychiatric liaison on a neoplastic inpatient service. *Int J Psychiatry Med* **4**:147–154, 1973.

Leigh H, Hofer M, Cooper J, *et al.*: A psychological comparison of patients in "open" and "closed" coronary care units. *J Psychosom Res* **16**:449–458, 1972.

Myers JK, Bean LL: *A Decade Later: A Follow-Up of Social Class and Mental Illness.* New York, John Wiley & Sons, 1968.

Raphael W: If I could alter one thing. *Ment Health (London)*, pp 1–5, 1965.

Roth JA, Eddy EM: *Rehabilitation for the Unwanted.* New York, Atherton Press, 1967.

Scott RA: *The Making of Blind Men: A Study of Adult Socialization.* New York, Russell Sage Foundation, 1969.

Smith H: Two lines of authority are one too many. *Modern Hospital* **85**:48–52, 1955.

Wesson AF: Hospital ideology and communication between ward personnel, in Jaco E (ed): *Patients, Physicians and Illness.* New York, The Free Press, 1958, pp 448–468.

CHAPTER 17

Therapeutic Dimensions

A 42-year-old married white man was admitted to the hospital with high fever. Subsequent workup showed that he had aspiration pneumonia (pneumonia due to aspiration of a foreign substance such as food into the lungs, usually in a state of intoxication or coma). History revealed and highlighted the fact that the patient had increased his alcohol intake considerably in the last two years. He had been divorced four years ago and remarried two years ago. His second wife had turned out to be an alcoholic.

In addition to aspiration pneumonia with secondary staphylococcal infection, liver function tests showed abnormalities indicating early liver disease, probably due to excessive alcohol consumption. The pneumonia was treated with antibiotics. The high fever was treated with aspirin and alcohol rubs. His wife was interviewed by the doctor and the social worker. As the pneumonia subsided, the doctor had a serious talk with the patient and his wife concerning the role of alcohol in the patient's medical condition. It was decided that both the patient and his wife should join Alcoholics Anonymous. Also, arrangements were made for them to see the social worker on a regular basis for couples therapy. They were also directed to take multivitamins.

Management plans must be directed at all three (the biological, the personal, and the environmental) dimensions. In the foregoing vignette, the main biological treatment for the disease, pneumonia, was antibiotics. To prevent the vitamin deficiency syndrome often occurring in alcoholism, multivitamins were also prescribed.

Alcohol rub for the fever was a treatment directed at the heat interchange between the patient and the physical environment. Air conditioning and humidification of the room are also examples of therapy in this dimension.

The physician was able to diagnose a disorder at the personal level in this patient—alcoholism (or the pattern of excessive alcohol intake). Further, he found that this disorder was shared, and probably encouraged, by the patient's wife. The management plans thus included treatment for alcoholism in the environmental and personal dimensions through Alcoholics Anonymous, the social worker, and couples therapy.

We will now briefly consider some common therapeutic modalities as they are directed primarily at each of the dimensions of the patient system. It will be clear, however, in each of the sections that the actual therapeutic effects interact extensively across dimensions.

Approaches in the Biological Dimension

Broadly considered, any therapeutic intervention works through the biological system, including interpersonal interventions and those directed at the personal dimension, since even symbolic transactions occur through perception and cognitive processes whose substrates are physicochemical. In the discussion that follows, treatment at the biological level is considered in a narrower sense, that is, biological treatment of the disease, such as treatment directed at eradicating its etiologic cause (e.g., the use of antibiotics, potassium administration to correct hypokalemia and surgical correction of tetralogy of Fallot). Most medications are used with the expectation that the biological effect will result in cure, reversal, or amelioration of the disease process. Despite such expectations of biological efficacy, physicians should recognize that many drugs work also through the expectancy effect (personal dimension). Furthermore, medications with proven biological effects may, in addition, have *side effects in the personal dimension* (Chapter 18). The side effects on the personality may be mediated through the drug's biological effect on the central nervous system or through its symbolic meaning. For example, although methadone is a potent analgesic biologically, some patients upon receiving it may become anxious because they identify it with drug addiction, and they may experience little pain relief, especially if it is administered without adequate explanation and reassurance. Many drugs cause psychological effects. (E.g., depression is a relatively common side effect of certain medications, such as reserpine, a drug used in management of hypertension.)

Surgery is a definitive intervention in the biological dimension. However, it is important to recognize that surgery also may have placebo effects. For a while many years ago, ligation of the internal thoracic artery was considered to be effective in the treatment of angina pectoris, and, in fact, many patients seemed to benefit from it. Eventually, however, the procedure turned out to be without long-term benefit. The beneficial effects experienced by patients were due to the placebo effect.

Some medications and surgical procedures have major interpersonal side effects (side effects in the environmental dimension). For example, foul-smelling ointments, loss of hair due to chemotherapy, and mutilating operative procedures may restrict the patient's social contact. With some biological treatments, such as the plaster cast, the patient's mobility is greatly compromised.

Surgical procedures are often associated with personal fantasies unrelated to their biological effects. For example, the frequent confusion between the kidney and genital organ functions may lead some patients to have fears concerning sexual potency after nephrectomy. Many women have the notion that their sexual enjoyment and libido will cease following simple hysterectomy. In fact, because of this expectation in some patients, there may be changes in sexual behavior and experience after hysterectomy even though the external genitals and ovaries are intact.

Physicians should *explore* the patient's fantasies and ideas concerning any proposed biological intervention and *clarify* them with adequate and lucid information.

Approaches in the Personal Dimension

Therapy in the personal dimension is geared toward the *patient's illness behavior, general health* (including habits), and the *meaning of illness* and psychological reactions to it. Reduction of the suffering aspect of the disease (illness) is essential for good collaborative work between the doctor and the patient. As we examined in Chapter 3, the immediate expectations of the patient in the consulting room are primarily concerned with reduction of suffering (personal dimension).

Biological treatment modalities that may be used for treatment in the personal dimension include *drugs, physical therapy,* and *electroshock treatment,* as well as psychotherapy and psychosocial interventions. Unlike biological treatment in the biological dimension, in which etiologic factors are the main target, biological treatment modalities in the personal dimension are primarily directed at modifying *feelings* and at general functional capacities and well-being of the patient. Accordingly, drugs used in symptomatic treatment, for example, to relieve pain and anxiety or to reduce fever and inflammation, are included in this category.

As discussed in Chapter 14, the *doctor–patient relationship* is a powerful therapeutic tool operating in the personal dimension. The placebo aspects of being treated by a doctor are often powerful, at least initially, no matter what the doctor actually does to treat the disease. Newly "discovered" medications and procedures often seem especially efficacious as a result of this effect—thus, the admonition, "You should treat as many patients as possible with new drugs while they still have the power to heal," which has been attributed to Trousseau, Osler, and Lewis (Shapiro, 1960). Physicians should be aware of this temptation and weigh the possible expectancy effect (beneficial) of a new medication against possible, yet unreported, adverse effects. The potency of the healing effect of the doctor–patient relationship can be increased by the physician's interest, empathy, and competence. It can be neutralized by a lack of interest in attempting to understand where the patient's distress and concerns are focused.

Psychotherapy in Medical Settings

Psychotherapy conducted by the physician consists of the application of psychological techniques within the context of the doctor–patient relationship, usually with specified and limited goals in mind. A more general and detailed discussion of psychotherapy is beyond the scope of this book. Interested readers should refer to standard psychiatric texts. The brief discussion that follows deals with psychotherapeutic principles and techniques which nonpsychiatric physicians should understand and be able to use effectively in clinical practice.

The doctor–patient relationship renders any and all actions and ministrations of the physician psychologically influential, whether they are explicitly intended to be or not. In turn, their psychological impact can and often does influence the course of illness and the patient's response to treatment. The physician who understands the psychological meaning of his work with patients can wittingly, judiciously, and deliberately utilize the psychotherapeutic potential inherent in the doctor–patient relationship in order to promote healing and maximize the beneficial effects of his medical treatment. Consider, for example, the psychological aspects of history-taking, physical examination, ordering of diagnostic tests, prescription of medication, and scheduling and conduct of follow-up visits.

The friendly and nonjudgmental, but, at the same time, professional interest and concern that are manifested toward the patient by the physician in the process of skillful *medical history-taking* provide an interpersonal base for reassurance and for the relief of tension that occurs in the patient when he can share with the doctor personal worries, problems, guilts, and anxieties that he had not shared with anyone previously and so had carried as private personal burdens. And, as the patient is encouraged to review possible contributing factors to disease, important facts concerning personal habits (smoking, alcohol, etc.), occupational stresses, interpersonal tensions, etc., may emerge that will be relevant to formulating the nature of the clinical problem and the therapeutic approaches that will be required to deal with it.

Similarly, it is easy, upon reflection, to appreciate the anxiety-relieving value of a thorough *physical examination*—skillfully and systematically conducted in an appropriate, dignified, and comfortable setting. This is important in setting the basic tone for the developing doctor–patient relationship. Readers might think back upon some of their own personal experiences as patients undergoing physical examination.

It is important for the physician not only to plan a program of *diagnostic procedures* in advance but also to share its rationale, strategy, and meanings with the patient. The physician's medical knowledge and skill are often crucially tested when he has to decide when and whether to dispense with further diagnostic tests. The way in which differential diagnosis is pursued can reinforce previous good developments in the relationship and can be particularly important in imparting to the patient the belief that the doctor is competent, concerned, and trustworthy.

When these initial steps have gone well, the patient's trust and confidence are based upon reality as well as upon positive transference phenomena which, of course, reinforce them.

At this juncture, the issue of *sharing information* with the patient and of *reassurance* warrants discussion. Reassurance should never be "hollow" or insincere; that is, the physician should not make explicit assertions that he knows to be unfounded. When it is necessary to spare the patient undue worry and anxiety, it is usually better for the doctor to carry the burden of leaving some things unsaid until such time as the patient may be ready to cope with them. Most often, the patient's fears are much worse than reality—providing the physician with considerable room for positive, explicit, factual explanations that will be reassuring. As we have noted earlier, sharing information is important, and in doing this, the doctor should take into consideration the patient's personality type, habitual defenses, and ways of coping in order to provide the information in a way that will be most helpful and useful to the patient (Chapter 15).

Hospitalization may be psychotherapeutic in several ways. In spite of the anxiety and adjustment process inherent in this major environmental change for the patient (see Chapter 16), hospitalization (if prepared for thoughtfully) means a definitive step for the patient in his commitment to fight the disease process. The hospital environment, once its disturbing features have been dealt with, provides the patient with a safe place where competent professionals will help him to get well. In fact, for some patients, the hospital may provide a needed temporary respite ("vacation") from pathogenic stressful life situations with which they have not yet been able to cope successfully. Complex and imposing hospital equipment may be seen as reassuring. Without trust in the physician and hospital (based on careful preparation and/or preexisting good relationship), the same equipment may be frightening. Hospitalization may provide legitimate opportunities for gratifying dependency needs, and this may relieve a chronic state of frustration or deprivation that may even have contributed to predisposition or vulnerability to disease. Some patients may, for the first time, gain a perspective on their lives and learn better ways of coping or relaxing during the course of hospitalization.

Follow-up appointments manifest that (1) the physician is interested in the patient's course and recovery and (2) the physician feels some hope about the patient's future and, in any case, will not abandon him. The latter is especially reassuring to seriously ill patients, including terminal cancer patients (Abrams, 1966). *Physical therapy* may provide a sense of mastery and hope for paralyzed patients. *Drugs,* as we have seen, are potent psychotherapeutic as well as pharmacotherapeutic agents. This is not only because of placebo effects. In addition to the fact that it is reassuring for the patient to know that there is a drug for his illness, the doctor's "giving" of the medication often gratifies basic dependency needs and is received in the context of the patient's trusting relationship with the physician. On the other hand, if drugs are given casually and haphazardly, the patient may consider the drug as a poor substitute for the physician's interest—an antipsychotherapeutic effect (see Chapter 18).

Psychotherapeutic *techniques* that may be used by the general physician in the context of medical management of patients include the following:

Reassurance. This consists of a general optimistic and hopeful attitude and specific statements based on data and/or experience designed to allay exaggerated or unfounded fears of the patient. For reassurance to be effective, the physician should know the sources of the patient's fears. They often are based on an incorrect understanding of the disease or proposed procedure.

Sharing Life's Problems. The doctor is a person in whom many patients can confide and to whom they can talk about things that they may feel embarrassed or fearful to discuss with anyone else. The simple act of verbalizing an emotionally taxing thought or situation can relieve chronic anxiety (and physiologic activation that accompanies it). After such verbalization, the patient may achieve a fresh outlook and be able to cope with the situation. The process of talking about an emotionally charged situation or thought, with expression of the emotion, has been called "ventilation"; we consider the term "sharing life's problems" to convey its nature more correctly.

Guidance and Advice. Judicious advice and guidance based on sound medical knowledge carries authority and often achieves readier acceptance by the patient than if it had been offered by a parent or employer. This is especially true when the advice is directed toward a possible contributing factor to disease, such as alcohol. For example, an alcoholic patient who has just recovered from an exquisitely painful episode of pancreatitis is more likely to heed the physician's advice (rather than a relative's) to join Alcoholics Anonymous.

Education. Through an educative process involving questions and answers and, possibly, reading material suggested by the doctor (bibliotherapy) the patient can learn about his medical condition and the doctor's strategy in treating it. This can reduce unnecessary anxiety and reinforce positive aspects of the doctor–patient relationship. This may also foster the adaptive defense mechanisms of sublimation and intellectualization (Chapter 5). Education may also be directed toward behavioral changes to reduce contributing factors to disease, for example, the dangers of smoking and the early warning signs of cancer requiring checkup.

Environmental Manipulations (see also the section on Approaches in the Environmental Dimension). When it becomes clear that certain stressful factors in the environment (occupational, interpersonal, etc.) are participating as serious vectors by precipitating or accelerating the disease process, it may be wise for the physician to suggest changes in the environment if such factors can be avoided (e.g., change of job and avoidance of mother-in-law's visits).

Limited Interpretations. This consists of judicious sharing with the patient the observation that certain stressful life situations are regularly associated with flare-up of disease or with incidence of symptoms. For example, the physician may note that many of a patient's attacks of migraine headache have regularly followed periods of intense pressured work in order to meet deadlines. The patient may be unaware of this fact, and, if confronted, may be able to rearrange work schedules to avoid repetitions of this situation or develop better ways of coping with the stress, for example, by finding tension outlets at such times in exercise or the practice of relaxation techniques. Obviously, the physician must know his patient quite well and have a good basic relationship in order to apply his own "insight" into the patient's problems in this way. The same holds true for environmental manipulation.

What may all of the foregoing accomplish, particularly for patients in whom psychosocial factors may play relatively minor roles as etiologic, pathogenic, or influencing factors? For many patients, the doctor's expectations of realizing direct positive benefits for the patient may be quite limited. Still, some very worthwhile limited goals may be realized:

1. Varying degrees of symptom relief
2. Giving up of secondary gain
3. Improvement in morale and overall quality of adjustment to illness, maintenance of hope
4. Improvement in general life adjustment, interpersonal relationships, and quality of life
5. Achievement of good compliance with the medical regimen

Noncompliance is a major problem in medical care (Sackett and Haynes, 1976), particularly in chronic diseases that are relatively asymptomatic for long periods, but nonetheless dangerous if untreated, for example, essential hypertension. Perhaps one of the major benefits of good psychologically oriented medical management is realized in prevention of serious noncompliance.

For patients in whom psychosocial stresses may play contributing etiologic, pathogenic, or influencing roles, some additional benefits may be realized to the degree that the measures discussed above enable the patient to manage his life more effectively (i.e., to avoid stressful situations, where possible and to understand, defend, and/or cope better); the rate of progession of the disease process may be slowed and complications and/or exacerbations delayed and possibly, in some cases, avoided.

Often, the physician who works in this way with patients will find that problems persist to the degree that a patient needs more advanced or specialized psychotherapy. This may be either because his life-adjustment problems are serious enough in their own right to require it or because the doctor judges that they are seriously aggravating the disease. Here is where another benefit of working in this way (psychotherapeutically) is realized—the patient can be expected to react positively to the suggestion that he have a consultation with a psychiatrist. The physician is in a position to make an effective and comfortable referral. For example:

> Mrs. Jones, it is clear from our discussions that your ulcer flared up when things got tense at home between you and your husband. The problems in your marriage that you are telling me about touch on issues that may be beyond my technical competence as an internist. But since they, like the foods you eat, etc., play an important part in healing or failure to heal, I think it would be a good idea for you to see Dr. Smith, a specialist in psychiatry, for a consultation. He has been helpful to me before in evaluating such situations and in helping to reach an opinion on the advisability of undertaking a course of psychotherapy. In any case, I will continue with your medical treatment and follow-up.

Such a referral does *not:* (1) say to the patient, "It is all in your head"; (2) reject the patient; (3) leave the patient without hope.

Formal Psychotherapy

Formal psychotherapy may be classified into individual, couple, family, and group psychotherapies on the basis of the number and type of patients treated. On the basis of theoretical orientation, it may be psychodynamically oriented (which may be again subclassified into Freudian, Jungian, Adlerian, Sullivanian, Horneyian, etc.), behavior-therapy-oriented (Skinnerian), "client-centered" (Rogerian), or "eclectic" (flexible combinations of the above). Medications, when needed, may be combined with any of these approaches. Classified on the basis of special techniques, there are psychoanalysis, psychoanalytically oriented psychotherapy, hypnosis, sodium amytal interview, behavior therapy (techniques such as desensitization, flooding, biofeedback), sex therapy, and others such as psychodrama and art therapy.

Most psychodynamically oriented psychotherapies can be classified along a spectrum from mainly "insight-oriented" to mainly "supportive" psychotherapies, although, almost invariably, they coexist with differing emphasis on one or the other aspect. The insight-oriented psychotherapies, as represented by psychoanalysis, aim at helping the patient develop understanding—explanatory concepts regarding the unconscious conflictual origin of his difficulties—that will aid in resolving conflict and permitting personality growth and more satisfactory life adjustment. Supportive psychotherapies (aspects) aim primarily at increasing the patient's defensive and coping abilities.

Self-Regulatory Techniques (Biofeedback, Relaxation Response, Self-Hypnosis). Biofeedback, relaxation and meditative techniques, and self-hypnosis are geared toward "self-regulation," that is, the maintenance of adaptive changes in the body through self-generated behaviors (Leigh, 1978). Through these techniques, the patient can control maladaptive or potentially maladaptive physiologic activation, produce a state of relaxation, and increase his coping abilities.

Biofeedback is a technique by which an individual learns to acquire control over bodily functions that are usually not controlled voluntarily, such as skin temperature, heart rate, blood pressure, and tones of certain muscles as recorded by EMG. This usually involves the use of electronic equipment that monitors the organ system to be controlled, whose activity is "fed back" to the patient in the form of signals indicating the success or failure of the attempted control. For example, blinking green lights from a polygraph may indicate a decrease in heart rate. The subject may then attempt to increase the frequency of the green light if he is to learn to decrease his heart rate. Biofeedback is based on operant conditioning principles.

Operant conditioning (sometimes called "instrumental" conditioning) was first described by B. F. Skinner in the 1930s (Skinner, 1938). Learning by operant conditioning, unlike Pavlov's classical conditioning (see Chapter 4), involves behaviors that are learned in response to *reward* or *punishment*. For example, a hungry rat in a cage equipped with a lever will, at some point, lean on the lever (spontaneously emitted behavior or "operant behavior"). If food is given to the rat each time it leans on the lever, the animal will increase the frequency of lever-pressing. The food in this case is a *positive reinforcer,* a stimulus that increases the probability of the operant behavior if the stimulus is given after it. A *negative reinforcer* is a stimulus whose *removal* following an operant behavior increases the probability of that behavior. For example, if a rat can turn off continuous electric shock by pressing a lever, the shock is a negative reinforcer for the operant response of pressing the lever.

Operant conditioning was initially considered to be a higher type of learning than classical conditioning, and the autonomic nervous system, being more primitive phylogenetically than the voluntary somatosensory nervous system, was considered to be incapable of operant conditioning. The pioneering work of Miller (1969) and his colleagues showed, however, that the autonomic nervous system could indeed "learn" from reward and punishment. For example, he was able to show that animals could, among other things, increase or decrease blood pressure and pulse rate, and increase or decrease glomerular filtration rate in response to reward. Biofeedback is the clinical application of this principle. Biofeedback has been shown to be effective in a variety of stress-related disorders such as migraine headaches, Raynaud's disease, certain cardiac arrhythmias, and tension headaches (Blanchard and Young, 1974; Task Force Reports of the Biofeedback Society of America, 1978).

The *relaxation response* is defined by Benson (1977) as a set of integrated physiologic changes that may be elicited when a subject assumes a relaxed position and engages in a repetitive mental action, passively ignoring distracting thoughts. The physiologic changes include decreases in oxygen consumption, heart rate, respiratory rate, and blood lactate; slight increases in skeletal muscle blood flow; and an increase in the EEG alpha waves. This response is presumed to be an integrated hypothalamic response that functions as a protective mechanism against overstress and as a counteraction against the fight–flight response (see Chapter 4).

The relaxation response was identified by Benson (1975) when he was studying the physiologic changes accompanying meditative techniques. Thus, the self-regulatory physiologic effects of meditative techniques are considered to be mediated by the relaxation response. The relaxation response seems to be a useful adjunct in the management of essential hypertension (Benson, 1977; Jacob *et al.*, 1977; Blanchard and Miller, 1977).

Self-hypnosis may also be used to bring about muscular relaxation and emotional tranquility. Hypnosis seems to elicit beneficial physiologic effects through vivid imagery and, in highly susceptible individuals, through a change in perception (Hilgard, 1965, 1975; McGlashan *et al.*, 1969). Self-hypnosis is also useful in pain control, habit control (such as smoking and overeating), and anxiety control (Spiegel and Spiegel, 1978). Interestingly, hypnoanesthesia is not reversed by naloxone, unlike acupuncture anesthesia or placebo anesthesia (Goldstein, 1976).

Approaches in the Environmental Dimension

Any treatment modality involves some environmental change, including the contact with the health care system for the patient. As noted above, simply being in the hospital is often helpful for the patient, because of both the expectations of forthcoming help and a sense of being "in good hands." Beneficial effects may also arise from the distancing of the patient from possibly pathogenic physical and/or interpersonal situations by admission to the hospital.

A change in the environment other than that of hospitalization may be indicated in some patients. Until recently, rest cure was an important treatment modality very commonly prescribed by physicians. We are all familiar with the revitalizing effects of a vacation away from home.

Environmental change may be necessary specifically to avoid pathogens, as in the case of severe allergies to endemic allergens. This may involve, for some patients, giving up pets, and for others, moving to a different climate.

Interpersonal changes may involve family (divorce, marriage, family planning, etc.), schools, occupations, or type of work. For example, a patient with serious heart disease may have to be transferred from a physically strenuous job to a less strenuous one.

Another interpersonal change may involve *changes in approach* to the patient. The hospital staff's learning how to approach a patient while taking into account his personality needs can result in a therapeutic environmental change. In the case of the sick Tarzan, this played a very important role in the management strategy (see Chapter 19).

Often, strains and tensions among the *staff* contribute to behavioral and psychological problems of patients. For example, when excessive staff turnover and low morale have generated interpersonal difficulties between members of the hospital staff, measures taken to improve morale and communication between and among the different groups (Chapter 16) will often, if successful, produce a better environment for patient care and amelioration of what appeared to be patient problems.

The *physical environment of the hospital* room can be therapeutic. A bright and cheerful physical environment contributes to a hopeful and optimistic psychological set. Respecting the patient's wishes concerning a multiple-bed or private room can increase his sense of control and so lessen anxiety (Leigh *et al.*, 1972).

It is essential that the hospital environment provide patients who have a tendency to be confused and irascible (Chapter 15), especially those with chronic organic brain syndrome, with cues for orientation; a large calendar, a clock, and a radio or television. The staff should also introduce themselves each time they touch the patient or perform procedures, since the patient may have forgotten that he is in the hospital and may develop delusions about what the staff is doing. Night-lights are also helpful for these patients, since they may become completely confused and agitated upon waking up at night in strange surroundings. Familiar objects from home (framed photographs, books, etc.) should be brought to the hospital and kept next to the patient's bed. Family and friends should be encouraged to visit. This will reduce the patient's anxiety by providing a sense of security and familiarity.

Summary

Management of a patient involves intervention in three dimensions: the biological, the personal, and the environmental. Therapeutic modalities geared primarily toward the biological system often have additional or side effects at the personal and interpersonal levels. The *doctor–patient relationship* is a powerful tool in therapeutic management in the *personal* dimension. Insight-oriented psychotherapy, in general, aims at helping the patient develop an explanatory perspective concerning his sufferings. Supportive psychotherapy is aimed at increasing the patient's coping ability here and now. Simply providing an opportunity for the patient to talk about his concerns and problems with the physician has major therapeutic impact. Many drugs and surgical procedures are used to alleviate discomfort and promote general health— measures directed at the personal dimension. *Environmental intervention* is *inherent* in any contact of the patient with the health care system, but especially in the case of hospitalization. Changes in approach to the patient can play an important role. For patients with a tendency to confusion, provision of a stable and orienting environment is an important aspect of treatment.

Implications

For the Patient

Therapeutic modalities geared toward the environmental and personal dimensions may have the most obvious impact for the patient. Therapeutic modalities geared toward the biological dimension, if the results are not immediately obvious, may not be adequately appreciated by the patient unless sufficient information is given. The patient's fantasies and ideas concerning all therapeutic modalities are determined by his unique experiences and cultural expectations. His ideas concerning the nature and efficacy of the proposed modality may be entirely at variance with the physician's (e.g., the efficacy of Laetrile, of electroshock therapy or of a particular school of psychoanalysis).

For the Physician

The physician should determine rational management approaches to the patient directed at the *three dimensions* by using the systems–contextual framework and the patient evaluation grid (PEG). The *priority of intervention* is determined on the basis of the gravity of the treatment objective and the immediacy of the problem. Physicians should be aware that the *doctor–patient relationship* is an important therapeutic tool in the personal dimension. We should also think about possible side effects of any proposed therapeutic modality in all three dimensions, for example, the side effects of a surgical procedure at the personal and interpersonal levels.

Psychotherapy is *not* a technique exclusively in the domain of the psychiatrist or psychotherapist. Whenever a physician talks with a patient, there is an element of psychotherapy.

For the Community and Health Care System

Medical education should emphasize the three dimensions of intervention for optimal treatment of patients. Physicians should be educated to play a central role in the three-dimensional management of patients. There has been a tendency for physicians to concentrate on the treatment of disease, while nurses and social workers have been concerned primarily with problems in the personal dimension and their interpersonal aspects. This is less than optimal, as medical knowledge and psychiatric skills taught to physicians are necessary in assessing the therapeutic needs of the patient in all these dimensions. The *primary evaluator* and *manager* of the patient should be the responsible physician, who can bring (and collaborate with) members of other disciplines and specialties into the specialized care of the patient.

Recommended Reading

Levine M: *Psychotherapy in Medical Practice*. New York, Macmillan, 1945. Although somewhat dated, this classic book shows the psychotherapeutic aspects of various ministrations by the general physician, as well as some techniques that can be used by more psychiatrically oriented physicians and psychiatrists.

Shapiro AK: A contribution to a history of the placebo effect. *Behav Sci* **5**:109–135, 1960. This is an excellent review of the prescientific doctor–patient relationship and the placebo effect in general. A highly recommended reading for any student of medicine.

Strain JJ, Grossman S: *Psychological Care of the Medically Ill: A Primer in Liaison Psychiatry.* New York, Appleton-Century-Crofts, 1975. A concise and useful book on the psychological management of medically ill patients. Certain specific clinical issues, such as hypochondriasis, the dying patient, and the surgical patient, are discussed, as well as the function of the liaison psychiatrist in the management of medically ill patients. A good supplementary reading for the student interested in comprehensive care.

References

Abrams R: The patient with cancer: His changing patterns of communcation. *N Engl J Med* **274:**317–322, 1966.

Benson H: *The Relaxation Response.* New York, William Morrow & Co, 1975.

Benson H: Systemic hypertension and the relaxation response. *N Engl J Med* **296:**1152–1156, 1977.

Blanchard EB, Miller ST: Psychological treatment of cardiovascular disease. *Arch Gen Psychiatry* **34:**1402–1413, 1977.

Blanchard EB, Young LD: Clinical applications of biofeedback training: A review of evidence. *Arch Gen Psychiatry* **30:**573–589, 1974.

Goldstein AL: Opioid peptides (endorphins) in pituitary and brain. *Science* **193:**1081–1086, 1976.

Hilgard ER: *Hypnotic Susceptibility.* New York, Harcourt Brace & World, 1965.

Hilgard ER: Hypnosis. *Annu Rev Psychol* **26:**19–44, 1975.

Jacob RG, Kraemer HC, Agras WS: Relaxation therapy in the treatment of hypertension: A review. *Arch Gen Psychiatry* **24:**1417–1427, 1972.

Leigh H: Self-control, biofeedback, and change in "psychosomatic" approach. *Psychother Psychosom* **30:**130–136, 1978.

Leigh H, Hofer M, Cooper J, et al.: A psychological comparison of patients in "open" and "closed" coronary care units. *J Psychosom Res* **16:**449–458, 1972.

McGlashan TH, Evans FJ, Orne MT: The nature of hypnotic analgesia and placebo response to experimental pain. *Psychosom Med* **31:**227–245, 1969.

Miller NE: Learning of visceral and glandular responses. *Science* **163:**434–445, 1969.

Sackett DL, Haynes R (eds): *Compliance with Therapeutic Regimens.* Baltimore, The Johns Hopkins University Press, 1976.

Shapiro AK: A contribution to a history of the placebo effect. *Behav Sci* **5:**109–135, 1960.

Skinner BF: *The Behavior of Organisms: An Experimental Analysis.* New York, Appleton-Century-Crofts, 1938.

Spiegel H, Spiegel D: *Trance and Treatment: Clinical Uses of Hypnosis.* New York, Basic Books, 1978.

Task Force Reports of the Biofeedback Society of America, *Biofeedback Self Regul* 3 (4), 1978.

CHAPTER 18

Drugs Affecting Behavior

1. A 20-year-old single woman who works as a secretary complained of a severe headache. Another secretary working in the same office gave her two aspirin tablets. When her headaches returned in two hours, she bought a bottle of aspirin and took three tablets. She did not have lunch because she felt sick but drank cup after cup of black coffee. Later, her supervisor advised her to go home and rest when she saw her taking another three aspirin tablets. At home, she continued to feel sick with both headache and nausea, but she could not rest because she had an important date with a new boyfriend. She took four more aspirins. She was brought to the hospital emergency room by her boyfriend when she developed severe nausea, abdominal pains, and dizziness in the evening.

2. "A man with advanced lymphosarcoma was included in an experimental study of the since-discredited drug, Krebiozen. After one administration, his tumors disappeared. When reports came out that the drug was ineffective, the doctor told the patient not to believe what he read and treated him with 'double strength' Krebiozen —actually an injection of water. The patient again experienced rapid remission. Then the AMA and FDA pronounced the drug worthless. The patient died within a few days."*

3. A 40-year-old housewife had been complaining for several years of shortness of breath and easy fatigability. She, however, would not consult a doctor and would demand attention from her husband and children. Eventually, her family treated her like an invalid, with a certain amount of contempt. She gained weight progressively and reduced her activity level. A few weeks ago, her dyspnea became so severe that she agreed to consult

---

*From Holden (1978). Quoted with permission. The vignette is based on a case history reported by Bruno Klopfer in Psychological variables in human cancer, *J Project Tech* **21**:331– 334, 1957.

a physician. Rheumatic mitral valve disease was diagnosed, and she was placed on a regimen of digitalis. Her dyspnea disappeared, and she lost weight dramatically. (The weight gain was largely edema—retention of fluids.) She again felt energetic and resumed her normal activities as an efficient housewife. Her relationship with family members improved and so did her sex life with her husband. She also became socially active again.

4. A 19-year-old single man was admitted to the psychiatric ward of the hospital. For the last several weeks, he had become increasingly with-drawn; he would stay up all night in his room, ostensibly listening to music, and sleep all day long. On the night of admission, his parents found him in his room, screaming at an imaginary person. He was quite incoherent and would not respond to his parents. On the psychiatric unit, he was given an intramuscular injection of chlorpromazine, after which he fell asleep. The following morning, the staff was able to converse with him rationally, although he would lapse into incoherent language from time to time. He was placed on a regular regimen of chlorpromazine.

5. A 60-year-old widow was admitted to the hospital because of severe low back pain. She appeared quite depressed and tearful upon admission. History revealed that she had been diagnosed as having a depressive syndrome (see Chapter 6) three years ago, and antidepressant medication had been prescribed. She was "continued" on the antidepressant drug in the hospital. Within ten days, she was much brighter, her tearfulness and hopeless feelings abated, and she slept better. Subsequently, it was found that she had not been taking the antidepressant medication regularly at home because she felt that the medication needed only be taken when she felt extremely depressed. Thus, after receiving again a regular regimen of antidepressants in the hospital, she showed dramatic improvement.

The vignettes illustrate the multiple effects of drugs in the three major dimensions. For example, aspirin taken for the relief of headache (vignette 1) was probably associated with the following sequence of events:

1. Salicylate, by inhibiting prostaglandin synthesis, reduces stimulation of pain receptors and, in addition, acts directly on certain brain areas involved in the processing of pain sensation. These actions affect biological components of the pain and lead to
2. Relief from the experience of headache (personal dimension), which leads to
3. The patient's buying a full bottle of aspirin (environmental–interpersonal interaction) when the headache returns. The association of aspirin with relief from headaches is a learned behavior (personal dimension).
4. Patient takes more aspirin, which results in irritation and possible ulceration of the gastroduodenal mucosa (biological).

5. Increased consumption of coffee (personal), perhaps related to anxiety and discomfort associated with interpersonal stress (personal, environmental), contributes further to the gastrointestinal irritation (biological).
6. The observation by her supervisor of her illness behavior (personal) and the aspirin-taking leads to her going home early (environmental change).
7. The date with her boyfriend increases her anxiety (personal), perhaps aggravating the headache, which, in turn, leads again to increased drug-taking, ultimately resulting in
8. Acute gastrointestinal disturbance and mild salicylate toxicity (biological), leading to hospitalization (environmental).

Drugs Affect All Dimensions of the Patient

Drugs are usually administered with a particular effect in the biological or personal dimension in mind. We may forget that drugs also have effects in dimensions other than those we have in mind. As illustrated in vignette 1, drug effects occur in many subsystems and in all dimensions: behavior of the person, of intracellular processes in neurons, and of other persons and systems in the environment.

The *pharmacologic action* of a drug is usually mediated by effects in the biological subsystem, and these often lead to changes that are perceived in the personal dimension. The analgesic effect of aspirin is an example. Sometimes a drug may simultaneously cause desirable changes in the biological dimension and undesirable changes in the personal dimension. Such undesirable side effects may be due to the pharmacologic effects of the drug on the central nervous system or to psychological responses to the drug's *symbolic meaning*. Patients with pain who do not respond to methadone, a potent analgesic, may ascribe conflictual symbolic meaning to this drug, which is also used for the management of addiction.

Most drugs have some pharmacologic central nervous system action. The physician must keep informed about the central nervous system effects of medications that he prescribes—patients often are concerned about how the drug will make them feel.

As would be expected, there may be complex interactions between drug actions, drug-taking behavior, and the patient's personality (see Chapter 15). Certain patients (e.g., with dependent, demanding personalities) may consider drugs as tangible evidence of the doctor's caring, while others (e.g., with orderly, controlling personalities) may view the taking of drugs as a threat to their autonomy. Guarded, suspicious patients may become distrustful of prescribed drugs, suspecting that they might be harmful—even poisonous—especially if unexpected side effects occur and if the doctor–patient relationship is less than optimal. Sedating drugs may be especially threatening to patients who have concerns about autonomy. Patients with long-suffering, self-sacrificing personalities who are "addicted" to the sick role may feel threatened by drugs that promise "cure." Patients with impulsive personalities may be erratic in drug-taking and may unexpectedly abuse or overdose on drugs. Patients with chronic memory deficits may not be able to self-administer drugs because they forget the dosage and schedule and when the medication was last taken. Serious accidental overdosage may occur in these patients.

The *placebo effect* is important to remember in prescribing any drugs. Placebos may act as powerful agents, exerting their effects through as yet incompletely understood central nervous system mechanisms associated with the psychological phenomenon of expectancy. The effects of placebos attest to the powerful influence that the brain can sometimes exert upon disease processes and the experience of illness (see vignette 2; see also Chapters 7 and 14 for further discussion of the placebo effect).

Drug effects that may be observed in the *environmental dimension* of the patient may be mediated in several ways. Some drugs cause changes in the *appearance* and *social attractiveness* of the patient, for example, staining of skin by tar ointments used in some dermatologic conditions, hair loss caused by cytotoxic agents, and the smell of paraldehyde. The social relationships of patients receiving these drugs may become restricted. Some drugs are used primarily to change the *physical environment,* such as antiseptics in the operating room and insecticides in the house. Antibiotics used indiscriminately may foster the development of drug-resistant strains of bacteria that are dispersed into and contaminate the environment.

In addition to direct effects on the environment, social attitudes toward certain drugs may indirectly influence the behavior of the patient's family and friends. For example, a patient who requires methadone for pain may be stigmatized because of the social symbolic association of methadone with addiction. A patient under "chemotherapy" may be treated by his friends or relatives in accordance with their ideas of how a *cancer patient* should be treated (whether or not the chemotherapy is, in fact, being given for cancer).

Other indirect effects of drugs in the environmental dimension can be mediated by changes in the *patient's behavior.* A medication causing a depressive syndrome as a side effect may indirectly lead to isolation of the patient from environmental supports because of social withdrawal; an antidepressant medication, on the other hand, may increase the patient's interaction with the environment.

To reiterate, any drug, no matter what its intended pharmacologic action might be, can exert effects in all dimensions—directly, through specific pharmacologic actions or symbolic meaning and, indirectly, through induced changes in behavior.

Another important consideration to bear in mind is the fact that *prescription* (or ordering) of a drug does *not* insure the taking of the drug. In one-quarter to one-half of all outpatients, the prescribed medication is not taken at all (Blackwell, 1973)! Factors influencing patient compliance with a medication regimen include the patient's understanding of the need for the drug, the duration and schedule of administration, perceived effects and side effects, the symbolic meaning of the medication, the patient's personality, and the status of the doctor—patient relationship (see Chapter 14). In the presence of a good doctor—patient relationship, patients are willing to continue drugs even if they do not seem to have an immediate beneficial effect and/or in spite of uncomfortable side effects. Open, comfortable communication channels between the patient and doctor will enable the patient to talk to the physician about side effects of the medication rather than to discontinue it without telling the doctor.

Even *shape, size,* and *color* of the medications have important effects on the likelihood of their being taken and on the safety of their use (Mazzullo, 1972). For example, pills of similar size and color can be confused, resulting in an overdosage of one of them. A larger pill often seems stronger to a patient than a smaller pill, regardless of its actual strength.

In the hospital, drugs are usually administered by the nurses in response to a physician's written order, and patients are generally not informed about the medication being given by the nurse. Even when the physician writes an order to continue the same medication the patient had been taking prior to admission, the hospital pharmacy may stock a different brand with a different shape and color. Difficulties and confusion can be avoided by discussing medications with the patient—those to be continued, whether the shape and color will be different, and whether new medications will be added.

Psychotropic Drugs

Some drugs are used primarily to change the patient's mood, thought processes, and/or behavior. Those medications whose primary pharmacologic action is on the central nervous system and which are used to produce changes in mood, thought processes, and/or behavior are called "psychotropic" drugs. It should already be obvious from the preceding section that psychotropic drugs are *not* the only medications that may have such effects. The psychotropic drugs, however, may be narrowly defined as a subset of drugs that act primarily and selectively on the central nervous system to produce relatively specific effects rather than general central nervous system stimulation or depression.

Psychotropic drugs may be broadly classified into (1) antianxiety drugs; (2) drugs affecting mood (antidepressants and lithium salts); (3) antipsychotic drugs; and (4) psychotomimetic drugs (those causing psychosis-like syndromes).

We will discuss very briefly general principles concerning the use of the first three classes of psychotropic drugs in clinical management. For detailed information, the reader should consult standard textbooks of pharmacology and psychiatry.

Antianxiety Drugs (Minor Tranquilizers)

As discussed in Chapter 4, anxiety is usually a signal of impending danger which may either be external or originate within the personality system of the patient. Ideally, the best treatment of anxiety is removing or avoiding the danger situation rather than decreasing the danger signal. Many anxiety situations are not amenable to relief by immediate intervention but may subside or undergo resolution given adequate time. It may be necessary and desirable in such cases to reduce overwhelming anxiety and so reduce also the strength of associated physiologic reactions that may themselves have pathogenic effects (see Chapter 4). Especially in hospitalized patients, excessive anxiety may interfere with recovery (e.g., in patients with myocardial infarction). As noted earlier, hospitalization and medical procedures in and of themselves almost always induce and aggravate anxiety.

Drugs commonly prescribed for their antianxiety effects include benzodiazepines, barbiturates, propanediol carbamates, antihistaminics, and antipsychotic medications in small doses.

Benzodiazepines such as chlordiazepoxide (Librium) and diazepam (Valium) are the most commonly used and abused. They seem to bind to specific receptors in the brain as well as, perhaps, to have effects similar to γ-aminobutyric acid (GABA) and glycine in the central nervous system (Squires and Braestrup, 1977; Snyder et al., 1977; Stein et al., 1977). They are effective in reducing anxiety but may be habit-forming and, in some individuals, may produce paradoxical agitation, confusion, or fatigue. Benzodiazepines can also be used as hypnotics (to induce sleep); they do not affect REM but decrease Stage 4 sleep. They also increase the seizure threshold.

Antipsychotic drugs (discussed below) also have antianxiety action and can be used in small doses (about one-tenth of the antipsychotic dose) to treat anxiety in nonpsychotic patients. One should be aware of infrequent but serious side effects of antipsychotic agents, such as tardive dyskinesia, when one considers using them (see below).

Barbiturates and *propanediol carbamates* (e.g., tybamate and meprobamate) are similar in action to benzodiazepines but perhaps more sedating and less specifically "anxiolytic." *Antihistaminics* are primarily sedating.

In addition to the drugs mentioned above, *narcotic analgesics* such as morphine are anxiolytic—especially in patients with severe pain or other physical distress such as shortness of breath. For such patients, adequate analgesia is also adequate treatment of anxiety.

A general principle in the use of antianxiety agents is that they should be used intermittently and for short periods of time because of their addictive potential. Concurrent comprehensive evaluation of the danger situation and/or a medical condition that may cause anxiety symptoms (Chapter 4) should be carried out, and the possibility of referral for counseling or psychotherapy should be considered. Self-control techniques of anxiety reduction, such as self-hypnosis, relaxation exercises and pursuing hobbies, are sometimes helpful and should also be considered.

Drugs Affecting Mood

Antidepressants. Drugs used in the treatment of the depressive syndrome are called antidepressants. When a depressed patient also shows signs of psychotic thought disorder (such as delusions), antipsychotic agents are often used in addition to antidepressants.

The antidepressants are not necessarily central nervous system stimulants. When an antidepressant is given to a normal person, the effect is usually sedation and drowsiness rather than euphoria. When it is administered to a patient with the depressive syndrome (see Chapter 6), in 80–90% of cases, there will be clear improvement, usually manifest in about two weeks' time, and often dramatic improvement by four to six weeks.

There are two classes of antidepressants: the monoamine oxidase (MAO) inhibitors and the tricyclic antidepressants. Both classes of drugs ultimately seem to cause an increase in the functional levels of biogenic amines in the brain, especially norepinephrine and serotonin. The MAO inhibitors are believed to act by reducing the intraneuronal breakdown of biogenic amines by MAO. The tricyclic antidepressants are currently thought to work primarily by inhibiting the reuptake of norepinephrine and/or serotonin at the nerve terminals, thus increasing their functional availability at the synapse (see Figures 10 and 12).

Tricyclic Antidepressants. Imipramine, desipramine, amitriptyline, protriptyline, and doxepin are examples of tricyclic antidepressants. Imipramine (Tofranil) seems to have a greater effect on norepinephrine-containing neurons, while amitriptyline (Elavil) has a greater effect on serotonergic neurons in usual therapeutic doses (Maas, 1978).

Tricyclic antidepressants have a number of *side effects,* especially due to their *anticholinergic* effects. They include dry mouth, blurry vision, urinary retention, tachycardia, and orthostatic hypotension. Cardiac arrhythmias may also occur due to sympathomimetic action. Desipramine, which blocks the reuptake of norepinephrine primarily, seems to have the least anticholinergic action (Snyder, 1977). Tricyclic antidepressants are also *sedating,* so that a hypnotic drug may not be necessary if the antidepressant is given at night. Tricyclics increase delta sleep and decrease REM. Amitriptyline appears to be more sedating than imipramine. Protriptyline seems to have little sedative property.

Tricyclic antidepressants interact with a number of other medications. For example, they reduce the potency of antihypertensive agents such as guanethidine by interfering with its uptake by the peripherial adrenergic neurons. Tricyclics should not be given with MAO inhibitors because of possible severe hypertensive crisis.

Tricyclic antidepressants are generally nonaddicting, and tolerance to the antidepressant effect does not develop, although the anticholinergic effects do become better tolerated.

Tricyclic antidepressants are toxic in large doses, primarily due to the anticholinergic effects and the cardiotoxic effect of an increase in the catecholamines in cardiac tissue. In prescribing tricyclic antidepressants, the possibility of overdose with suicidal intent should be considered.

In addition to treatment of depression, tricyclic antidepressants may be used to treat enuresis in childhood, severe obsessive–compulsive disorders, and phobic anxiety states.

MAO Inhibitors. Phenelzine (Nardil), tranylcypromine (Parnate), and isocarboxazid (Marplan) are examples of MAO inhibitors. Unlike tricyclic antidepressants, MAO inhibitors, especially tranylcypromine, may have amphetamine-like central-nervous-system-stimulating properties in addition to their antidepressant effect. The antidepressant effect of MAO inhibitors is considered to be related to the drug's entering into stable combination with the enzyme MAO, thereby irreversibly inhibiting its action.

MAO inhibitors are potent REM suppressants. They can also lower blood pressure, although their anticholinergic effects are much less potent than those of the tricyclic antidepressants (Snyder, 1977).

A major consideration in the use of MAO inhibitors is that they *interact* with a number of *foods* and *beverages,* as well as with other medications. In general, any sympathomimetic drugs and foods containing sympathomimetic amines, particularly *tyramine,* can cause a *hypertensive crisis* in conjunction with an MAO inhibitor. Cerebrovascular accidents may occur during the hypertensive crises. Foods containing tyramine include cheese, beer, wine, pickled herring, chicken liver, aged meats, sausage, broad-bean pods, coffee, yeast, and canned figs. Many nonprescription drugs contain sympathomimetic agents. MAO inhibitors potentiate the effects of biogenic amine precursors like L-dopa. *Meperidine* is *contraindicated* and can cause marked hyperpyrexia. MAO inhibitors can interfere with the detoxification mechanisms of many drugs, including barbiturates, alcohol, anticholinergics, and tricyclic antidepressants. Patients on MAO inhibitors should be cautioned not to take any other medication without consulting the physician and should be given a *list of foods and medications* that should not be taken concurrently.

There is some evidence that "atypical" depressives who do not show a classical depressive syndrome but whose depression is severe enough to warrant drug treatment may benefit from MAO inhibitors more than from tricyclic antidepressants. This population includes patients with depressive and hypochondriacal symptoms (Robinson *et al.*, 1978). In view of the myriad interactions with foods and other drugs, however, treatment with MAO inhibitors should be considered with extreme caution and used only when the physician is satisfied that full compliance with the instructions will occur.

In addition to treatment of depression, MAO inhibitors have been used to treat phobic anxiety states and narcolepsy (utilizing the REM-suppressant action).

Lithium Salts. Lithium salts were used in the 1940s as a salt substitute for cardiac patients. Deaths occurred due to lithium poisoning, and the use of lithium salts was discontinued until the reintroduction of lithium as an antimanic drug in the 1960s. Lithium is currently used as a carbonate (Li_2CO_3). Lithium carbonate is effective in the *treatment of acute mania* (improvement in 70–80% of patients within 10–14 days) and as a maintenance drug in the *prevention* of manic attacks (Goodwin and Ebert, 1973). Lithium is also effective as a maintenance drug in reducing the number and intensity of recurrent unipolar depressive episodes (Baldessarini and Lipinski, 1975). This may be especially helpful in patients who have already shown recurrent episodes of depression (see Chapter 6).

The mechanism of action of lithium seems to be attributable to its being an "imperfect substitute" for other cations such as sodium and potassium and to its alteration of the intracellular microenvironment necessary for hormone action (Singer and Rotenberg, 1973). The latter involves interference with the hormone activation of adenyl cyclase or the action of cyclic AMP.

How lithium reverses and prevents mania and how it prevents depressive episodes are not completely known. Lithium may correct the tendency toward increased intracellular sodium concentration in affective disorders (see Chapter 6). There is evidence that lithium may exert antagonistic actions at catecholamine-mediated synapses in the brain. On a short-term basis, lithium increases serotonin turnover in the brain. With chronic administration, however, the turnover rate becomes normalized. Lithium initially increases norepinephrine turnover in rat brain, but, on a long-term basis, the norepine-phrine synthesis is normal. Lithium may increase the intraneuronal release of norepinephrine to be metabolized by MAO and decrease its extraneuronal release. Lithium inhibits basal and norepinephrine-activated adenyl cyclase (Gerbino et al., 1978).

Lithium may also decrease the synthesis and release of acetylcholine and affect the metabolism of GABA and glutamates in the brain (Baldessarini and Lipinski, 1975). The overall clinical effect of lithium seems to be stabilization of moods.

In using lithium carbonate, it is necessary to *monitor* the plasma *lithium concentration* on a regular basis. The therapeutic range is 1.0–1.5 mEq/liter initially, and for maintenance, 0.6–1.0 mEq/liter. The plasma level of lithium should *never* exceed 2 mEq/liter! The blood level should be drawn preferably 12 hours after ingestion of the last dose. Lithium should be administered in divided doses to maintain, as much as possible, steady blood levels.

Lithium can cause fatigue and muscular weakness. Toxic signs include nausea, vomiting, diarrhea, slurred speech, and ataxia. Other side effects include nephrogenic diabetes insipidus, goiter with hypothyroidism, and EEG changes.

Lithium should be administered *with extreme caution* to patients on a sodium-restricted diet, because lithium excretion is slow and severe toxicity may occur. Lithium decreases the pressor effect of norepinephrine.

Antipsychotic Drugs (Major Tranquilizers, Neuroleptics)

A number of drugs are now available for the treatment of psychotic states, including *schizophrenia*. They generally fall into one of the following cat-egories: phenothiazines, butyrophenones, thioxanthines, dibenzodiaze-pines, and rauwolfia alkaloids.

The phenothiazines are representative of the antipsychotics. Synthesized in 1883, phenothiazine was first used in the 1930s as an antihelminthic, urinary antiseptic, and insecticide. Promethazine, a phenothiazine, was used as an antihistamine, sedative, and, in the early 1950s as premedication for anes-thesia. The introduction of chlorpromazine as an antipsychotic agent in the late 1950s and its wide acceptance in the 1960s revolutionized psychiatric treatment for schizophrenia.

All drugs that belong to the category of antipsychotic agents have, to a greater or lesser extent, certain features in common, as represented by chlor-promazine.

Central Nervous System Effects. All antipsychotics except rauwolfia alkaloids *block dopamine receptors* in the brain (see Figure 11). The dopamine receptor blockade in the dopaminergic mesolimbic system by the antipsychotics is considered to be the main mechanism of the antipsychotic effect. Dopaminergic blockade in the nigrostriatal tract by the antipsychotic agents can result in extrapyramidal symptoms, including parkinsonian features, dystonias, and the serious side effect of *tardive dyskinesia*. Tardive dyskinesia is a syndrome that is marked by characteristic involuntary movements of the mouth, tongue, and other parts of the body. It is considered to be due to the development of "receptor hypersensitivity" of the postsynaptic neurons (see section on Behavioral Effects). Dopaminergic blockade is also probably responsible for the increase in prolactin levels in patients receiving antipsychotics, since dopamine normally inhibits prolactin release from the pituitary. Increased prolactin levels may cause gynecomastia and lactation. Rauwolfia alkaloids such as reserpine probably exert antipsychotic action through depletion of biogenic amines in the neurons, including dopamine, norepinephrine, and serotonin. Antipsychotic agents also block the reuptake of norepinephrine and serotonin in the brain but do not affect GABA.

At the hypothalamic level, antipsychotic agents inhibit the release of growth hormone and may antagonize the release of the hypothalamic prolactin-release-inhibiting hormone. Hypothalamic temperature regulation may be interfered with by antipsychotics, and *hypothermia* may ensue.

Antipsychotics seem to increase the "filtering activity" of the reticular activating system in the brain stem, reducing the inflow of stimuli in a selective fashion (see Figure 7). Antipsychotics have varying degrees of antiemetic action through an action on the chemoreceptor trigger zone. Chlorpromazine (Thorazine) and prochlorperazine (Compazine) have relatively high antiemetic action.

Antipsychotic agents slow the EEG pattern but also *lower the seizure threshold*. Drug-induced seizures are common among patients with preexisting seizure disorders or with a tendency to seizures.

Autonomic Nervous System Effects. Antipsychotic agents have varying degrees of *anticholinergic* activity, *anti-α-adrenergic* activity (direct receptor block), *adrenergic* activity (through blockade of reuptake of catecholamines), and *antihistaminic* activity. Chlorpromazine may reverse the pressor effects of epinephrine. Postural hypotension occurs more commonly with chlorpromazine than with more potent (and thus used in small doses) piperazine-ring phenothiazines such as prolixin or butyrophenones. Thioridazine (Mellaril) may cause ejaculatory incompetence in male patients. In high doses, thioridazine may also cause retinitis pigmentosa.

Behavioral Effects. Antipsychotic drugs have a *specific effect* on psychotic individuals in reversing or reducing the psychotic symptomatology, including the thought disorder, autism, hallucinations, paranoid ideations, withdrawal, and blunted affect. Agitation or belligerence is also reduced. These effects tend to occur over the course of several weeks in schizophrenia. Psychotic states due to any disease process, including organic psychosis as well as schizophrenia, often respond to antipsychotics.

In addition to the specific antipsychotic effect, the antipsychotic agents also have varying degrees of *sedative action*. Characteristically, the sedation caused by antipsychotic agents is accompanied by a feeling of indifference to environmental events and psychomotor slowing. This phenomenon has been called the "neuroleptic syndrome," and the antipsychotics, *"neuroleptic drugs."* Antipsychotic drugs are also called "major tranquilizers," in comparison to the antianxiety agents like benzodiazepines, which are called "minor tranquilizers."

In experimental animals, antipsychotic agents impair *conditioned avoidance learning*. This test is often used for screening drugs that might possess antipsychotic effects. Minor tranquilizers do not have this effect. Sleep caused by a sedating antipsychotic drug such as chlorpromazine is easily arousable.

All antipsychotic agents reduce spontaneous *motor activity* in humans and animals. In large doses, this blends into the *parkinsonian* picture of rigidity, loss of associated movements, and tremors. Some patients may develop catalepsy (waxy flexibility) with the administration of large doses of antipsychotics. *Akathisia* is an extrapyramidal symptom caused by some antipsychotics. It is characterized by a marked increase in motor activity, restlessness, and a literal inability to sit still. This as well as other extrapyramidal symptoms can be effectively reversed with anticholinergic agents or antihistaminic agents such as benztropine (Cogentin) or diphenhydramine (Benadryl). A relatively rare but serious side effect with prolonged use is *tardive dyskinesia*. This syndrome is often irreversible.

The side effects of antipsychotics, in addition to those already mentioned, include hepatic microsomal enzyme induction, obstructive jaundice, cardiac arrhythmias, EEG changes, blood dyscrasias, photosensitivity, and skin rash.

Indications and Precautions. In the presence of a psychotic state, antipsychotic agents are indicated to control the psychotic symptoms. In psychosis associated with an underlying medical disease (see Tables 8 and 9), treatment of the underlying disease should accompany symptomatic treatment of the psychosis with antipsychotic agents. The choice of drug depends, to a large extent, on the side effects to be avoided or taken advantage of. For example, an agitated patient might receive a more sedating phenothiazine such as chlorpromazine, while a psychomotor-retarded, depressed, psychotic patient might do better with a less sedating drug. For details concerning the side effects of individual antipsychotic drugs, the reader, as noted earlier, is referred to standard textbooks of psychiatry and pharmacology.

Summary

Although drugs are usually administered to effect a particular change in the biological or personal dimension, all three dimensions, including the environmental– social dimension, are affected by drugs.

The pharmacologic action of a drug is usually mediated by changes in the *biological dimension,* which may eventually cause changes in the *personal dimension* (e.g., analgesia). The personal dimension may be affected, additionally, by the *symbolic meaning* of the drug. The *placebo effect* is a potent and often beneficial effect that accompanies the use of any drug and may augment its action. The *environmental dimension* of the patient may be affected by drugs directly (e.g., foul odor in the breath of a patient taking paraldehyde) or indirectly (through the symbolic meaning of the drug to others or through the behavioral change of the patient).

Prescribing a drug is *not* equivalent to its actual administration. Up to one-half of outpatients do not take prescribed drugs. The factors affecting *compliance* with a drug regimen include (1) the quality of the doctor– patient relationship; (2) the shape, size, and color of the drug; (3) the patient's information about the drug; and (4) the personality of the patient.

Psychotropic medications are drugs whose primary pharmacologic action is on the central nervous system to produce relatively selective changes in mood, thought processes, and/or behavior. They include *antianxiety drugs, drugs affecting mood, antipsychotic drugs,* and *psychotomimetic drugs.*

The *benzodiazepines* are the most commonly used *antianxiety* agents. While they are usually effective, they may produce paradoxical agitation in some individuals. They increase seizure threshold and reduce delta sleep. They are also sedating and may be used as hypnotics (especially flurazepam). The benzodiazepines are habit-forming with prolonged use. Antianxiety agents should be used judiciously and, generally, temporarily.

The *tricyclic* antidepressants *imipramine* and *amitriptyline* are the most commonly used antidepressants. The tricyclics seem to block the reuptake by the presynaptic membrane of released norepinephrine and/or serotonin, which causes an increase in the functional levels of these amines at the synapse. The antidepressants require time to work fully—usually, at least 10– 14 days are necessary before the effects are manifested. The most common side effects of tricyclics are sedation and anticholinergic effects.

There are many drug interactions with *monoamine oxidase inhibitors,* and many foods, especially those containing the pressor amine tyramine, interact with the MAO inhibitors, causing serious hypertension. Meperidine is contraindicated in a patient receiving an MAO inhibitor.

Lithium carbonate is effective as an *antimanic* agent and also in preventing recurrent unipolar depressions. The plasma lithium level must be monitored in patients receiving lithium. The therapeutic range is 0.6–1.5 mEq/liter. Lithium should be administered with extreme caution to patients on sodium-restricted diets.

The *phenothiazines* and *butyrophenones* are representative *antipsychotic* agents. Their action seems to be the blockade of dopamine receptors, and they appear to increase the filtering activity of the reticular activating system. They tend to be sedating, and some have antiemetic action. They lower the seizure threshold and impair conditioned learning in animals. Autonomic side effects include orthostatic hypotension and anticholinergic effects. Neurologic side effects include pseudoparkinsonism, akathisia, and tardive dyskinesia.

Implications

For the Patient

Properties other than the specific pharmacologic action of the drug may be of primary importance to the patient, for example, the size, color, shape, and name of the drug as well as the price. The symbolic meaning of the medication also plays an important role in the patient's perception and expectations of a drug. Many patients do not comply with a drug regimen. This may be due to a number of reasons, the most important being the lack of a trusting doctor–patient relationship and associated lack of communication. The side effects of medications, although not alarming to the doctor, may be quite frightening to the patient if unexpected. Some patients attach extraordinary significance and importance to taking drugs and may become dependent upon them.

For the Physician

Physicians should recognize that drugs affect all dimensions of the patient, regardless of the desired specific pharmacologic action. In discussing and prescribing a medication, the physician should take into account the patient's personality type, previous experience with drugs, and expectations and symbolic meanings of the proposed drug. Specific questions must be asked to obtain such information. Good compliance with a drug regimen rests on a good doctor–patient relationship and an open channel of communication. The significance of the nonpharmacologic aspects of drugs, such as the size, shape, and color of a pill, should be recognized and understood by the physician. Explanation concerning possible side effects of a medication is essential in reassuring the patient and maintaining a good doctor–patient relationship.

The physician should be familiar with the effects of any planned medication in all dimensions of the patient and also with its interaction with other drugs and substances (as tyramine-containing foods and MAO inhibitors).

For the Community and Health Care System

The community should be educated about the fact that drugs have many actions, some of which may be dangerous in themselves or in interaction with other drugs and substances. The public should learn to use medications only in consultation with a physician. Medical education should emphasize that any drug affects all three dimensions of the patient. Emphasis should also be placed on the nonpharmacologic aspects of drugs, such as the shape, color, name, and symbolic meaning. Unrealistic and exaggerated claims by some pharmaceutical companies concerning their products should be regulated.

Recommended Reading

Goodman LS, Gilman A: *The Pharmacological Basis of Therapeutics.* New York, Macmillan, 1975. This is the standard textbook of pharmacology. We would especially suggest the chapter by Byck on drugs and the treatment of psychiatric disorders for a more detailed treatment of the subject. An excellent reference for all questions concerning drugs.

Hansten PD: *Drug Interactions.* Philadelphia, Lea & Febiger, 1976. (Paperback). A very useful reference. Various drug interactions are presented in a tabular form.

Jarvik ME (ed): *Psychopharmacology in the Practice of Medicine.* New York, Appleton-Century-Crofts, 1977. A multiauthored volume. Unlike that edited by Lipton *et al.* (see below), this is oriented more toward the primary physician. Concise but comprehensive.

Lipton MA, DiMascio A, Killam KF (ed): *Psychopharmacology: A Generation of Progress.* New York, Raven Press, 1978. An up-to-date, comprehensive, and authoritative multiauthored book on various aspects of psychopharmacology, including basic biochemistry, neurophysiology, neurotransmitters, animal behavior pharmacology, and clinical psychopharmacology. An excellent reference book for the relatively advanced reader. The book is huge (1731 pages, including index).

References

Baldessarini RJ, Lipinski JF: Lithium salts: 1970–1975. *Ann Intern Med* **83:**527–533, 1975.

Blackwell B: Drug therapy: Patient compliance. *N Engl J Med* **289:**249–252, 1973.

Gerbino L, Oleshansky M, Gershon S: Clinical use and mode of action of lithium, in Lipton MA, DiMascio A, Killam KF (eds): *Psychopharmacology: A Generation of Progress.* New York, Raven Press, 1978, pp 1261–1275.

Goodwin FK, Ebert MH: Lithium in mania, in Gershon S, Shopsin B (eds): *Lithium: Its Role in Psychiatric Research and Treatment.* New York, Plenum Press, 1973, pp 237–252.

Holden C· Cancer and the mind: How are they connected? *Science* **200:**1369, 1978.

Maas JW: Clinical implications of pharmacological differences among antidepressants, in Lipton MA, DiMascio A, Killam KF (eds): *Psychopharmacology: A Generation of Progress.* New York, Raven Press, 1978, pp 955–960.

Mazzullo J: The nonpharmacologic basis of therapeutics. *Clin Pharmacol Ther* **13:**157–158, 1972.

Robinson DS, Nies A, Ravaris CL, *et al.:* Clinical pharmacology of phenelzine. *Arch Gen Psychiatry* **35:**629–635, 1978.

Singer I, Rotenberg D: Mechanisms of lithium action. *N Engl J Med* **289:**254–260, 1973.

Snyder SH: Antidepressants and the muscarinic acetylcholine receptor. *Arch Gen Psychiatry* **34:**236–239, 1977.

Snyder SH, Enna SJ, Young AB: Brain mechanisms associated with therapeutic actions of benzodiazepines: Focus on neurotransmitters. *Am J Psychiatry* **134:**662–665, 1977.

Squires RF, Braestrup C: Benzodiazepine receptors in rat brain. *Nature* **266:**732–734, 1977.

Stein L, Belluzzi JD, Wise CD: Benzodiazepines: Behavioral and neurochemical mechanisms. *Am J Psychiatry* **134:**665–669, 1977.

CHAPTER 19

Some Illustrative Patients

In this chapter, we will present the evaluation and management of three illustrative patients, beginning with the case of the sick Tarzan, whose history and portions of a verbatim interview with whom were presented in Chapter 13. All of the cases presented in this chapter, including the "sick Tarzan," are actual case histories. Of course, some identifying data have been changed for reasons of confidentiality.

The Management of the Sick Tarzan*

We are now prepared to formulate a comprehensive three-dimensional management plan for our patient, armed with information and insights from all of our previous chapters. In rereading the case history, it should become clear that there is a discrepancy in the model of illness between the patient and the doctor. For example, "My doctor thinks I had a heart attack. All I need is to get back my strength, which I lost from being in here too long." In fact, the patient believes, "Once you start laying in bed without moving and letting your blood move, you might as well bury yourself." Once we understand the patient's own unique theory concerning illness and ways of recovery, we can understand why it is so important for the patient to become active and why he may feel compelled to try to lift his bed.

His commitment to activity, however, is not necessarily unamenable to reason. He, in fact, believes that, perhaps, being too active and not "resting a minute" after sexual intercourse with his wife might have caused his disease ("I didn't give my heart a chance to rest").

*Please reread Chapter 13.

The doctor, then, might consider attempting either to change the patient's model of illness to correspond with his own or to modify it just enough to allow optimal medical treatment to proceed. In order to make this decision, the physician has to assess why and how strongly the patient's model is held. In Tarzan's case, the importance of activity was emphasized over and over again, as if it were a prophylactic against death. It becomes clear during the interview that the patient had used activity as his most characteristic life-style and that he felt very proud of his strength and "bigness": "I've got a *big* chest so I can take in a lot of air"; "I don't drink small amounts of anything"; "In my youth, I was so strong that . . . I had to wrestle with four or five fellows at one time"; "I was what they called a natural strong man"; and so on. To a man with this kind of self-image, feeling weak and ill must be a terribly uncomfortable state. And this was exactly what he felt: "[B]ut today I feel sorta weak. . . . I think it's because they don't let me move my blood in the hospital." The patient's need for activity now is not simply a logical outcome of his general belief concerning health maintenance, but it also has a defensive quality—he needs to overcome his feeling of weakness from being inactive.

The physicians, with the help of the psychiatrist, decided to attempt to modify the patient's model rather than to change it completely. Strongly held beliefs that serve defensive functions are not easily given up, and the emergency nature of the medical condition militated against an attempt that might possibly have resulted in a rupture of the doctor–patient relationship. To attempt to change his activity orientation would have been an attempt to change his long-term (background context) personality and coping style.

The patient's apparent denial of heart disease itself ("My doctor thinks I had a heart attack") was not complete: "I didn't give my heart a chance to rest." If he does not deny the presence of disease, he does deny the emotional upset that one might expect to be associated with it: "*Nothing bothers me. . . . I don't let nothing bother me.*" Behind this denial, we get a glimpse of great suffering in the past—he apparently had thought that he had cancer in his 30s but was told that "it was all from nerves." Since then, he adopted an attitude of "nothing bothers me." Although this attitude may not be conducive to the patient's preparing for danger situations in a deliberate fashion, the ability to deny anxiety and fear may be helpful, if used in moderation, once on the coronary care unit (see Chapter 16). So long as the patient's behavior is not maladaptive due to the denial, denial can be a protective mechanism. The question in this case might be how to change the behavior (e.g., lifting up the bed) without frightening the patient excessively, as would happen if one confronted him with the consequences of extending the heart lesion. If his denial were not functioning, we might again have a patient who is, as he described he had been when he thought he had cancer, worried, with pains in his head and diarrhea lasting for years.

The patient gives a good indication that an important person to recruit as a collaborator in the management may be his wife: "She wants me to stay home with her on Saturdays, I stay home with her." We notice that the patient is rather boastful, especially concerning his strength and, perhaps, masculine prowess. He did not respond well to nurses' reproaches concerning his activity. Perhaps an authoritarian approach threatens his sense of masculinity and need to be in control. His need for control, which goes along well with his activity orientation, is pretty clear throughout the interview itself, including, "And, someday, you fellas are going to come to the same conclusion—that moving the blood is the most important thing of all."

The patient came into conflict over authority with the nursing staff about who can give orders to whom. This resulted in his increased anxiety and the need for more activity to reassure himself that he did have control after all. In part, the authoritarian attitude of the nursing staff may be related to the rigidly authoritarian nursing hierarchy generally found in hospitals and the "double bind" in which nurses often find themselves (Chapter 16). It is unthinkable that a patient should wish to violate orders deliberately!

Actually, there were indications that the patient was having difficulties adjusting to the coronary care unit as early as the second day of admission. For example, he was found sitting up in a chair and was agitated at night and "arrogant." He asked for large doses of Valium. Because of a communication gap, however, the nurses' observations were not known to the doctors, who might have attempted to understand the patient's source of increasing anxiety.

To summarize, then, we have a patient who has an activity-oriented, controlling personality and who feels threatened about being immobile in bed in the coronary care unit. He has difficulties with nurses over authority but has a supportive wife, for whom he would do "anything." He has documented serious heart disease and is in pain and danger of his life. He has a strong belief that he has to "move blood" to survive.

On the basis of the discussion above and the PEG of sick Tarzan (Figure 33), the following three-dimensional management plans were worked out.

Biological Dimension

1. Adequate pain relief with narcotic analgesics (meperidine, 50 mg intramuscularly every three hours): Pain relief is necessary for myocardial rest and gives the patient a sense of control.

2. Decrease diazepam, as large doses of tranquilizers may make the patient feel weak and drowsy.

3. Other necessary treatment of the MI and PVCs.

59 yrs, ♂, married, president of a small company, 2 daughters, ages 26 and 24

CONTEXTS

DIMENSIONS	CURRENT (Current States)	RECENT (Recent Events and Changes)	BACKGROUND (Culture, Traits, Constitution)
BIOLOGICAL	Chest pain Nausea Relevant physical data Dx MI Diazepam, procainamide Meperidine	Borderline hypertension (7-8 years, no meds)	Hx of heart disease and cancer in family
PERSONAL	Nausea Pain Thinks pain due to indigestion Believes exercise essential for survival	Increased smoking (3-4 yrs) Increased drinking (3-4 yrs)	No previous hospitalization Has a "strong man" image Uses denial as a defense Hx of "nerves" — thought he had cancer, decided to deny — "nothing bothers me" Active, "take charge" type of personality boastful, dramatic Believes in exercise
ENVIRONMENTAL	ICU Bedrest Nurses Wife Very attached to wife; will "do anything for her" Being in hospital means business associates will be in charge	Father d. of MI 6 yrs ago Mother d. of pulmonary edema (3 yrs ago) 2 daughters married within last 4 yrs, live in another state Sex immediately before MI hospitalization	Middle class Italian, Catholic backround High school education Many relatives died of cancer Father was very authoritarian executive of a small company for 25 yrs

Figure 33. PEG of the sick Tarzan.

Personal Dimension

1. Treatment of pain with narcotic analgesics as above.
2. Nausea ceased to be problematic spontaneously.
3. Allow "moving blood" without compromising treatment: A schedule of token toe exercise was devised so that the patient could "move the blood" without having to strain the heart trying to lift up the bed. Taking into acccount the active, controlling, and taking-pride-in-being-a-strong-man personality, this plan was presented as follows:

DOCTOR: I think we can suggest a good exercise for this purpose. However, I wonder if I can ask you to do something that's very difficult for a strong and big man like you—in fact, this may be the most difficult thing that anyone can ask of you—but, since you have a lot of strength, you might be able to do this.

PATIENT: Well, maybe I can try. I can do anything you know. What is it, Doc?

DOCTOR: For a very strong and active man like you, staying in bed for a few days is one of the most difficult things for anyone to ask you to do. But your heart needs the rest so that it can heal. While you are in bed, you can still move your blood by doing an exercise—you can move your toes up and down, which will pump the blood all the way through the toes. But I am not sure that you have the patience and strength to do this difficult thing. . . .

PATIENT: Well, Doc, I think I can try. I am an impatient man, but when I know that I am moving my blood, I can become the most patient man on earth.

In the long run, the patient was able to give up smoking and reduce drinking when these were presented to him as challenges to his willpower and strength to promote his health.

Environmental–Interpersonal Dimension

Perhaps the most important intervention occurred in this dimension, because it involved changing the approach of the medical and nursing staff to the patient and his wife. The psychiatrist consultant coordinated this educational task.

1. The primary physician was instructed how to be able to present the approach he used concerning "moving blood" (see above). The patient was offered pain medication regularly, but he could decline to take it if he had no pain (reverse p.r.n. schedule).
2. The patient's wife was mobilized to be a collaborator in management. For this reason, she was invited to sit down with the doctor and nurses and

jointly discuss the patient's progress—and compliance with the regimen. If the patient seemed to become too active, such as tending to sit up or get out of bed, the wife would go to him and say, "You know that it's important for me that you are strong and well. It worries me a lot when the doctors get worried about you and your getting out of bed; please stay in bed for a few more days—for me." She turned out to be a good collaborator, not only in ensuring compliance with the treatment, but also in reporting to the doctors and nurses about any change in the patient's state, level of anxiety, and sedation, so that medications could be adjusted on the basis of her observations.

3. Taking into account the talkative, boastful aspect of the patient, the members of the nursing staff were encouraged to listen to him and communicate that they were impressed by his strength. The nurses were able to understand that he needed to feel extra strong because otherwise he would feel so weak and afraid. As the nurses listened to him, they found him to be a rather charming "tall-story" teller, with whom it was rather enjoyable to converse. When the nurses had to be firm with him, they asked him to comply because otherwise they would "get into trouble." This appeal was usually heeded by him, because it gave him a sense of masculine chivalry—to do things so that a nurse would not get into trouble.

As his medical condition improved, he was given as much control as possible over his activity, including setting his own schedule for shaving and bathing. He was allowed out of bed as soon as possible and transferred out of the coronary care unit as soon as the physical condition allowed. Upon transfer from the coronary care unit, the nurses on the medical ward were alerted to his unique needs, and he was prepared for the transfer carefully.

The concerted efforts by everyone concerned—doctors, nurses, and wife—were successful, and the remainder of his hospital stay was uneventful.

The Case of the Catatonic Patient with Enlarged Ventricles*

History and Course

This 27-year-old white married woman was admitted to the medical service for treatment of severe ulcerative colitis. She was a high-school graduate and the mother of two children. Upon arrival at the hospital, she was mute and immobile.

The family stated that the patient had complained of "racing thoughts"

*Originally published in a somewhat different form in Leigh H: Good outcome in a catatonic patient with enlarged ventricles. *J Nerv Ment Dis* **166**:(2): 139– 141, 1978. Copyright 1978 by Williams & Wilkins Co. Portions reprinted with permission from the publisher.

and a feeling that she was going "crazy" beginning several weeks prior to admission. In fact, the patient had stopped taking prednisone (a synthetic cortisol-like drug) which was given her for the colitis, because she felt it was making her "crazy." It was restarted, however, and she was receiving relatively high doses (60 mg/day) of prednisone for three weeks prior to hospitalization. She had no previous psychiatric history.

In the hospital, she was mute and unresponsive and showed waxy flexibility—that is, her limbs would remain indefinitely in any position in which they were put. Her eyes were open, and she appeared vigilant, occasionally grimacing at people in her room. The physical examination on admission revealed an emaciated and diaphoretic young woman with labile hypertension (170–130/120–90 mm Hg), tachycardia (90–125/min), and fever (rectal temperature, 100–101°F). Laboratory findings showed anemia (hematocrit, 29–27%), hypokalemia (2.2 mEq/liter), and hypomagnesemia (1.6 mEq/liter). All other values, including thyroid studies, were within normal limits.

Upon admission, she was placed on a regimen of hydrocortisone, 100 mg intravenously four times a day. Serum potassium and magnesium abnormalities were corrected by administration of sodium and potassium without visible improvement in the patient's mental status. An automatic computerized tomographic axial scan (ACTA), which visualizes the brain structures on X ray, was performed on the second day of hospitalization and revealed "grossly enlarged lateral, third, and fourth ventricles with no evidence of cortical atrophy"—that is, a structural abnormality of the brain was found. A repeat ACTA scan three days later confirmed enlarged ventricles with no evidence of a tumor which might have caused this abnormality. An EEG revealed moderate, generalized, bilateral rhythmic slow-wave activity with no focal or epileptic features—an indication of generalized slowing of brain function. At this time, the most likely diagnosis was considered to be subacute sclerosing panencephalitis, a very grave condition for which there is no specific treatment.

She would occasionally manifest severe tremors of all her extremities which were sometimes mistaken for convulsions by the nursing staff. She was placed on small doses (2 mg) of perphenazine, an antipsychotic phenothiazine, three times a day, with some improvement. She would occasionally "wake up" from her stuporous, immobile state and converse with the staff, but then she would lapse back into the catatonic state. During the lucid intervals, she was apparently responding to visual and, occasionally, auditory hallucinations.

Throughout her hospital course, she had stools positive for blood and developed episodes of frank gastrointestinal bleeding with marked evidence of toxicity. An emergency total colectomy was performed in the sixth week of hospitalization.

After the colectomy, all vital signs and laboratory findings returned to normal, and the hydrocortisone was gradually tapered off. Her mental status improved gradually such that five weeks after the colectomy, she was competely oriented and showed good recent and remote memory. She did serial 7s well, and her calculations and abstractions were within normal limits (see Chapter 10 for a discussion of the mental-status examination). Her judgment was good. Her affect was normal, and she related with the staff quite well. Tremors, waxy flexibility, and hallucinations were no longer present. She was eager to go home and return to her family and stated that she had no recollection of the events that had transpired during the period she was in the hospital until the time she recovered from the surgery. She did not remember any of the conversations she had with the physicians during her lucid periods, nor did she remember any of the hallucinations she had before surgery. A repeat ACTA scan performed at the time of discharge from the hospital, two and one-half months after surgery, still showed enlarged ventricles of the same magnitude.

Comments

The PEG constructed shortly after admission is found in Figure 34. The management plan for this patient involved discussing all aspects of the case with her husband, the important supportive person. This was especially important, because the patient, being mute and immobile, could not sign any forms for hospitalization or surgery and was not in any state to discuss management plans with the physicians. Treatment of the catatonic syndrome involves first an evaluation and treatment of the possible causes (see Table 9). Symptomatic treatment with antipsychotic medications (such as perphenazine) may be necessary. Possible causes of the catatonia included, in the biological dimension, hypokalemia, hypomagnesemia, steroids (hydrocortisone, prednisone), and the structural abnormality of the brain (enlarged ventricles on the ACTA scan). The toxicity from ulcerative colitis and fever may also contribute to this picture. The electrolytes (potassium, magnesium, etc.) were corrected, and the ulcerative colitis was initially treated with high doses of steroids without much change in the mental status. This left the possibility that (1) the steroids given to treat the colitis might be contributing to the mental state, (2) the structural abnormality of the brain on ACTA was indicative of a brain pathology that was causing the catatonic state, such as subacute sclerosing panencephalitis, or (3) the catatonic syndrome was primarily a psychiatric disorder, for example, schizophrenia, that might be only secondarily related to the biological abnormalities found.

In view of the negative family and past history of psychiatric disorder, and the outgoing, sociable personality of the patient, it seemed less likely that the patient had schizophrenia. Although the encephalitis was a possibility, no

27 yrs, ♀, white, married, housewife, 2 children

DIMENSIONS	CONTEXTS		
	CURRENT (Current States)	RECENT (Recent Events and Changes)	BACKGROUND (Culture, Traits, Constitution)
BIOLOGICAL	Labile hypertension Tachycardia Fever Anemia Electrolyte imbalance Hypokalemia Hypomagnesemia Steroids ACTA – enlarged ventricles Ulcerative colitis	Ulcerative colitis for 3 yrs Prednisone 60 mg (3 wks)	No family history of psychiatric illness
PERSONAL	Catatonic syndrome Mute	Racing thoughts (several wks) Felt she was "going crazy" for a few weeks – stopped Prednisone Prednisone restarted (3 wks ago)	No past psychiatric history Pleasant, sociable person
ENVIRONMENTAL	Came in ambulance accompanied by husband	Married five years Two children Husband supportive	High school graduate Middle class Protestant Two siblings well Parents living and well No psychiatric history in family

Figure 34. PEG of the catatonic patient with enlarged ventricles.

specific measures could be applied to treat it. In retrospect, and in view of the good outcome, this was probably not the cause of catatonia.

Following colectomy for the ulcerative colitis, the patient was withdrawn from the steroids. Simultaneously, her mental status improved. Thus, most likely, the steroid medications given to treat her medical disease contributed significantly to her abnormal mental status.

The patient's limited response to antipsychotic medication illustrates the nonspecific nature of antipsychotic treatment, that is, regardless of the etiology, psychosis can be symptomatically treated with these medications. In certain situations where steroid medications are life-saving, the psychiatric side effects may have to be treated with antipsychotic drugs while the steroid medications are maintained.

Many physicians felt initially that this patient had an irreversible process in the brain. Such thinking led some clinicians to despair of effective therapy and even to suggest the futility of colectomy in "such an obviously brain-damaged patient." The subsequent course of this patient indicates, however, the value of correcting any treatable source of a multifactorial problem.

While the structural brain abnormality might have been associated with the brain's vulnerability to catatonia, it could not have been the major "cause" of the problem. This case draws our attention to the fact that every effort should be made to identify and treat *all* possible etiologic and contributing factors in a seriously ill patient.

The Case of the Suicidal Terminal Cancer Patient*

History

This 35-year-old white woman, a physician's wife and the mother of three children, was admitted to the intensive care unit of the hospital. She was found comatose in her bed by her husband upon coming home from work late at night. An empty bottle that contained secobarbital, a sleeping medication, was found next to her bed. Prior to the suicidal attempt, the patient was being treated with radiation and chemotherapy for a cancer of the breast with widespread metastases.

Four years prior to the present admission, a lump in her left breast was detected on a routine physical examination and was subsequently diagnosed as malignant. Two years following the radical mastectomy, another cancer was

*Originally published in a somewhat different form in Leigh H.: Psychotherapy of a suicidal, terminal cancer patient. *Int J Psychiatry Med* **5**:173–182, 1974. Copyright 1974 by Baywood Publishing Co. Portions reprinted with permission from the publisher.

detected in the right breast, necessitating another radical mastectomy. Approximately one year prior to the current admission, there was evidence of spreading of the cancer to the bone and behind the eyes. The spreading cancer was treated with chemotherapy, radiation therapy, and removal of both ovaries, since breast cancer tends to spread less when female hormones are absent. She also received steroids and pain medications for the severe pain she developed in her back and leg due to the spreading of cancer to the bones. The side effects of these treatments were grogginess, baldness, and facial puffiness, and there was growth of a moustache due to the absence of female hormones and the masculinizing effect of steroid hormones. The steroids also made her feel "high" and euphoric sometimes.

She was an intelligent and attractive (in spite of the bodily changes of late) young woman who felt defeated and depressed. With the appearance of signs of spread of the cancer, she progressively withdrew from her social activities and her work as a social worker. She was feeling guilty about being a burden to her family and frightened about the possibility of being a "vegetable." For fear of burdening her family, she did not discuss her feelings of frustration and sadness. She wrote in her diary, which was found by her husband when she attempted suicide, "In order to maintain my equilibrium and not burden others, I'll try to be my own therapist and write down my feelings and thoughts about myself." In it, she expressed feelings of being "out of battle" and of not being involved. She had feelings of depression whenever she had pain but occasional euphoria due to steroids and pain medications: "It is crazy to feel okay with what I have, but I am ready to take my exit pills tomorrow, if necessary."

Evaluation of the environmental–interpersonal dimension through interviews with her and her husband confirmed the initial impression that she had a supportive and concerned family. Her husband, however, had guilty and conflictual feelings because he could not spend as much time as he felt he needed to with his wife because of his busy schedule as a cardiologist. He was also uncertain about how to prepare his children for the eventual death of their mother. The suicidal attempt was a great shock to him and increased his guilt feelings toward her. The patient's mother lived in a city some distance away. The patient saw her occasionally but had a very ambivalent relationship with her. Her father, described as an ineffectual person, died as the result of an accident when the patient was in her teens. She had a younger sister who was a housewife in another town.

Her oncologists were highly competent and empathic but tended to expect their patients to deny the serious nature of the disease. They were very proud, for example, that all of their patients with terminal cancer had a bright emotional outlook and "smiled at everybody." Of course, this patient's suicidal attempt belied this notion and came as a great shock to them.

The patient characterized herself as having been a fighter, for whom activity and mastery were very important. She had a full-time job and was a skillful tennis player. Pain and prolonged suffering, however, made her feel exhausted, weak, and defeated. She seemed to have used the defenses of activity and intellectualization successfully in the past, but of late, they seemed to be less effective in the face of pain and continuing progression of disease. She found that trying to smile and deny the presence of the serious illness, as her doctors seemed to want her to do, was more depressing to her. She wished that she could talk about her pessimistic thoughts with her doctor but felt that this would be a burden to the doctor.

Evaluation

On the basis of information available at the time of evaluation, a PEG was formulated, as in Figure 35. The immediate need of the patient was, of course, treatment of the overdose during the hospitalization, evaluation of the patient's suicidal potential and prevention of it, and evaluation of the family situation and mobilization of support.

In terms of relatively long-term management, two problems had to be considered: the metastatic cancer and the depression and suffering of the patient and family. In the environmental dimension, the husband's guilt feelings about not spending enough time with his wife (recent context) had to be dealt with. In view of her ambivalent feelings about her mother and sister, they were not considered to be a great resource for interpersonal support. She was not a religious person and did not wish the involvement of the clergy.

In the personal dimension, encouraging activity and intellectualization within the limits of physical capacity would be useful in view of her personality style, coping style, and defense mechanisms. A plan of collaborative treatment of her illness would be more likely to succeed than blanket reassurances with a "trust me" attitude. Her occupation as a social worker and her diary indicated that she would probably use and benefit from psychotherapy, although she had not yet sought it. In the recent context, the presence of pain was an important factor in making her feel out of control, defeated, and discouraged. A regimen of adequate pain medication was planned. If the disfiguring side effects of treatment were put in the context of tangible signs of a fight against cancer, they might be less depressing given this patient's personality, somewhat like the combat scars of old and proud veterans. Also, antidepressant medication should be considered for this patient.

In the biological dimension, treatment of the cancer should, of course, continue. As much information as possible about the expected effect of the treatments and the progress should be shared with the patient.

35 yrs, ♀, married (to an M.D.), social worker, 3 children

CONTEXTS

DIMENSIONS	CURRENT (Current States)	RECENT (Recent Events and Changes)	BACKGROUND (Culture, Traits, Constitution)
BIOLOGICAL	Massive overdose of barbiturates Terminal metastatic breast cancer Steroids Pain medications	Lump in breast 4 yrs ago – radical mastectomy Recurrence in remaining breast – radiation, then mastectomy 2 yrs ago Metastases to orbit & bones (1 yr) Chemotherapy, radiation, steroids, oophorectomy (within last yr)	Family history of cancer – aunt
PERSONAL	Suicidal attempt Fear of immobilization	Pain ↑ 1 yr Baldness, appearance change, jaundice (about 6 mos) Feeling defeated in recent mos Futility over recurrent disease Fear of burdening family and doctor – recent mos	Social worker Attractive, intelligent A fighter, activity & mastery important Orderly, controlling type Intellectualization Counterphobic maneuvers
ENVIRONMENTAL	Husband & 3 children are supportive No suicide note Oncologists	Husband – busy physician feels guilty for not spending more time Oncologists expect patient to be cheerful	Father died when patient in teens Controlling and ambivalently experienced mother Mother preferred sister (who lives in another town) Jewish, middle class

Figure 35. PEG of the suicidal terminal cancer patient.

Course of Management

The patient was initially managed in the hospital until she recovered fully from the effects of the overdose. During this period, her suicidal potential and depression were evaluated by the psychiatrist in collaboration with the primary physician. It was decided that, although the suicidal attempt was serious, it was a reaction to the patient's feeling out of control and at an impasse with the oncologists about communicating her concerns. Thus, with improved communications and psychotherapy, she might cease to be suicidal. A considerable amount of depression was present, and amitriptyline therapy was instituted. Her family was evaluated by the psychiatrist, and it was decided that the psychiatrist would see the patient regularly—daily while in the hospital and once a week after discharge—and that her husband would also be seen by the psychiatrist on a biweekly basis to discuss his own feelings of guilt. This would also provide him with the opportunity to discuss various concerns of his including the preparation of their children for the eventual loss of their mother.

As these plans were set in motion, the patient was discharged from the hospital as the acute medical condition resolved. She kept her appointment with the psychiatrist diligently. The psychiatrist maintained close contact with the primary physician and the oncologist, discussed with the patient any new symptoms and plans of therapy, and encouraged her to communicate directly with the oncologists. She no longer felt that she had to always smile at them.

The psychiatrist, with the support of her primary physician and oncologist, encouraged her to return to work as much as she could tolerate (which was about half-time) and also to write down her experiences in fighting cancer. Writing this chronicle was a substitute activity for a more strenuous one, like playing tennis, and also served the function of being a record of her valiant fight against this serious disease.

She wanted to discontinue the amitriptyline soon after it was begun because of its side effects, especially sedation—she felt more out of control when feeling groggy. It was discontinued, and the patient's depression lifted without medications as she gained a greater sense of control.

Psychotherapy was initially aimed at increasing her coping ability through discussing how she might cope with possible stressful events, such as increasing side effects from treatment (e.g., baldness). The idea that the side effects might be seen as something like battle scars was accepted by the patient with relief and determination. Soon, however, she wanted to explore her unconscious conflicts and meanings concerning her disease, cancer. She discussed in detail her ambivalent relationship with her mother, who had always been inconsistent and inconsiderate of her. She remembered experiences of being reprimanded by her mother for any independent activity and her mother's attempts to control her every activity, including what time in the morning she could get up and what she should eat. She sought relief from this unhappy relationship by going to college away from home. Her father was ineffectual and did not interfere with her mother's controlling attitude.

In the course of psychotherapy, the meaning of the cancer became clear to her—it represented an alien, evil force that was attempting to control her life, change it, and, ultimately, extinguish it. In many ways, she saw her cancer as a symbol of the kind of overwhelming force that, like her mother, seemed to want to control her and subjugate her completely. As she began to see cancer as an alien object, she was able to feel that she might be able to win over it, as she had been able to gain her independence from her mother. The process of gaining independence from her mother was a protracted one in which, at times, she had to give in, but, at other times, she was able to achieve greater independence. She began to see her struggle with the cancer in a similar vein. She resolved not to feel completely defeated by one or two setbacks.

She decided to live and plan for relatively short and discrete periods—a few months at a time. She felt a certain degree of mastery in *willing* herself to live for the discrete intervals.

During the seven-month period of outpatient psychotherapy, she seldom mentioned pain or physical discomfort and stayed away from prolonged discussions concerning her medical treatment. In fact, she seemed to want to believe that whatever physical symptoms she felt had a psychogenic origin and could be dealt with in psychotherapy. However, she recognized this as wishful thinking and did not neglect to take medications and treatments for the disease. The psychiatrist was in close contact with the oncologists throughout this period and made sure that the patient was complying with the medical regimen. Although she had free use of narcotic analgesics, she used them very sparingly, because she did not like their sedating side effects.

The disease progressed relentlessly in spite of the combined efforts of the primary physician, surgeon, oncologists, and psychiatrist. As spread of the cancer to the brain was discovered, she began to feel dizzy and had constant nausea. She still continued psychotherapy and was able to talk about her sadness over her disappearing youth and mourn for her unfinished plans, but then she hoped that her husband would remarry soon after her death—almost as if to continue her happy marriage.

As she became too ill to be able to come to the psychiatrist's office, her care was left primarily to her family. She chose not to be hospitalized during the final phase of the illness. The psychiatrist talked with her regularly on the telephone, when she would tell him about the amount of work she was able to do at home in spite of the symptoms. During the final weeks of her life, her husband was almost constantly with her, having taken partial leave from his work. He continued to see the psychiatrist regularly, and several times after her death, for support, discussion of plans and sharing his thoughts and feelings.

Comments

This case illustrates how a terminal cancer patient found herself at an impasse of communications with her caretakers. As a result of complex interactions between her personality, her disease, its symbolic meaning, physical and emotional pain, and the effects and side effects of treatment modalities, she was driven to a suicidal attempt.

Management plans based on a systematic evaluation of the patient were three-dimensional and effective. The patient's life was prolonged, and she died a natural death—but, above all, the eight and one-half months of life she lived after the suicidal attempt were *gratifying* to her. She died like the fighter that she had always been, and she died feeling that she had fought well to the very end, fighting as a team with her doctors and her family.

CHAPTER 20

Summary and Perspectives

Staying alive is something that we do automatically. Health is usually taken for granted; ordinarily, we become aware of it only when something goes wrong, that is, when we experience signals of bodily malfunction, symptoms and signs of disease. While the nature of life itself remains a mystery, a great deal is known about the processes and mechanisms involved in living systems (Miller, 1978).

General systems theory proposes that the universe is composed of a hierarchy of concrete systems (Von Bertalanffy, 1968; Miller, 1978). The latter are accumulations of matter and energy that are organized into interacting, interrelated subsystems existing in a common space–time continuum. A patient is a *living system* composed, in turn, of biological subsystems. He is also part of a surrounding suprasystem (ecosystem). The living system is an *open system;* matter–energy and information pass back and forth and across the system. General systems approach avoids the dichotomy between mind and matter. What have been called ''mental'' and psychological are conceptualized as manifestations of the information-processing subsystems, while what have been called ''somatic'' and physiologic are conceptualized as manifestations of the matter–energy-processing subsystems of the living system. Of course, both systems are made of matter–energy. The health care system is also an open system, into which patients enter, in which they are treated, and which they ultimately leave.

Living systems are amazingly complex. For example, an individual person in his life space can be thought of as a virtually infinite series of mutually interactive systems arranged in such a way that (1) one single system may function individually as a *unit* or as a part (subsystem) of a larger system (suprasystem); (2) there are two-way interactions between and among adjacent and related unit systems and suprasystems and subsystems; in these transactions, both interactants are affected and changed; and (3) change in any unit or group of units eventually may affect functioning in all other parts of the aggregate. It's a good thing we do it automatically!

Each of us constitutes an individual or unit living system, existing in an environmental system. Both the individual person and the surrounding environment can be regarded as subsystems of a biopsychosocial suprasystem. Although energy and information can flow freely in both directions between the person and his environment, the person nonetheless maintains a separateness which is evidenced by the fact that the total energy level in the living person is higher than that of the surrounding environment (Schrodinger, 1962). This fact, in one sense, defines what it means biologically to be alive, that is, to maintain a dynamic equilibrium that sustains differential energy levels between the organism and the surrounding environment in an open energy system (negative entropy). When life ceases, the energy differential disappears.

Physical integrity of the living person is maintained by a series of interacting boundaries which begins at the interface between person and environment (e.g., skin, mucosal lining of body orifices, epithelial lining of lung, and sensory apparatus of the nervous system) and extends progressively deeper and deeper within the individual's interior and specialized subsystem (see Figure 36). Energy transactions with the physical components of the environment consist of a chain-like series of physicochemical reactions starting at or rela-

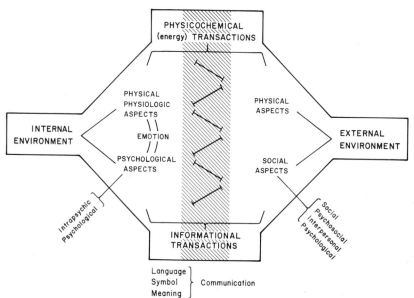

Figure 36. Interacting boundaries between the person and the environment.

tively near to the surface of the body and extending inward all the way to intracellular processes.

Psychosocial integrity of the person is maintained by a series of articulations with the interpersonal and social environment. In this sphere, transactional exchanges of information or meaning are mediated by symbols, including language. Patterns of sensory stimuli that are conducted into the individual via the peripheral nerves or special sensory organs are processed by the brain into *meanings* against the background matrix of memory and other cognitive processes. These as yet poorly understood brain processes and functions are grouped together as belonging with the realm of the "mind" (psychological processes).

Emotions participate in both of the foregoing series of articulations—both in the energy transactions ("physiologic") and in the meaing transactions ("mental"). Thus, emotions bridge the physical and symbolic aspects of environment with the physiologic and mental aspects of the person.

The famous French physiologist Claude Bernard pointed out that the internal environment of the body must be maintained in a constant, steady state in order for optimal life processes to occur. The myriad elaborate and intricate chemical and physiologic regulatory mechanisms that are involved in stabilizing the *milieu intérieur* are referred to collectively as *homeostasis,* a term coined by the American physiologist Walter Cannon (1932). The collection of dynamic physiologic processes that maintain the constant internal environment (which supports health and its accompanying sense of well-being—that we so much take for granted) in the face of challenging inconstancy of the external environment is called *adaptation. Health* can be regarded as a state of *successful and effective adaptation,* and *illness* as *maladaptation.* Adaptation to both physical and psychosocial aspects of the environment encompasses transactions between the person and the environment and among the components within the person. The latter may serve either or both of two purposes: (1) to maintain internal constancy despite environmental challenge and/or (2) to initiate and implement action that would change the environment or accommodate it. All of this is integrated, coordinated, and mediated by the nervous system and the neuroendocine apparatus. Psychological and social challenges in the environment are perceived, evaluated, and reacted to by the organism through the multiple operations of the brain which we call by the collective term "mind."

So, with respect to both the physical and psychosocial dimensions of the environment, we can see that the brain serves as the control center for physiologic and psychological mechanisms. The environment, the person as a unit, and the components of the person are, so to speak, connected by and in the brain, which serves to regulate the person's physiologic and behavioral adaptation to environmental challenge.

Environmental challenges can be thought of as *stresses* that create a demand for adaptive work on the part of the organism; they may be physical or symbolic in nature. Their detection and processing as well as the ultimate responses to them in the form of internal readjustments and/or behavioral output into the environment are mediated by neural and endocrine structures. The extent and vigor of response reflect the *strain* that was created within the organism in reaction to stress. Some of these responses are primarily physical or physiologic, for example, regulation of the pH of the blood; others are primarily psychological, for example, writing poetry. There is also a vast spectrum of life processes that expresses themselves (and are mediated) in both the physiologic and the psychological spheres. The most prominent of these, of course, are the emotions.

The intriguing "intimate-but-separate" nature of the relations between the inside and outside of living systems has stimulated interesting philosophical reflections about reciprocating influences of each upon the other in evolution and development. In his essays, Lewis Thomas (1974) discusses in a highly imaginative and stimulating way some implications of resemblances between the cytochemistry of cells and the oceanic saline environment in which living matter had its origin. For example, he speculates that the mitochondria in our cells might be the descendants of some primitive bacteria that entered the primordial cells eons ago and stayed there in a symbiotic relationship with the cells. On the other hand, the advent of photosynthetic cells changed the course of evolution of the earth through the production of oxygen, which, in turn, determined the course of evolution of living systems on earth. He also finds striking similarities between the single cell and the earth as an entity.

Similar analogies can and have been drawn between the nature of social structures and institutions on the one hand and some aspects of personality structure on the other, for example, based on similarities between (external) moral and ethical standards of behavior as reflected in law and religion and internal psychological "structures" such as conscience (superego) and the emotion of guilt. It may not be too farfetched to speculate that these internal and external analogues evolved from an interactive process, that is, psychological processes influencing and shaping developing social conventions and, in turn, being influenced and shaped by society. Some students of semiotics postulate similar reciprocal relationships between structural characteristics of the central nervous system and structures of the environment that determine patterns of sensory input. Noam Chomsky, a linguist, postulates that meanings as expressed in language are dependent upon functional substructures inherent in the organizational nature of the central nervous system (Chomsky, 1978). All of these ideas do seem to converge in suggesting a mutually interactive developmental lineage between the inside and the outside of living organisms.

To summarize, a person is comprised of, and is a part of, a virtually infinite series of systems and subsystems. These systems and subsystems can be broadly grouped into two organizations—the person and the environment. The *physical environment* includes terrain, climate, fauna, flora, and environmental toxins. The *social environment* consists of significant individuals, families, small groups, communities, cities, states, and nations, all embedded in and influenced by a variety of cultures and subcultures—present and past.

The person can be viewed as subdivisible into organ systems, individual organs, cells, and intracellular sybsystems. The *meaning system,* a function of the brain, defines the person's psychosocial integrity. Transactions or changes in any part of the personal system ultimately can be expected to affect all other parts of the system. For example, a change in the salt content of drinking water in the environment will ultimately affect hormones regulating electrolyte and fluid balance, function of cells in the kidney, function of the cardiovascular-renal system, and, finally, thirst and water-seeking behavior.

All of the systems we have discussed exist in *time* as well as in space. The environment and the person have a past, present, and a future. Progress though time is a continuing evolutionary process. At any given moment, the systems express what has gone before, and what transpires in the present will affect the state of the systems in the future. To understand the current state (including maladaptation) of any of these systems, knowledge of the past is helpful and often necessary. People undergo continuing development and maturation. The life cycle, the process of individuals' change over time, can be divided into phases, each of which has its unique adaptive tasks (Erikson, 1963; Levinson, 1978). At any point in time, the person exhibits remnants of past patterns of function as well as current patterns that have been built upon the older ones which have been modified in the course of development—a process called epigenetic development. To understand the environmental past, we turn to history, geology, archaeology, and cultural anthropology. To understand the person's past, we look to his or her genetic endowment and developmental life history, that is, a review of life experiences and their impact upon developmental processes and maturation. This historical perspective has relevance in clinical diagnosis—the current or immediate state of balance between pathogenic vectors and the resistance of the individual to the pathogenic challenge will reflect and be influenced by what has transpired before in relevant subsystems. This is the reason that the medical history starts with the current chief complaint and proceeds to the history of the present illness (a chronicle of developing symptoms and signs) and, from there, to past medical history, review of systems, and family history. In this volume, we have expanded this theme to propose a clinical diagnostic method for tracing biological, personal, and environmental dimensions in terms of the present, the recent past, and the distant past (background).

States of adaptation or maladaptation (health or disease) have biological, psychological, and social aspects, and, to be fully understood, they must be described with respect to all three systems: (1) the biological system, (2) the personal (psychological) system, and (3) the environmental system.

Keeping all of this in mind, review what actually occurs in a routine medical encounter, for example, the first time a patient and physician meet in the consulting room. Each of the individuals constitutes a biopsychosocial system. When the two come together, a therapeutic doctor–patient relationship is established, and around this dyadic relationship a whole series of subsystems forms and evolves in support of the care of the patient. This new complex system will include individuals and groups who are significant members of both the patient's and the physician's psychosocial spheres. This means family and friends of the patient and the myriad individuals and organizations drawn from the health care system, including other physicians, nurses, social workers, and allied professionals (physical therapists, aides, etc.). The interactions will occur in clinics, offices, hospitals, wards, and special treatment units in the hospital and will require activities of administrative and financial organizations such as hospital administration, health plans, insurance, and government subsidiaries. Since transactions at all interfaces affect all parts of the system, the physician will have to deal with relevant biological, psychological, and social vectors as he carries out his job. Because of this, the behavioral sciences provide important and critical facts and concepts which are basic and necessary for satisfactory understanding and management of these complexities of medical practice. It has been our goal in this volume to introduce and sensitize the readers to what we think may be the most immediately relevant information from the behavioral sciences and to show how it may be integrated with relevant biological and physiologic principles in understanding health, disease, and clinical practice. Of course, such a goal cannot be fully achieved in an introductory textbook. We hope that we have stimulated the readers' thoughts, whetted their appetites, and started them on the road toward developing their own approaches.

References

Cannon WB: The Wisdom of the Body. New York, WW Norton & Co, 1932.
Chomsky N: Language and unconscious knowledge, in Smith JH (ed): Psychoanalysis and Language. New Haven, Yale Universities Press, 1978, pp 3–45.
Erikson EH: Childhood and Society. New York, WW Norton & Co, 1963.
Levinson DJ, Darrow CN, Klein CB et al.: Seasons of a Man's Life. New York, Alfred A Knopf, 1978.
Miller JG: The Living Systems. New York, McGraw-Hill, 1978.

Schrodinger E: *What is Life? The Physical Aspect of the Living Cell.* Cambridge, Cambridge Universities Press, 1962.
Thomas L: *The Lives of a Cell: Notes of a Biology Watcher.* New York, The Viking Press, 1974.
Von Bertalanffy L: *General System Theory.* New York, George Braziller, 1968.

Index